A Modern Approach to the Perimenopausal Years

New Developments in Biosciences 2

Walter de Gruyter
Berlin · New York 1986

A Modern Approach to the Perimenopausal Years

Editor
Robert B. Greenblatt, M. D.

Co-Editor
Renate Heithecker

Walter de Gruyter
Berlin · New York 1986

Editor
Robert B. Greenblatt, M. D.
Professor Emeritus of Endocrinology
Medical College of Georgia
Augusta, Georgia 30912
U.S.A.

Co-Editor
Renate Heithecker
c/o Schering AG
Department of Clinical Endocrinology
and Fertility Research
Müllerstrasse 170–178
D-1000 Berlin 65

This book contains 62 illustrations and 44 tables.

Library of Congress Cataloging-in-Publication Data

A modern approach to the perimenopausal years.
(New developments in biosciences ; 2)
Proceedings of a conference held in 1985 in Berlin.
Includes bibliographies and index.
1. Menopause--Congresses. 2. Estrogen--Therapeutic use--Congresses. I. Greenblatt, Robert B., 1906– . II. Heithecker, Renate, 1946– . III. Series. [DNIM: 1. Climacteric--congresses. 2. Menopause--congresses. W3 NE865 v.2 / WP 580 M689 1985] RG186.M63 1986 618.1'75 86-16699
ISBN 0-89925-184-6 (U.S.)

CIP-Kurztitelaufnahme der Deutschen Bibliothek

A modern approach to the perimenopausal years / ed.: Robert B. Greenblatt. Co-ed.: Renate Heithecker. – Berlin ; New York : de Gruyter, 1986.
(New developments in biosciences ; 2)
ISBN 3-11-010937-9
NE: Greenblatt, Robert B. [Hrsg.]; GT

3 11 010937 9 Walter de Gruyter · Berlin · New York
0-89925-184-6 Walter de Gruyter, Inc., New York · Berlin
 Typesetting and Printing: Buch- und Offsetdruckerei Wagner GmbH, Nördlingen. – Binding: Lüderitz & Bauer GmbH, Berlin. – Cover design: Rudolf Hübler. – Printed in Germany.

Contents

2.2 Hormonal treatment

2.3 Risk-benefit evaluation of hormonal therapy

2.4 Special aspects in premenopausal women

Opening remarks

H. Hannse

Of the 19 papers to be read at this symposium, a total of eight deal with the hormonal treatment of climacteric disorders and the risks and benefits of such treatment. This type of therapy has its origins in developments which occurred nearly 60 years ago – i.e. the first epoch-making research on steroid hormones. Permit me to briefly review the contributions made to this field of endocrinology during its early years in Germany and, in particular, at Schering here in Berlin.

Research on sex hormones has been going on at Schering since 1923, the year in which Prof. Schoeller became director of our main laboratory. In the same year, inspired by the investigations of the Viennese gynecologist Steinach, the pharmacologist Prof. Dohrn, who had been with Schering since 1902, initiated the first attempts to extract hormones from biological material. But it was not until 1925 when the Allen-Doisy test became known that the foundations for precise hormone research were laid in Berlin. Originally starting material used was placentas, the hormonal activity being in the lipoid fraction. Even in those early days it was possible, with the aid of highly purified extracts, to treat female climacteric disorders successfully. As a result of this work. Schering was able to introduce Progynon, the first estrogen preparation, in 1928.

The gynecologists Aschheim and Zondek, who were working at the Berlin Charité at that time, discovered that ovarian hormone activity was at this highest level in the follicular fluid. For this reason they named the as yet unknown hormone Folliculin: at that time, people assumed that there was only one female hormone. Soon, these two researchers also discovered that the urine of pregnant women und pregnant mares was a much richer source of folliculin, a discovery which was the prerequisite for further research into sex hormones and for the manufacture of hormone preparations for wide-spread therapeutic use.

Prof. Schoeller and his co-workers suspected that folliculin belonged to the sterol group. This suspicion led, in 1928, to collaboration with Butenandt, a young assistant to Prof. Windaus in the Department of Chemistry at the University of Göttingen, who was working with this class of compounds. By 1929, this cooperation between academia and industry had already led to the isolation of the follicular hormone; a short time later, the structure of estrone was elucidated. Schering was responsible for collecting large quantities of the urine of pregnant women and drawing out a raw extract, while the university laboratory undertook the further concentration and purification. Prof. Butenandt, who at that time was involved in an exciting race against other groups in Amsterdam and St. Louis, later referred to the discovery of estrone as the birth of steroid hormones.

In 1933, Schering also succeeded in synthesizing estradiol by hydrogenating estrone; this was two years before this most potent of the natural estrogens was isolated from follicular fluid. The first economically practicable synthesis of estrone and estradiol was accomplished by Inhoffen in Schering's main laboratory. In 1938 he succeeded in synthesizing estradiol from the abundantly available cholesterol by way of dehydroepiandrosterone acetate. A further epochal synthesis can also be ascribed to Inhoffen, namely that of ethinylestradiol in 1938. This was the first highly potent oral estrogen, and it is still the most widely-used estrogen component in hormonal contraceptives.

Aschheim and Zondek were the first to realize that ovarian activity is stimulated by a hormone of the so-called anterior lobe of the pituitary gland. Taking this as their starting-point, the Schering researchers Hohlweg and Junkmann discovered the regulation of the anterior pituitary function by the hypothalamus and the cybernetic regulatory mechanism based on gonads, pituitary gland and diencephalon. Their results were first published in 1932.

Similar pioneer work was done in the gestagen field: in 1929, after the Allen-Corner test became known, efforts to isolate the corpus luteum hormone from pig ovaries began, once again in collaboration with Butenandt. The isolation of the pure substance, the structural elucidation and the synthesis of progesterone were all accomplished by Butenandt, Hohlweg and Westphal, and Inhoffen synthesized the first orally effective gestagen ethisterone in 1938.

Building upon these developments, in 1932 the Berlin gynecologist Kaufmann succeeded for the first time in bringing about proliferation and transformation of the endometrium and, subsequently, artificial menstruation in a castrate, using a sequential regimen of estrone benzoate and a highly purified corpus luteum extract from Schering.

The essential foundations for the hormonal treatment of female climacteric disorders, which is one of the subjects of today's and tomorrow's programm, were laid here in Berlin in those early days. Today, some 57 years after the in introduction of our company's first estrogen preparation, we at Schering are extremely pleased to be able to hear a group of international experts give their assessments of the hormonal therapy of climateric disorders which was introduced at that time.

Prologue

R. B. Greenblatt

Dr. Hannse, on behalf of all of us present I wish to thank Schering for making this meeting possible. I also wish to express my appreciation for your comprehensive historical review of the steroid hormones that have become the cornerstone in treatment of the illness so common to women, and to Dr. Lachnit our collective gratitude for organizing this wonderful symposium. It is a tribute to the doctors the world over that the menopause is at last receiving the recognition that is its due. Shakespeare set the tone for this symposium when he wrote about the woman in her middle years:

> "Age cannot wither her, nor custom stale her infinite variety".

Let us, as physicians, cherish this goal.

I am honored to preside at this international symposium on "The modern approach to the perimenopausal years". I should like to use my prerogative to plead for an extended view of the climacteric which includes not only vasomotor disturbances and atrophic vaginitis but also the metabolic changes in bone and skin, the influence of serum lipids on cardiovascular disease, and the role that altered cerebral neurohumors play in psychological disorders. I also wish to impress on you that the menopause is not a short event in a woman's progression through life but a condition to be endured from the moment the ovaries begin to falter to the very last of life. As a woman's life span increases so do the problems of the perimenopausal period. Nervous system disruptions connected with the climacteric were formerly attributed to nature's inability to rid the body of "evil humors". New concepts of the intricacies of the hypothalamic-pituitary-ovarian axis give lie to such poetic speculation about the femine mystique.

Each woman passes through three epochs in her progression through life. The first, from birth to adolescence is in preparation for the second, the years of fecundity. The third ends her potential for reproduction. Thus, she enters the menopause, the permanent cessation of menstruation. Now, in her advancing years, she is protected from the stresses and tribulations of child bearing, for which, unfortunately, she pays a price, the loss of estrogen production by the ovaries.

Until Gardanne published his treatise in 1816, "L'âge critique de la femme", very little had appeared in medical annals or in the world's literature about the change of life. The Bible relates how Sarah's personality changed when "it ceased to be with Sarah after the manner of women". A quatrain retrieved from a 4th C. monastery speaks of an aging woman's irascible and canine attributes:

"Quid irasceris
Quid sicut canis iactus te
Quid sicut lepus resilis?
Quisce".

Shakespeare poignantly described Lady Macbeth's "thick coming fancies that keep her from her rest", and the "written troubles of the brain" which came to the fore at a time when environmental stresses were piled on existing biologic deviations. Macbeth pleads with the doctor to give her "some sweet oblivious antidote".

Paracelsus, the controversial 16th C. physician, rekindled an old belief in presenting his doctrine, "similia similibus curantur" (like cures like). More than 300 years elapsed before Brown-Sequard (1889) reported on the rejuvenating effects of injections of pasteurized testicular extracts which he himself took and Murray (1891) effectively prevented the myxedema of hypothryoidism by oral administra-

Table I Note response of a 46-year-old woman who complained of 20 hot flashes per day in a double-blind study who was subjected to an estrogen, an estrogen-androgen, an androgen and a placebo.
Reproduced from Robert B. Greenblatt et al. J. of Clin. Endocrin. 10:1547, 1950

Miss R.N., w.f. 46. Surgical castration. Hot flashes–20 per day.					
AE	1	2	3	4	
May	×				Complete relief. Smear 3 plus.
June		×			Complete relief. Smear 3–4 plus.
July					Hot flashes returned 1 wk. after stopping AE-2.
Aug.			×		75% relief, libido increased. Smear 2–3 plus.
Sept.			×		Same, occasional hot flash. Smear 3 plus.
Oct.				×	Hot flashes 20 per day, nervous. Smear 2 plus.
Nov.			×		Hot flashes stopped. Bled 2 days. Increased libido.
Dec.			×		Same. Slight hair growth. Bled 2 days.
Jan.		×			Complete relief.
Feb.	×				Complete relief, greater calm. Smear 3–4 plus.
Mar.		×			Best of all. Complete relief, increased well-being.

Patient stated preference for AE-2 because of improved well-being and libido in addition to control of hot flashes.

tion of thyroid gland. About this time, sufficient scientific evidence became available to show that loss of ovarian function (by ovariectomy or ovarian senescence) was responsible for many of the distressful symptoms of the menopause. Thus, in 1893, Regas injected ovarian extracts subcutaneously into a patient with menopausal psychosis and affected a cure. Then in 1899, Glass demonstrated that the grafting of ovaries in previously ovariectomized women re-established menstruation, sexual desire, and a sense of well-being. Encouraged by such results, ovarian slices were implanted under the rectus muscle of the abdomen in the hope of assuaging severe menopausal symptoms.

During the first third of this century the oral administration of dried ovarian residue was prescribed fairly extensively. If any amelioration of hot flushes was experienced by some women on such substances, it was purely a placebo effect. The belief was current that such a preparation would act as effectively as the well-established use of oral thyroideum siccum. In 1950, my group at the Medical College of Georgia published, in the *Journal of Clinical Endocrinology,* the results of a double-blind study using a potent estrogen, an estrogen-androgen preparation, an androgen, and a placebo and found that 97% obtained relief of hot flushes with the estrogen and 16% with placebos. We now know that placebos may provoke the secretion of endorphin, a cerebral hormone which has sedating properties. Surprisingly, of the four preparations, the estrogen-androgen was preferred by most (Tables I & II).

Table II Results of the double-blind study revealed that 97% responded well to the estrogen, while 16% responded to the placebo. Most of the patients preferred the combination estrogen-androgen preparation because of the increased well-being and improvement of libido. Reproduced from Robert B. Greenblatt et al. J. of Clin. Endocrin. 10:1547, 1950
Analysis of response to therapy with AE preparations in 74 private patients and 28 clinic patients with 284 courses of therapy

	Courses of therapy		Percentage of patients				
Therapy	Private	Clinic	With nausea	With increased libido	With acne, hoarse-ness, or hirsutism	With intact uterus and bleeding following treatment	With no improve-ment
AE-1							
Diethylstilbestrol, 0.25 mg.	67	21	30.5	12.3	0	34.2	3.1
AE-2							
Diethylstilbestrol, 0.25 mg.							
Methyltestosterone, 5.0 mg.	54	19	4.0	23.5	13.2	30.5	10.4
AE-3							
Methyltestosterone, 5.0 mg.	44	19	5.2	42.0	12.8	0.98	23.6
AE-4							
Placebo	36	24	3.6	1.8	0	0	83.8

Table III Free serum tryptophan is much lower in depressed than in non-depressed menopausal women. Following the administration of estrogens there is a rise in serum tryptophan usually accompanied by a lessening of depression.

Free and Total Tryptophan in Depressed and Non-depressed Menopausal Women	Free	Total
Depressed menopausal patients	3.76*	34.66*
	±0.09	±0.89
	n = 136	n = 136
Non-depressed menopausal patients	5.12	44.8
	±0.34	±2.87
	n = 20	n = 20

P = < 0.05

The use of estrogens, not only for the treatment of vasomotor disorders but also for the treatment of the psychosomatic aspects (depression, anxiety, migrainoid headaches, frigidity) as well as metabolic derangements (osteoporosis, lipidemia, thinning of the skin), needs no apology. Recent work has demonstrated without a question of a doubt that estrogen is of value in preventing bone loss, though demineralization may follow rapidly after discontinuation of therapy. On the other hand, bone integrity will be, more or less, maintained as long as treatment is continued. Such observations seem to suggest that those women with a tendency toward the development of osteoporosis, i.e., Caucasian, slender women with

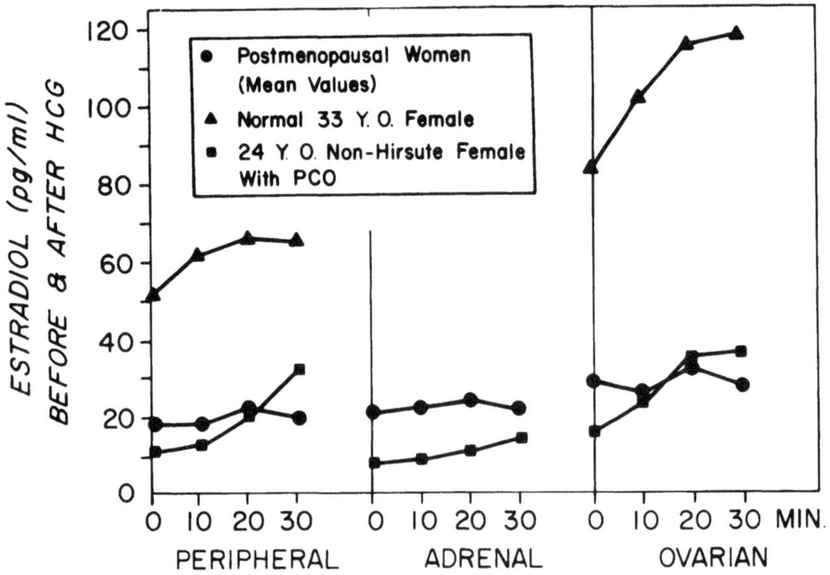

Fig. 1 Serum estradiol values rose perceptibly following i.v. administration of 5,000 i.u. of hCG in ovarian vein blood of a normal female but not in the adrenal and ovarian vein blood of 4 menopausal women and one 24-year-old woman with the polycystic ovary syndrome.

sedentary occupations, require hormone replacement therapy (HRT) for all their postmenopausal years. Perhaps Robert Wilson, the author of *Feminine Forever,* was not as foolish as the "establishment" made him out to be.

Although the many myths about estrogen's harmful effects and the exaggerations about its tumorigenic properties have not been completely laid to rest, it is fair to say that it is now generally admitted that the benefits far outweight putative risks. I am in full agreement with many of my distinguished colleagues that limiting therapy to only the treatment of accepted symptoms of estrogen deprivation i.e., vasomotor and atrophic vaginitis, militates against the use of hormonal preparations for many distressing symptoms associated with the menopause. Symptoms such as nervousness, depression, insomnia, migrainoid headaches, loss of sexual drive and dyspareunia may not be hormone dependent but are frequently hormone responsive. Our

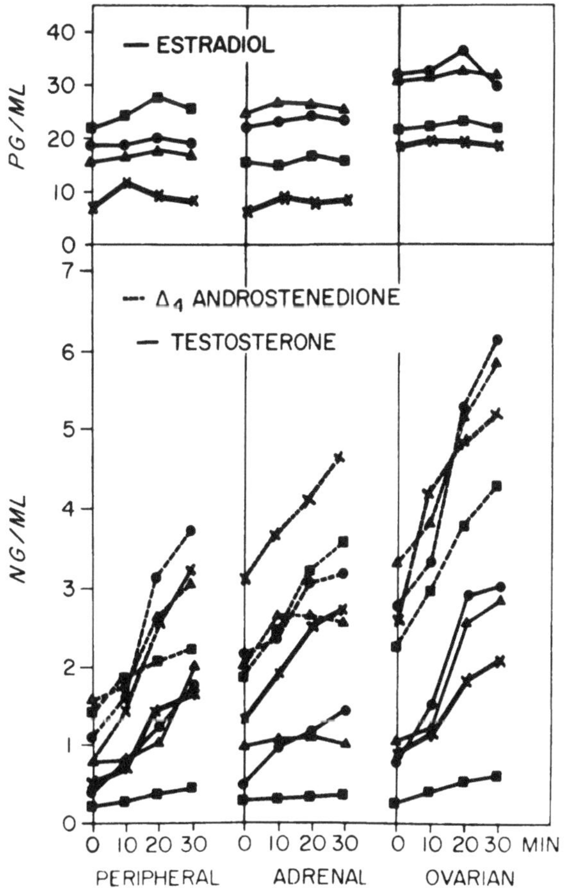

Fig. II Following 5,000 i.u. of hCG I.V. estradiol levels in plasma obtained from peripheral, adrenal and ovarian blood remained unchanged but △ 4 androstenedione and testosterone levels rose.

own studies on the influence of estrogens on free serum tryptophan levels confirmed the findings of Aylward. Low tryptophan levels rose while signs of depression lessened in a considerable number of patients (Table III). There is some evidence of reduced levels of 5-hydroxytryptamine (sertonin) in the brain and cerebrospinal fluid of depressed patients. Free tryptophan may also be low in these patients. It is believed that estrogens displace the albumen-bound tryptophan thus freeing the unbound portion which then becomes accessible to the brain and increases 5-hydroxytryptophane synthesis. Neurohumors and transmitters in the brain are influenced by circulating hormones. It has long been known that oophorectomy increases, and administered estrogens decrease, brain norepinephrine in animals.

Before closing my introductory remarks and calling on Professor Egon Diczfalusy, the illustratious chairman of this mornings panel, I should like to make one more point, and this is that the menopausal ovary does not *de novo* produce the primary hormone E_2, not even following stimulation with intravenous injections of 5000 i.u. of hCG. However, ovarian secretion of $\triangle$ 4A and testosterone are enhanced (Fig. I & II). Androgens evidently play a role in the body economy of women. It would appear then that the administration of an androgen, in judicious amounts, should not be considered to cause antiphysiologic or pharmacologic mayhem. Recall that only the male canary normally sings; when testosterone is administered to the female canary, she too will sing.

1 Physiology and pathophysiology of the perimenopausal years

Some aspects of oogenesis, follicular growth, and endocrine involution

W. Nocke

1. Introduction

The aging of the ovary is a slowly proceeding involution process which starts during the premenopausal years of the female life. It includes a series of marked morphological alterations in the organ itself, which result in a gradual decline and final cessation of the generative and endocrine functions of the ovary. According to Rössle & Roulet (1941) the mean weight of the ovary already begins to decrease at the age of thirty years. The direct and indirect endocrine consequences of the involution process display a varity of clinical manifestations which may be of much concern to the quality of life and to numerous aspects of the physical and psychic health of the woman. The last uterine bleeding before the definite cessation of menses is referred to as the menopause. This is generally considered complete after one year of amenorrhoea. The time thereafter is termed the postmenopause.

In the female organism there is an interplay between the germ cells, the surrounding somatic tissue and its related endocrine activity, and the neuroendocrine system. The presence of germ cells is a prerequisite for the differentiation of the associated somatic tissue since in the absence of germ cells follicles fail to develop. On the other hand, the somatic tissue is indispensable for nutrition and development of the germ cells. Furthermore, the follicular structure which arises from the surrounding tissue of the germ cells provides the vehicle for ovulation and the source for steroid hormone biogenesis (Baker, 1971). Finally, intraovarian events are controlled by the neuroendocrine system, which itself is regulated by ovarian signals, so that an integrated circuit of regulations operating between the hypothalamus, the pituitary gland, and the ovary is established.

Thus, if we regard the aging of the ovary as a decline of its cyclical endocrine activity with progressing age, both the evolution and the involution of the processes mentioned and, in particular, the cyclical follicular dynamics throughout the female life must be considered.

2. Fate of germ cells throughout female life

Various aspects of the transformation from the primary germ cell to the fertilized egg have been reviewed by many investigators (e.g. Baker, 1963, 1971, 1972; Mauléon, 1969; Franchi, 1970; Franchi & Baker, 1973; Lindner et al., 1974; Zuckerman & Baker, 1977; Weir & Rowlands, 1977; Edwards 1980; Channing et al., 1982; Tsafriri et al., 1983; Bomsel-Helmreich, 1983; Szöllösi & Gerard, 1983).

2.1 Primordial germ cells, oogonia, primary oocytes

Germ cells are first identifiable in the yolk sac epithelium at about 4 weeks following fertilization, i.e., 6 weeks after the onset of the last menstrual period[1]. Some 1000–2000 primordial germ cells arise from extragonadal sites, migrate either by active amoeboid movements or via the blood stream into the developing ovary, and arrive at the genital ridges by about 7–8 weeks of gestation. They rapidly multiply by mitotic division, resulting in some 600.000 "stem" cells at 10 weeks of gestational age. Since at this time the gonad is clearly defined as an ovary, these cells may be termed *oogonia.* Starting at about 9 weeks of gestation, an increasing proportion of oogonia stop further cleavage and enter the meiotic prophase, thus becoming *primary oocytes,* whereas the remaining oogonia continue to divide mitotically (Ref.: Baker, 1963, 1971, 1972; Franchi & Baker, 1973; Zuckerman & Baker, 1977).

2.2 Elimination of germ cells by atretic degeneration

As has been estimated by Baker (1963), the process of germ cell multiplication in both fetal ovaries reaches a maximum count of some 6,8 million cells at 22 weeks of gestation, consisting of 4,8 millions of primary oocytes and 2 millions of residual oogonia *(Fig. 1).*

Thus, at midgestation the fetal ovaries still contain a mixed population of germ cells, predominantly primary oocytes. Before birth, the vast majority of germ cells is eliminated from the ovaries by a complex process of degeneration commonly termed *atresia,* which affects oogonia, oocytes, and their associated follicle cells. According to Franchi & Baker (1973), atresia is defined as a loss of oocytes (or follicles) from the ovary other than by ovulation. From midgestation until birth the number of germ cells is reduced by about 5 million. Almost half of the oocytes remaining at birth show signs of atretic degeneration, so that only about 1 million intact cells survive.

---

1 Data on the gestational age are expressed as weeks after onset of the last menstrual period.

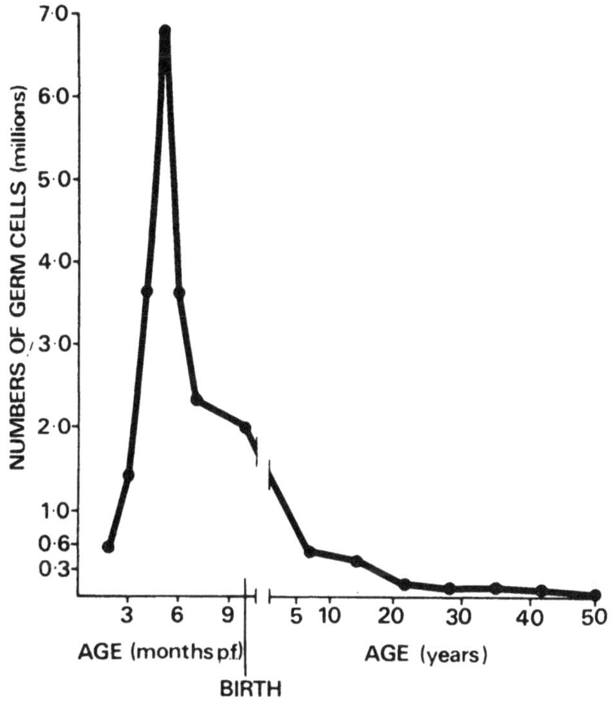

Fig. 1 The numbers of germ cells in human ovaries (paired) from 2 months after fertilization to menopausal age. (With permission from Baker, 1963).

The degeneration of germ cells also continues, to a lesser extent, when the oocytes become enclosed in primordial follicles and is carried on throughout the entire female life, pregnancies and lactation included. At the age of 7 years about 300.000 oocytes have survived, but 40% of them show definite signs of degeneration. Finally, when the woman approaches the menopause at the age of 45–50 years, only a few hundred of primary oocytes are present in both ovaries (Ref.: Baker, 1963, 1971, 1972; Franchi & Baker, 1973; Weir & Rowlands, 1977).

2.3 Meiosis

In order to reach full maturation, the primary oocyte has to undergo the process of meiosis, which consists of two different cell divisions. The first, a reduction division, results in the *secondary oocyte* and an abortive polar body, both of which contain a haploid set of chromosomes. The meiotic transformation of the primary to the secondary oocyte is arrested at a certain stage. Late follicular growth is delayed for prolonged periods, i.e., for, at least 13 years, until early puberty, or, at the most, for 50 years until near the menopause. This means that the "resting stage" of meiosis is maintained throughout the entire intraovarian lifespan of the primary oocyte until it is eventually selected for ovulation. When this happens, a resumption of meiosis is triggered by an LH surge some 36–48 hours prior the ovulation. Much more probable, however, is the termination of the meiotic arrest of the primary oocyte by atretic degeneration, rather than by selection for ovulation. Baker (1971) has pointed out that the term "resting stage" is no longer tenable since it has been shown that the period of arrested development is accompanied by profound changes of the mammalian oocyte which are responsible, at least in part, for its growth and maturation.

The second more rapid meiotic maturation division is mitotic and requires ovulation and fertilization for its completion. It results in the ovum or the zygote containing a rearranged diploid set of chromosomes, and the extrusion of a second, diploid polar body.

The prophase of the first meiotic division consists of five different stages (leptotene, zygotene, pachytene, diplotene, and diakinesis), which the primary oocytes under go to a varying extent. The "resting stage" of meiosis occurs at the diplotene stage. Passing through the meiotic prophase up to the diplotene probably requires several weeks. At term, 65% of the primary oocytes have reached the diplotene, and within several weeks after birth oogonia and pre-diplotene stages of primary oocytes have completely disappeared.

Thus, both ovaries of the newborn female start postnatal life with about 1 million of intact germ cells of a single type, namely primary oocytes retaining arrest at the diplotene stage of the meiotic prophase. Since oogonia are eliminated, a "neoformation" of germ cells is precluded. The "stock" of primary oocytes of an individual can therefore only decline with age (Ref.: Baker, 1963, 1971, 1972; Mauléon, 1969; Franchi, 1970, Franchi & Baker, 1973; Zuckerman & Baker, 1977; Bomsel-Helmreich, 1983; Szöllösi et al., 1983; Tsafriri et al., 1983).

3. Formation and growth of follicular structures, and endocrine implications

During the meiotic prophase, somatic cells associate with the primary oocyte thus forming the franulosa, the theca interna, and the stroma cell layer of the final follicular structure. All of these cell types are involved in ovarian steroid hormone biogenesis. The formation of follicular structures, and its further growth and maturation is commonly classified into four or more development stages. However, since the transition between stages is fluent, they are diversely defined by different authors (Ref.: Baker, 1971; Franchi & Baker, 1973; Zuckerman & Baker, 1977; Hodgen et al., 1983).

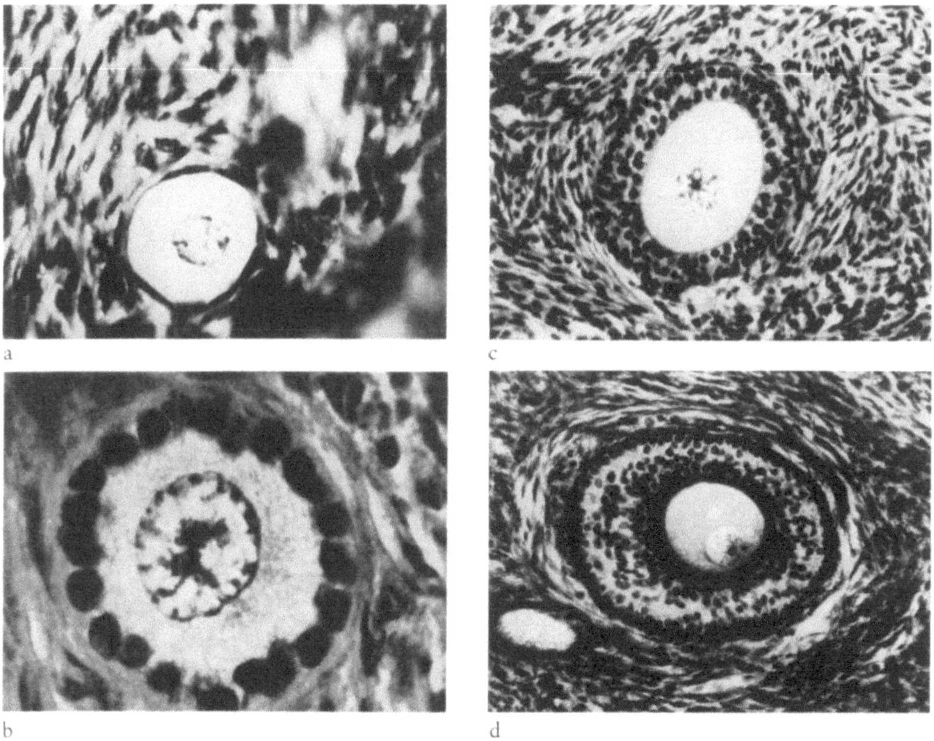

Fig. 2 Different developmental stages of human folliculogenesis between the primordial and the Graafian follicle. (With permission from Shettles, 1960). For details cf. text 3.

(a) In the *primordial follicle* the primary oocyte is surrounded by an incomplete single layer of flattened granulosa cells which is formed in the majority of germ cells before birth when the oocyte is "resting" at the diplotene stage of the meiotic prophase.

(b) In the *primary follicle* the primary oocyte is growing and now surrounded by a complete single layer of enlarged granulosa cells of cuboidal or columnar structure.

(c) In the earlier stages of the *secondary follicle,* the growing primary oocyte reaches its final size of 100–130 μm in diameter and is embedded into about for compact layers of granulosa cells, which arise from rapid mitotic division and are now termed the membrana granulosa (or stratum granulosum). Between the primary oocyte and the membrana granulosa, the zona pellucida (or oolemma) is formed. In the figure, within the nuclear chromatin reticulum a single nucleolus is present. Around the membrana granulosa, but separated by a basement membrane, the theca cell layers are formed by a concentric arrangement of the stroma cells. The innermost layer becomes vascular and generates large glandular cells forming the theca interna. The theca externa, which is not clearly separated from the theca interna and retains mainly fibroblastic tissue, is formed by the outermost layer. The secondary follicle reaches a diameter of about 200 μm.

(d) In a more advanced stage of the *secondary follicle,* the rapid mitotic proliferation of the membrana granulosa continues, and the transformation into a tertiary follicle is started by the production of follicular fluid. Within the granulosa layers fluid-filled cavities are formed and enlarge rapidly.

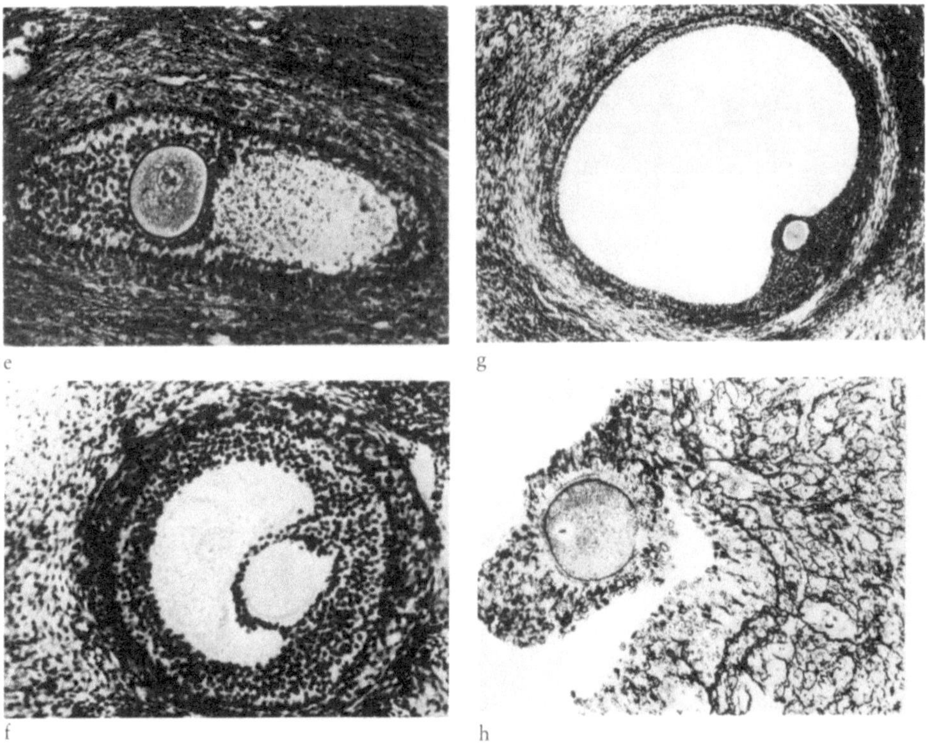

(e) In the earlier stages of the *tertiary follicle,* the fluid-filled cavities within the granulosa layers become confluent, and the formation of the antrum folliculi begins. The primary oocyte is in an excentrical position outside the early form of the antrum.

(f) In a more advanced stage of the *tertiary follicle* (antral follicle) the primary oocyte, surrounded by granulosa cells, is placed at the follicular wall thus forms the cumulus oophorus. The cross-section shows a typical semilunar shape of the antrum folliculi. The theca interna is markedly extended and the glandular cells are growing. A network of lymphatic vessels develops in both the theca interna and the theca externa. The tertiary follicle measures 10–14 mm in diameter. The primary oocyte is still "resting" in the meiotic prophase.

(g) The tertiary follicle, increasing rapidly in volume and reaching a final diameter of 20–25 mm, has now become a preovulatory *Graafian follicle.* The granulosa cells of the cumulus oophorus are reduced and form the corona radiata. Both the granulosa and the theca layers are attentuated. This stage coincides with the surge of pituitary LH, which induces the resumption of meiosis 36–48 hrs. prior to ovulation. The first meiotic division results in a haploid secondary oocyte with an attached haploid polar body and is completed some hours before ovulation.

(h) The *cumulus oophorus* of the late Graafian follicle becomes elevated and separates itself more and more from the follicular wall, so that the oocyte, embedded in its residual cumulus cells, floats freely in the antrum. At the time of ovulation, the oocyte is readily released and drained out with the follicular fluid. The egg is kept in the stage of a haploid secondary oocyte until ovulation and undergoes the second (mitotic) meiotic division only after fertilization.

3.1 Primordial follicles

The first step of folliculogenesis is the formation of the primordial follicle by the surrounding of the primary oocyte with an incomplete single layer of flattened granulosa cells *(Fig. 2a)*. This occurs at the diplotene stage of the "resting" meiotic prophase of the primary oocyte, i.e., in the majority of germ cells before birth, and is independant from pituitary gonadotrophins. Since in primordial follicles the rate of atretic degeneration is reduced, the embedding into granulosa cells appears to fulfil metabolic requirements of the differentiating oocyte. The topical origin of the granulosa cells is still controversely discussed. However, according to Franchi & Baker (1973) they most probably originate from the "sex cords" which grow down from the coelomic epithelium of the undifferentiated gonad.

3.2 Primary follicles

The primary oocyte grows in the primary follicle *(Fig. 2b)* and is surrounded by a complete single layer of enlarged granulosa cells of a cuboidal or columnar structure. The transformation of primordial into primary follicles which is still independant from pituitary gonadotrophic stimulation, is started before, or shortly after, birth and continues throughout female life until the postmenopause. The numbers of primary follicles do not fluctuate during the menstrual cycle until they reach the stage of gonadotrophin dependency when they either progress to the secondary stage or, much more probably, undergo atretic degeneration. It should be mentioned that some authors extend the term primary follicle to the point of presence of more than one layer of granulosa cells and the formation of the zona pellucida and that others do not differentiate between primordial and primary follicles.

3.3 Secondary follicles

The secondary follicle *(Fig. 2c)* reaches a diameter of about 200 µm, and its covering consists of about four compact layers of granulosa cells, which are now termed the membrana granulosa (or stratum granulosum). The cells originate entirely from hypertrophy and rapid mitotic division within the original single cell layer of the primary follicle; no further cells are added from the surrounding tissue. The primary oocyte increases in volume to its final size of 100–130 µm diameter. Between the primary oocyte and the membrana granulosa, the zona pellucida is formed. This is important for metabolic processes in the oocyte and in the cleaving egg during fertilization and pre-implantation.

Around the membrana granulosa but separated by a prominent basement membrane, a concentric arrangement of the stroma cells initiates the formation of the theca cell layers. The innermost layer generates large glandular cells forming the theca interna, which is the predominant source of oestrogen biogenesis during the follicular phase of the cycle. The theca interna becomes vascular, thus surrounding the follicle by a refined network of capillary vessels. The arterial capillaries provide the avascular membrana granulosa and the oocyte with nutrients. The venous capillaries drain, the steroid hormones secreted from the theca cells into the ovarian hilar veins and thereby into the general circulation. The outermost layer forms the theca externa, which ist not clearly separated from the interna and retains more fibroblastic tissue than cellular structures.

The progression of primary follicles to the secondary stage requires stimulation by gonadotrophins, in particular by FSH. The transformation occurs from the late luteal phase of a cycle until the early proliferative phase of the following cycle, when a broad elevation of basic FSH concentration in peripheral blood is present. It has been estimated that in macaca mulatta (Koering, 1969) about 20 primary follicles enter the development to the secondary stage in each ovulatory cycle, however, all but two become atretic before completion. One of the two residual follicles also normally undergoes atresia at an intermediate stage of about 1 mm diameter. Thus, only one out of 20 primary follicles becomes a secondary follicle and is selected for a development into the tertiary stage.

Follicular growth to the secondary stage may also occur in early childhood and prepuberty, induced by an irregular basic secretion of pituitary FSH, or even in late fetal ovaries, probably induced by a diaplacental transfer of maternal FSH. However, the ultimate stages of follicular growth, which include full maturation, resumption and completion of meiosis and ovulation, require an established hypothalamic-pituitary-ovarian axis and are therefore not reached before completion of puberty. Thus, before puberty, follicles reaching an advanced primary or secondary stage of development are inevitably destined to atresia. However, the vast majority of growing follicles of any stage of maturation are predetermined for the same fate even after the endocrine system is fully established.

3.4 Tertiary follicles

In the one residual secondary follicle, the most striking event is the FSH-controlled formation of the antrum folliculi, which is accompanied by a rapid increase in volume *(Fig. 2d, e, f)*. Fully developed tertiary stages are therefore also known as antral follicles, and secondary stages as pre-antral follicles.

The tertiary stage of development is initiated in the late secondary follicle *(Fig. 2d)* by a rapid mitotic proliferation of the membrana granulosa whereby the nuclei of the granulosa cells become more granulated. Follicular fluid (liquor folliculi) is produced by secretion of the granulosa cells and by transudation from the theca interna capillaries, giving rise to the formation of fluid-filled cavities within the granulosa layers. These enlarge rapidly, flow together and thus form the antrum folliculi *(Fig. 2e)*. The primary oocyte, which remains surrounded by granulosa cells, is placed into an excentrical position forming the cumulus oophorus. At this stage, cross-sections of the tertiary follicle show a typical semilunar shape *(Fig. 2f)*. Concomitant changes of the theca layers include a marked extension and growth of the glandular cells in the interna, and the development of a network of lymphatic vessels in both the theca interna and externa.

The tertiary follicle which is fully developed around day 7 of the cycle becomes the "dominant" follicle (cf. Hodgen et al., 1983) selected to enter final maturation

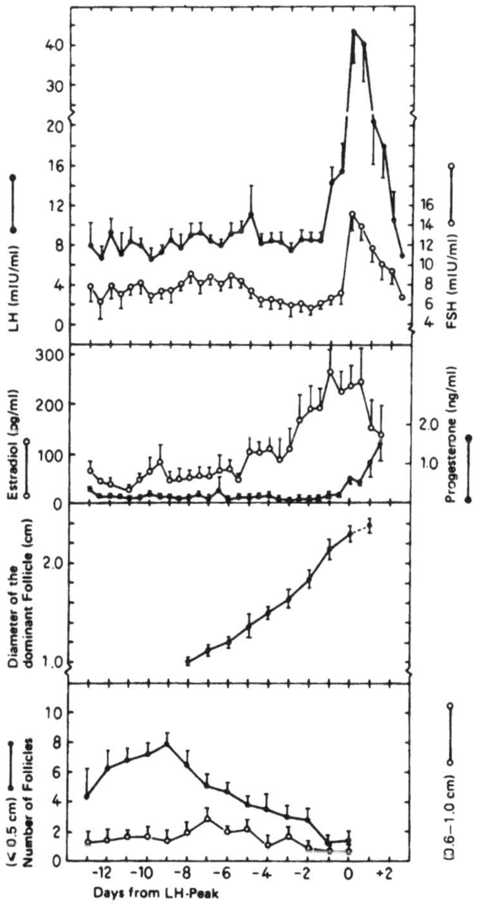

Fig. 3 Pattern of LH, FSH, estradiol-17β, and progesterone secretion, ultrasonographically determined growth of the dominant follicle, and number of follicles during the normal menstrual cycle, normalized to the day of the LH surge as day 0. Each point represents mean ± SEM of 7 observations. Blood samples were drawn twice daily, ultrasonography was performed once daily. Note the parallel increase of serum estradiol and of the diameter of the dominant follicle and the concomittant decline of FSH levels and number of small follicles. (With permission from Leyendecker & Wildt, 1983).

before ovulation. It measures 10–14 mm in diameter and can be identified by ultrasonography 6–8 days prior to the midcyclic LH surge (Leyendecker & Wildt, 1983; Wildt et al., 1983). At this time, the ovarian secretion of oestradiol-17β begins to rise; it surpasses the level of 100 pg/ml 5 days before the LH peak. According to the negative feedback regulation, FSH decreases *(Fig. 3)*.

3.5 Graafian follicles

As it approaches the point of ovulation, the tertiary follicle increases rapidly in volume, reaching a final diameter of 20–25 mm when the preovulatory LH peak occurs (Wildt et al., 1983). The structure has now become a Graafian follicle and is definitely selected for ovulation *(Fig. 2g)*.

The granulosa cells of the cumulus oophorus are reduced and form the corona radiata. The cumulus separates from the follicular wall so that the primary oocyte, embedded in its residual cumulus cells, floats freely in the antrum. Both the granulosa and the theca layers of the follicular wall are attenuated *(Fig. 2h)*.

The LH-induced resumption of meiosis occurs some 36–48 hours prior to ovulation. It starts with the completion of the meiotic prophase, i.e., by the passing of the primary oocyte from the arrested diplotene into the diakinesis stage of the meiotic prophase. This is followed by the first meiotic division, which results in a *haploid secondary oocyte* with an attached haploid polar body and which is completed some hours before ovulation. In most mammalia, the secondary oocyte remains in this stage until ovulation has occurred and undergoes the second (mitotic) meiotic division only after fertilization.

As it approaches ovulation, the Graafian follicle becomes visible at the ovarian surface in the form of a conical protrusion (thecal conus) with a stigma at the summit. This is penetrated, probably by enzymatic proteolytic digestion, at the moment of ovulation. The secondary oocyte is drained out with the follicular fluid and is picked up by the Fallopian tube.

The concomitant endocrine events *(Fig. 3)* occur in the following sequence: The growth of tertiary and Graafian follicles is accompanied by a steep increase in the secretion of estradiol-17β, which surpasses a serum concentration of 150 pg/ml about 60 hours before the LH peak. This level is considered the critical threshold for an estradiol-induced positive feedback effect on the LH release. The latency period of this reaction has an estimated duration of about 48 hours. Thus, LH begins to rise 48 hours after estradiol has passed the 150 pg-threshold in the presence of a dominant follicle of 22 mm in diameter. The increase of progesterone starts 24 hours later and passes the concentration of 1 ng/ml serum 48 hours after the beginning of release of LH, indicating the onset of luteinization (for details and references cf. Leyendecker et al., 1972, 1975, 1976; Nocke & Leyendecker, 1972a, 1972b; Wildt & Leyendecker, 1981, 1983; Wildt et al., 1983; Knobil & Wildt, 1983).

4. Perimenopausal involution of the hypothalamic-pituitary-ovarian endocrine system

During the premenopausal years the cyclical events described above gradually reduced until postmenopausal amenorrhea is established. The process is obviously initiated by a progressive functional impairment of the ovarian link within the regulatory circuit operating between the hypothalamus, the pituitary gland, and the ovary itself. Thus, the involution of the endocrine system originates from the ovary. As a consequence, the control of the endocrine events becomes more and more dearranged, and clinical manifestations such as menstrual disorders and finally the cessation of bleedings and of fertility follow.

In the stage of the premenopausal transition, regular menstrual bleedings may still occur for a long time, even though a stepwise dearrangement of ovarian function is already in progress. The menstrual pattern before regular bleedings cease varies widely. It may comprise the entire range of cyclical disturbances with or without ovulation, and includes the slight luteal dysfunction at the one end of the scale, and the abrupt onset of amenorrhoea on the other end. The great variation of endocrine implications in premenopausal menstrual disorders is essentially comparable to that described in younger as well as in elderly women by several authors (cf. Brown et al., 1959; Brown & Matthew, 1962; Hammerstein, 1969, Leyendecker et al., 1975).

A remarkable example of an acute dearrangement of a cycle has been observed by Cooke (1976) in a 37 year old patient *(Fig. 4)*. After clomiphene treatment, an abrupt transition of normal LH and FSH concentrations to postmenopausal levels occurred, indicating a rapid exhaustion of the ovarian response. The excessive rise of LH and FSH was associated with a steep decrease of estradiol and with the onset of hot flushes.

In addition to the functional ovarian impairment, a concurrent age-related endocrine involution at the hypothalamic and/or at the pituitary level has also been suggested from animal experiments. Some authors claim a decreased responsiveness of the pituitary to GnRH, while others consider the hypothalamus as the main site of aging involved in the termination of fertility in senescent animals. The overall results are contradictory and not transferable to the human female. Furthermore, few of the experiments have included ovarian steroid replacement in their design (cf. review by Butcher & Page, 1981).

One of the best known endocrine events in postmenopausal women is the striking increase of pituitary gonadotrophin production, in particular of FSH, as measured either in urine or in the circulating concentrations in peripheral blood. It has been demonstrated that pituitary gonadotrophin production already increases several years before the menopause. It was also reported (cf. Pincus et al., 1955; Kaiser & Daume, 1965) that the urinary estrogen excretion declines in premenopausal women. A typical study is summarized in *Fig. 5*. From the results, a gradual decrease

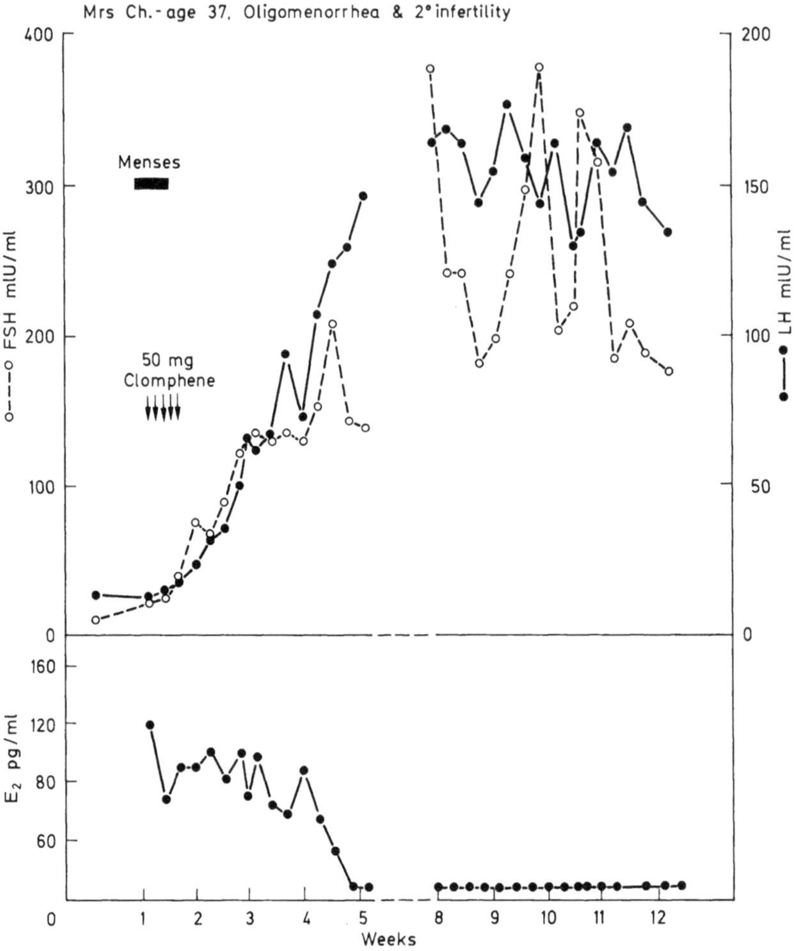

Fig. 4 Acute transition from normal LH, FSH, and estradiol concentrations to postmenopausal levels following clomiphene treatment. (With permission from Cooke, 1976).

of total urinary estrogens with progressing age was evident, as compared with the normal mean excretion during the cycle. The decline was significant (P = 0,05) at 2,5 years before the menopause. In the same women urinary gonadotrophins were measured by bioassay. The mean excretion was significantly (P = 0,05) increased more than 2,5 years before the menopause: there was an almost fivefold increase as compared to the maximum excretion during ovulatory cycles.

A long-held hypothesis deduced from studies of this kind was that the pituitary gonadotrophins in premenopausal women increase due to a reduced negative feedback effect as a consequence of a decline in ovarian estrogen secretion. However, a premenopausal decrease in ovarian estrogen secretion was not unequivocally confirmed. It has therefore been suggested that a declined sensitivity of the negative

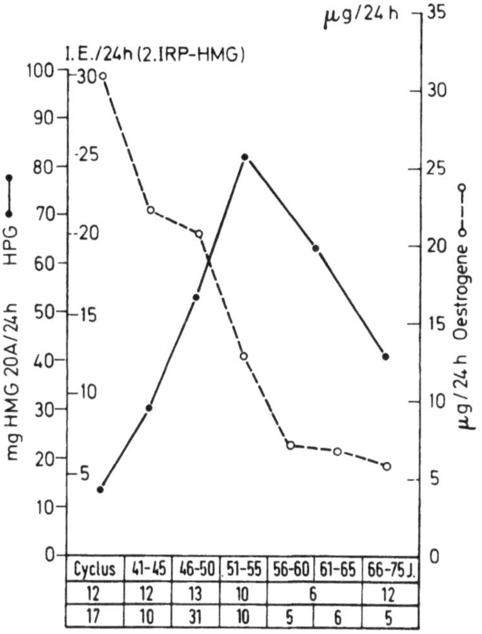

Fig. 5 Mean urinary excretion of pituitary gonadotrophins (HPG) and total estrogens (estrone + estradiol-17β + estriol) in women between 41 and 75 years of age as compared to the normal excretion during the menstrual cycle (drawn from data of Kaiser & Daume, 1965). (With permission from Nocke & Leyendecker, 1970).

Table 1 Serum concentrations of FSH (µg/dl) and estradiol-17β (ng/dl) in ovulating women by age groups at different stages of the menstrual cycle (data from Reyes et al., 1977).

hormone	phase of the cycle	age group (years)			
		20–29	34–39	40–44	45–50
FSH	early follicular	26	35	49	80*
	late follicular	18	18	33*	39*
	periovulatory	23	35	30	62*
	luteal	8	14	22*	27*
	premenstrual	10	16	15	47*
estradiol-17β	early follicular	2	3	3	5*
	late follicular	9	11	12	13
	luteal	8	8	8	6

* P <0,05 as compared to 20–29 years of age

feedback system rather than a decrease in estrogen secretion might be responsable for the rise in pituitary gonadotrophins (cf. Dilman, 1971). It has also been proposed that an inhibin-like ovarian hormone may be a factor in the control of pituitary FSH secretion (cf. Sherman & Korenman, 1975; Sherman et al., 1976). *Table 1* shows results from a study of the serum concentrations of FSH and estradiol-17β in women with menstrual cycles between 20 and 50 years of age (Reyes et al., 1977). The authors reported an increase in circulating FSH with advancing age at different stages of the menstrual cycle, in particular during the early follicular phase; no increase in LH was observed. In contrast to a current opinion, serum levels of estradiol were increased during the early and late follicular phase with progressing age, but this was significant (P = 0,05) only in women over 45 years in the early follicular phase. These results obviously do not support the view that the reduced negative feedback effect is due to impaired estrogen secretion. However, they are compatible with either a reduced sensitivity of the neuroendocrine system or the existence of an inhibin-like ovarian substance secreted independently of estradiol.

The experiments shown in *Fig. 6* to *Fig. 8* were conducted in order to study the negative and positive feedback effects of estradiol and progesterone in postmeno-

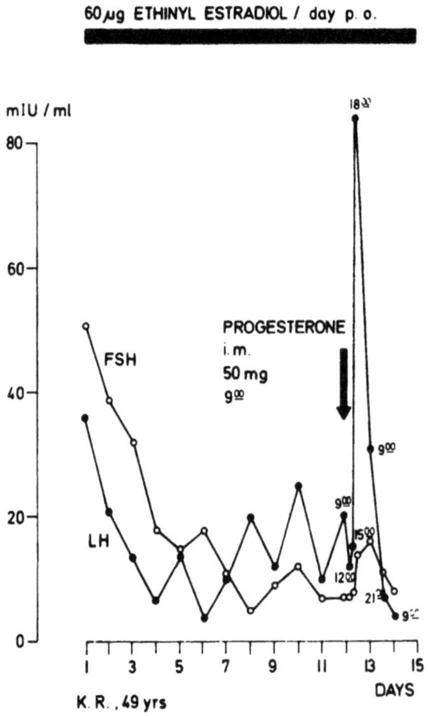

Fig. 6 Ethinylestradiol-induced negative, and progesterone-induced positive, feedback-reaction in an oophorectomized postmenopausal woman. (With permission from Leyendecker et al., 1972).

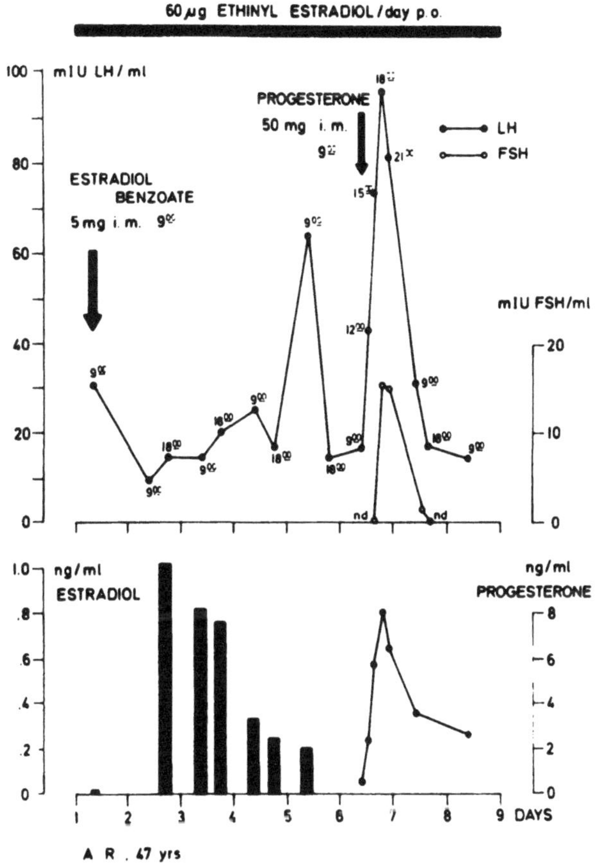

Fig. 7 Subsequent estradiol benzoate- and progesterone-induced positive feedback-reactions in an oophorectomized postmenopausal woman. (With permission from Leyendecker et al., 1972).

pausal women. By applying an appropriate pretreatment with ethinyl estradiol followed by singly injections of estradiol benzoate and/or progesterone, we attempted to simulate the endocrine situation of the preovulatory phase of the cycle. Abrupt LH surges were induced by injections of either progesterone *(Fig. 6)* or estradiol followed by progesterone *(Fig. 7)*. However, when the sequence was reversed and progesterone injected first, the subsequent injection of estradiol failed to induce a release of LH secretion *(Fig. 8)*, thus indicating the inhibition of an estradiol-induced positive feedback-reaction in the presence of progesterone (for details cf. Leyendecker et al., 1972; Nocke & Leyendecker, 1972a, 1972b). Comparable responses were obtained in young eugonadal women when a similar experimental design was applied (Leyendecker et al., 1976).

The results, therefore, do not support the hypothesis of an impaired neuroendocrine responsiveness against the negative and positive feedback effects of estradiol and progesterone in postmenopausal women.

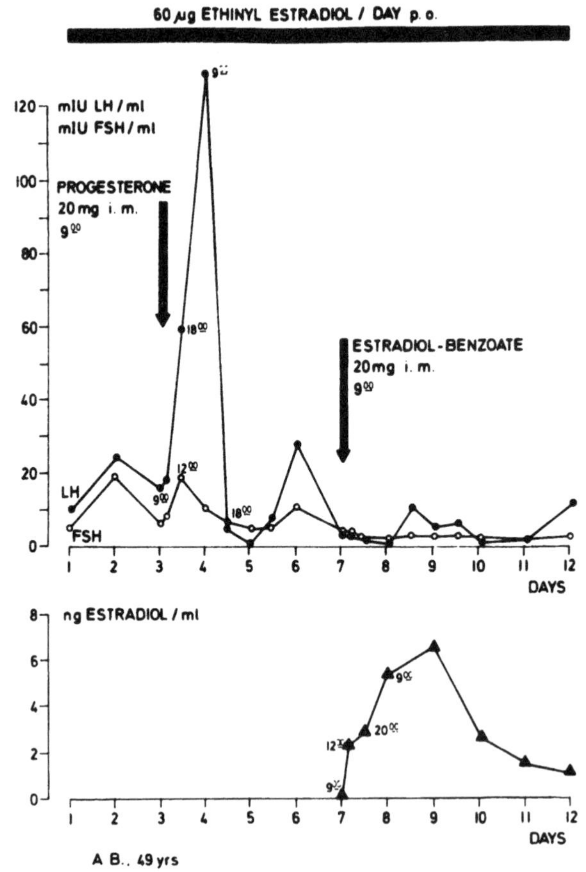

Fig. 8 Progesterone-induced positive feedback-reaction in a postmenopausal woman. The subsequent injection of estradiol benzoate failed to induce a second release of LH. (With permission from Leyendecker et al., 1972).

5. Postmenopausal steroid hormone production from ovarian and non-ovarian sources

Although the cyclical activity of follicular structures has expired in postmenopausal ovaries, this does not necessarily imply the entire cessation of steroid hormone secretion and production. From urinary excretion studies, it has, in principle, been known for almost 20 years that some postmenopausal women still excrete small but significant amounts of estrogens and other steroid metabolites and that these steroids may decrease following oophorectomy. On the other hand, following oophorectomy, pituitary gonadotrophin excretion may increase, thus indicating, indirectly, an ovarian secretion of estrogens or their precursors (Procopé, 1968; Procopé & Adlercreutz, 1969; Nocke, 1969).

For example, in a total of 264 postmenopausal women mentioned in the literature, a mean total urinary estrogen excretion between 5,0 and 26,2 µg/24h was reported. The women were 50–85 years of age and 1–26 years postmenopausal. When the subjects suffering from various diseases were excluded, the "normal" mean excretion was between 5 and 10 µg/24h. A comparison of a total of 205 postmenopausal women with 125 oophorectomized women showed significantly higher mean urinary excretion rates for estrogens in the former group by a factor of 1,2–2,9, and for gonadotrophins in the latter group by a factor of 1,2–1,9 (Nocke & Leyendecker, 1970).

In oophorectomized women, the residual urinary estrogen excretion may be further decreased by adrenocortical suppression or adrenalectomy, and elevated by administration of ACTH (Bulbrook et al., 1958a, 1958b; Bayer et al., 1958a, 1958b, 1960, 1961; Procopé, 1968; Procopé & Adlercreutz, 1969; Breuer, 1969).

A significant urinary estrogen excretion has been shown to exist particularly in postmenopausal women with cortical stromal hyperplasia of the ovary. and with ovarian tumors such as cystadenomas which are not considered to be endocrinologically active. The steroid mostly involved in postmenopausal estrogen production seems to the estrone, which is considered to be mainly a peripheral metabolite of ovarian and adrenal C_{19}-steroids. From an extensive study of this topic Procopé (1968) concluded

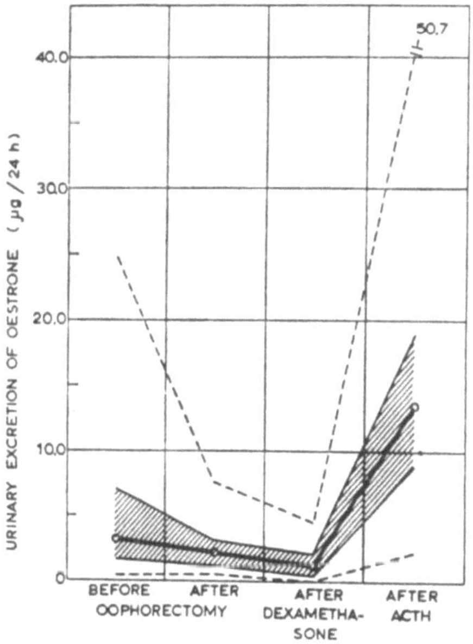

Fig. 9 Urinary estrone excretion in postmenopausal women before and after oophorectomy, after dexamethasone suppression, and after ACTH stimulation of the adrenals. The decrease after dexamethasone administration was significant (P<0,01), and the increase after ACTH administration highly significant (P<0,001). Median values, quartiles, and range of 34 subjects. (With permission from Procopé, 1968).

a) that in postemenopausal women with a normal age-related ovarian histology, urinary estrogens are mainly of extraovarian origin;
b) that in postmenopausal subjects with various degrees of estrogen effects (vaginal smear, endometrium), with ovarian cortical stromal hyperplasia, and with ovarian tumors commonly considered not endocrinologically to be active, particularly cystadenomas, the estrogens or their precursors are produced by the ovaries;
c) that in oophorectomized postmenopausal women urinary estrone or its precursor(s) is, to a significant extent, of adrenocortical origin.

This can be illustrated by some observations. In *Fig. 9* the changes in urinary estrone excretion after administration of dexamethasone ($P<0{,}01$) and of ACTH ($P<0{,}001$) were significant (Procopé, 1968).

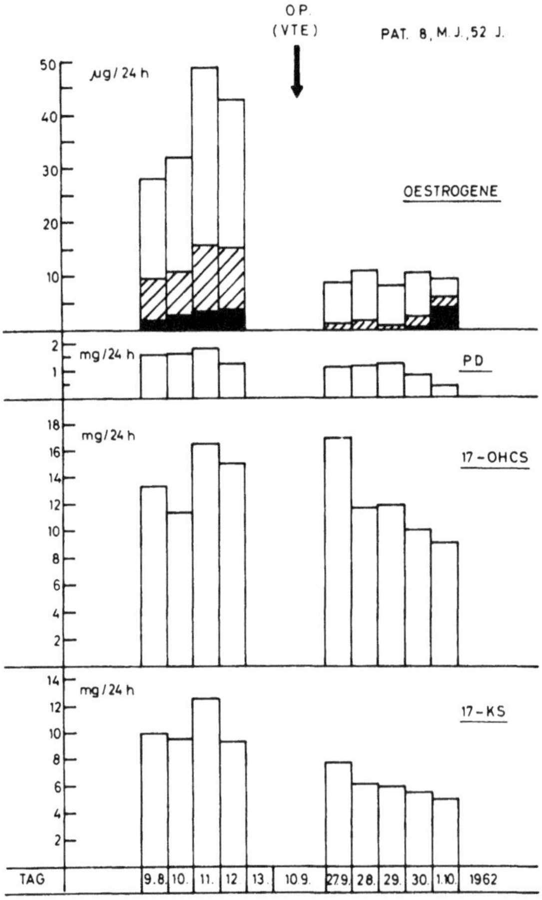

Fig. 10 Urinary excretion (from above) of estriol, estrone, estradiol-17β, pregnanediol, total 17-hydroxycorticosteroids, and total 17-oxo steroids in a 52 year old menopausal patient with endometrial carcinoma before and after oophorectomy. (With permission from Nocke, 1969). *Methods:* Brown et al. (1957); Nocke (1961); Norymberski et al. (1953); Appleby et al. (1955).

In the patient shown in *Fig. 10,* 52 years of age and 7 months after her last menstrual bleeding, a considerable persisting urinary estrogen excretion was decreased to 26% of the control level following oophorectomy. The mean preoperative/postoperative differences were significant ($P<0{,}01$) in total estrogens, estrone and estriol, but not in estradiol-17β. There was a twofold ($P<0{,}05$) increase in urinary gonadotrophin excretion following operation (Nocke, 1969).

In the five patients shown in *Table 2,* aged 53–63 years of age and 4–10 years postmenopausal, a small estrone excretion (0,5–2,0 μg/24h) was decreased by 6–48% following oophorectomy. The differences were significant in 4 of the 5 cases (Nocke, 1969).

Table 2 Preoperative vs. postoperative urinary excretion of estrone in five postmenopausal women with endometrial carcinoma (Nocke, 1969).

patient	urinary estrone (μg/24h)		mean differences		
	ante op. $\bar{x} \pm s$ (N)	post op. $\bar{x}' \pm s'$ (N')	%	t	p
1	0,84 ± 0,05 (4)	0,55 ± 0,65 (4)	−35	2,679	<0,05
2	0,49 ± 0,07 (4)	0,46 (1)	− 6	0,291	>0,70
3	0,96 ± 0,37 (4)	0,50 ± 0,15 (5)	−48	2,528	<0,02
4	2,04 ± 0,28 (5)	1,15 ± 0,12 (4)	−44	5,933	<0,001
5	1,90 ± 0,04 (3)	1,43 ± 0,07 (5)	−25	7,966	<0,001

$\bar{x}$, $\bar{x}'$ mean value
s, s' standard deviation
N, N' number of duplicate determinations
p probability of t (N+N'−2 degrees of freedom)
Methods: Brown & Blair (1960); Nocke (1961).

Table 3 Urinary excretion of estrone (E_1), estradiol-17β (E_2), estriol (E_3), total estrogens ($E_1+E_2+E_3$), total 17-oxo steroids (17-OS), total 17-hydroxycorticosteroids (17-OHCS), pregnanediol (PD), and pregnanetriol (PT) in a 72 year old patient bearing a large benign pseudomucinous cystadenoma of the left ovary before and after bilateral oophorectomy (Nocke, 1969).

condition	urinary steroid fraction ($\bar{x} \pm s$)							
	estrogens (μg/24h)				17-OS	17-OHCS	PD	PT
	E_1	E_2	E_3	total	(mg/24h)	(mg/24h)	(mg/24h)	(mg/24h)
ante op. (3)	5,2±0,6	17,8±12,4	5,4±2,9	28,3±15,6	11,0±1,2	14,3±0,2	2,33±0,19	1,08±0,12
post op. (3)	2,3±0,9	3,9± 2,7	1,1±0,5	7,2± 3,4	6,2±1,3	6,7±1,1	0,38±0,45	0,42±0,03
ratio ante op. / post op.	2,3	4,6	4,9	3,9	1,8	2,1	6,1	2,6
analysis of F	20,582	3,608	6,646	5,299	31,848	141,429	314,467	87,137
variance P	<0,05	>0,05	>0,05	>0,05	<0,01	<0,001	<0,001	<0,001

Methods: Brown et al. (1957); Nocke (1961); Norymberski et al. (1953); Appleby et al. (1955); Nocke (1970).

In a woman 72 years of age *(Table 3)* presenting with an ovarian pseudomucinous cystadenoma and uterine bleeding, a decrease of total urinary estrogens to 25% of the control levels was observed after removal of the ovaries. The differences, however, were significant only with estrone and the C_{19}- and C_{21}-steroid metabolites. Separation of the individual C_{19}-steroids by gradient elution chromatography *(Fig. 11)* suggested that the tumor might have produced some androgens. As shown in *Table 4,* the biological negative feedback activity of the steroids secreted or produced by the tumor was indicated by a 6,6 fold increase of pituitary gonadotrophin excretion following the operation (Nocke, 1969). These results may be compared to an *in vitro* study using the microsomal and soluble fractions from a papillary serous cystadenocarcinoma of a 54 years aged postmenopausal woman with virilization (Plotz et al., 1966). The authors demonstrated the transformation of 4-^{14}C-progesterone to androstenedione and testosterone, of 7-^{3}H-17α-hydroxypregnenolone to dehydro*epi*androsterone and androstenedione, and of 7-^{3}H-pregneneolone to dehydro*epi*androsterone.

The urinary estrogen excretion persisting in oophorectomized women may be significantly decreased or even abolished after cortisone treatment (*Fig. 12;* Bayer et al., 1961; Breuer, 1969) and after adrenalectomy (*Fig. 13;* Bulbrook et al., 1958b),

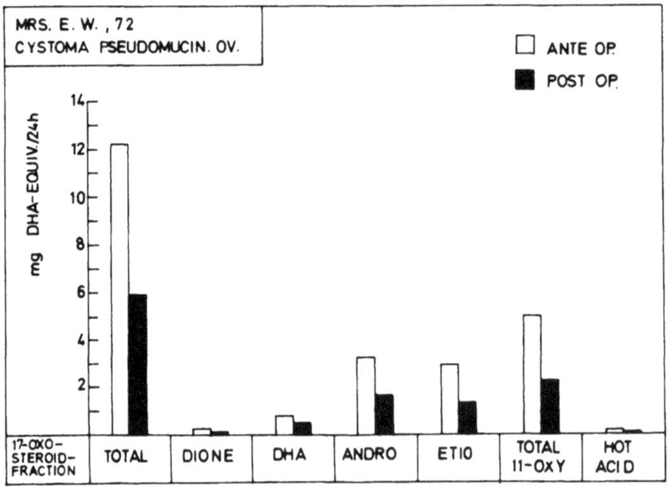

Fig. 11 Urinary excretion of the individual 17-oxo steroids in a 72 year old patient with a pseudomucinous cystadenoma of the left ovary before and after bilateral oophorectomy. (With permission from Nocke, 1969).
Method: Kellie & Wade (1957).

Dione	androstane-3, 17-dione + etiocholane-3, 17-dione
DHA	dehydro*epi*androsterone
Andro	androsterone
Etio	etiocholane-3α-ol-17-one
Total 11-oxy	total 11-oxo- and 11β-hydroxy-17-oxo steroids
Hot acid	steroid fraction hydrolyzed by boiling with 10% HCl

Table 4 Increase of urinary pituitary gonadotrophin (HPG) excretion in a 72 year old patient following removal of a pseudomucinous cystadenoma of the left ovary (Nocke, 1969).

condition	design of assay[2]			urinary HPG-excretion		statistics[2]			
	U + S	N	J	HMG-U/ 24h[3]	IU/24h[4]	fiducial range (P = 0,05)	g_c	λ_c	L_c
ante op.[1]	1 + 3	3	3	5,8	2,4	59–167%	0,016	0,163	6,13
post op.[1]	3 + 3	3	3	38,1	15,9	70–144%	0,016	0,163	6,13

1 Urine pool of 3 consecutive days
2 *Methods:*
extraction: Johnson (1958)
design and statistics: Borth et al. (1957); Borth (1960)
bioassay: Levin & Tyndale (1937)
3 HMG-20A
4 2nd IRP-HMG

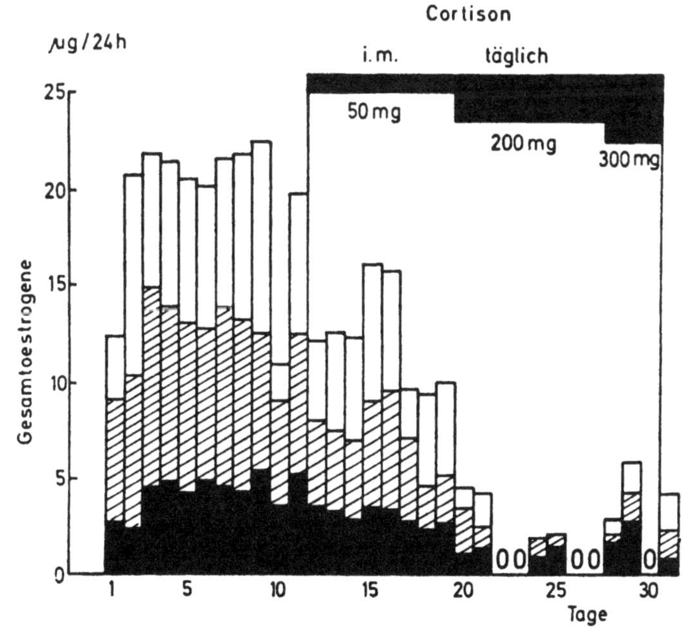

Fig. 12 Urinary excretion of (from above) estriol, estrone, and estradiol-17β in a 46 year old oophorectomized patient before and after cortisone treatment. (With permission from Breuer, 1969). *Methods:* Brown et al. (1957); Nocke (1961).

and considerably increased after administration of ACTH, but not of HCG or PMS (*Fig. 14;* Bayer et al., 1960; Breuer, 1969). It appears reasonable to conclude, therefore, that urinary estrogens, or their precursors, excreted in oophorectomized women are of adrenocortical origin.

Several authors have studies the transformation of various radioactive steroid substrates into estrogens by postmenopausal ovaries *in vitro.* Using ovarian dissec-

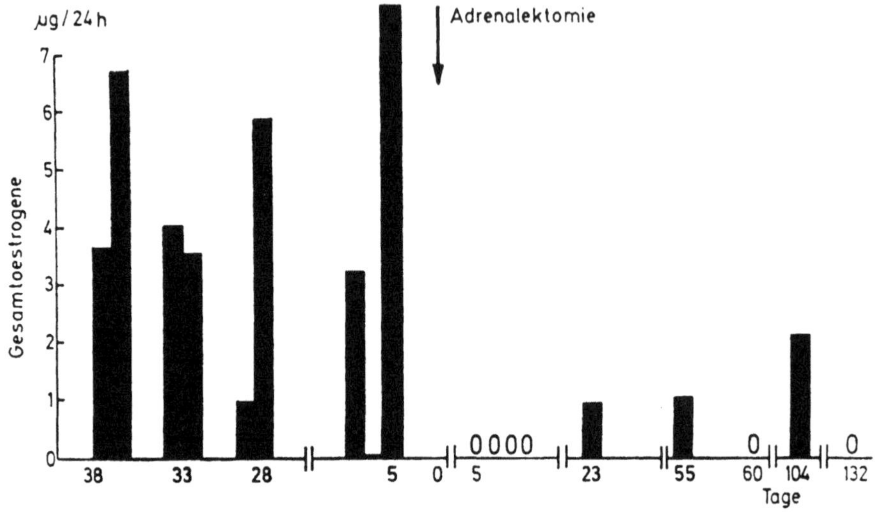

Fig. 13 Urinary excretion of total estrogens (estrone + estradiol-17β + estriol) in a 48 year old oophorectomized patient before and after bilateral adrenalectomy (*case 1* from Bulbrook et al., 1958b). – (With permission from Breuer, 1969).
Method: Brown et al. (1957).

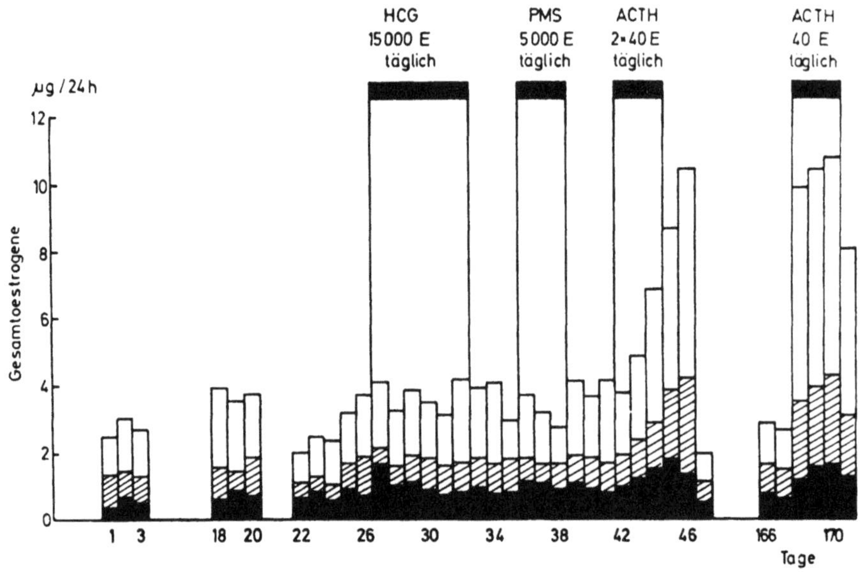

Fig. 14 Urinary excretion of (from above) estriol, estrone, and estradiol-17β in a 34 year old oophorectomized patient before and after administration of HCG, PMS, and ACTH. (With permission from Breuer, 1969).
Methods: Brown et al. (1957); Nocke (1961).

tions in the presence of ovine FSH and of several cofactors, Forleo & Collins (1964) identified small amounts of estradiol-17β with 4-^{14}C-progesterone and 4-^{14}C-testosterone, and of estrone and estradiol with 4-^{14}C-androstenedione as a substrate. Plotz et al. (1967) incubated the combined microsomal and water soluble fractions from ovarian tissue homogenates of 22 postmenopausal women with TPNH as a cofactor. Traces or small amounts of estrone and estradiol-17β were identified in one experiment with 4-^{14}C-pregneneolone, and in two experiments with 4-^{14}C-testosterone as a substrate. The ovaries contained a cortical stromal hyperplasia and belonged to women with adenomatous endometrial hyperplasia. Using stromal tissue from menopausal and postmenopausal ovaries, Mattingly & Huang (1969) found a transformation into estrogens of 2% with 7-^{3}H-pregneneolone, and of 4% with 7-^{3}H-androstenedione as a substrate.

A more detailed understanding of the postmenopausal ovarian and extraovarian steroid biogenesis *in vivo* was provided by determinations of steroid hormones in peripheral and ovarian vein blood under various conditions, such as before and after endocrine ablation, or following selective suppression and stimulation of a certain gland. Judd et al. (1974a) reported a decrease of testosterone and androstenedione in the peripheral blood of postmenopausal women following oophorectomy and concluded that the ovarian testosterone secretion may be larger in postmenopausal than in premenopausal subjects. In another study by Judd et al. (1974b) comparing the levels of androstenedione, testosterone, estrone, and estradiol in peripheral vs. ovarian vein blood, the mean levels in the ovarian effluent were found higher by a factor of 15 in testosterone ($P<0{,}01$), of 4 in androstenedione (n.s), and of 2 in both estrone and estradiol ($P<0{,}05$). These data definitely show a secretion of testosterone by the postmenopausal ovary, and also provide some evidence for a small secretion of estrone and estradiol-17β. However, since the absolute amounts of estrogens are very small, the authors suggested that, as suggested by Siiteri & MacDonald (1973), circulating estrogens in postmenopausal women arise predominantly from a peripheral conversion of androstenedione to estrone. Since reliable data on the ovarian perfusion rate are lacking, the data do not permit a conclusion about the ovarian contribution to peripheral blood levels of steroid hormones in postmenopausal women.

Vermeulen (1976) reported an extensive study on the blood levels of eight steroids in postmenopausal women under basal conditions, after adrenocortical stimulation (ACTH) and suppression (dexamethasone), and after ovarian stimulation (dexamethasone and HCG). Estrone, estradiol, testosterone, dihydrotestosterone, androstenedione, dehydro*epi*androsterone, progesterone, and 17α-hydroxyprogesterone were determined. The levels obtained were compared to the concentrations found during the follicular phase of the cycle, and with those found in oophorectomized postmenopausal women. The following conclusions may be drawn from this study:

a) Progesterone and 17α-hydroxyprogesterone are almost exclusively, and dehydro*epi*androsterone is predominantly, of adrenal origin. A small but significant amount of dehydro*epi*androsterone is also secreted by the postmenopausal ovary.
b) Androstenedione, testosterone, and dehydrotestosterone are of mixed adrenocortical and ovarian origin. The postmenopausal ovary is probably the direct or indirect source of about 50% of testosterone, and of 30% of androstenedione circulating in peripheral blood.
c) The estrogens appear to be of predominantly adrenocortical origin. They probably arise mainly from a peripheral aromatization of C_{19}-steroids secreted by the adrenal cortex, but to a smaller extent also by the ovary. This does not entirely exclude that certain postmenopausal ovaries which contain structures of particular tissue may also directly secrete small amounts of estrogens.

The peripheral conversion of androgens into aromatized C_{18}-steroids has been studied extensively (MacDonald et al., 1967; Longcope, 1971; Schindler et al., 1972; Grodin et al., 1973; Siiteri & MacDonald, 1973; Hemsell et al., 1974; Nimrod & Ryan, 1975). The main results can be summarized as follows:

a) The principal estrogen produced in postemenopausal women is estrone, which is predominantly derived from a peripheral aromatization of circulating androstendione. Neither the adrenal cortex nor the ovary contributes significantly to the total estrogen production in asymptomatic postmenopausal women by direct glandular secretion.
b) Incubations with adipose tissue *in vitro* using androstenedione and 19-hydroxyandrostenedione as a substrate have shown a conversion mainly into estrone, whereas testosterone is mainly converted into estradiol-17β.
c) The *in vivo* conversion of circulating androstenedione into estrone shows a highly significant progression with advancing age.

6. Summary

The aging of the primate overy is a gradually progressing process of many years duration. The process results in the involution of the capacity to generate follicular structures. The principal endocrine consequence is the cessation of those hormonal events showing a cyclical pattern because they are correlated to follicular growth and regression.

However, a certain non-cyclical endocrine activity of the ovary is maintained until advanced age, although on a much reduced level. This capacity is provided by extrafollicular tissue of somatic origin, in particular the stroma cells. These structures continue to secrete small amounts of testosterone and androstenedione, which are both reversibly interconvertable in many peripheral tissues. Added to the secretory products of the adrenal cortex, the circulating androgens are, *via* androstenedione, aromatized to estrone, which, by a reversable reduction at carbon 17, also gives rise to small amounts of the biologically more active estradiol. This peripheral conversion takes place mainly in adipose tissue, and is progressive with increasing body weight and advancing age.

Under certain exceptional circumstances, there also may be a small direct secretion of estrogens by the postmenopausal ovary.

Acknowledgement. The author is indebted to Mrs. Marlen Przybilka for preparing the photographs, and to Mrs. Doris Vornberger for typing the manuscript.

7. References

Appleby, J. I., G. Gibson, J. K. Norymberski, R. D. Stubbs (1955): Indirect Analysis of Corticosteroids. 1. The Determination of 17-Hydroxycorticosteroids. Biochem. J. **60**, 453–460.

Baker, T. G. (1963): A quantitative and Cytological Study of Germ Cells in Human Ovaries. Proc. Roy. Soc., London, Ser. B, **158**, 417–433.

Baker, T. G. (1971): Electron Microscopy of the Primary and Secondary Oocyte. *In:* Raspé, G. (ed.): Schering Symposium on Intrinsic and Extrinsic Facots in Early Mammalian Development, Venice, 1970. Pergamon Press-Vieweg, Advances in the Biosciences **6**, Oxford, Edinburgh, New York, Toronto, Sidney, Braunschweig; pp. 7–27.

Baker, T. G. (1972): Oogenesis and Ovarian Development. *In:* Balin, H., S. R. Glasser (eds.): Reproductive Biology. Excerpta Medica Foundation, Amsterdam, New York; pp. 398–437.

Bayer, J. M., H. Breuer, W. Nocke (1958a): Die Ausscheidung der Oestrogene im Urin beim Mammacarcinom vor und nach Ovariektomie sowie in spontaner Postmenopause. Ein Beitrag zur Frage der adrenalen Oestrogene. Langenbecks Arch. u. Dtsch. Z. Chir. **288**, 84–95.

Bayer, J. M., H. Breuer, W. Nocke, W. Richter (1958b): Die Oestrogen-Ausscheidung im Urin beim Mamma-Carcinom nach verschiedenen therapeutischen Maßnahmen. Bull. Soc. Internat. Chir. **17**, 146–155.

Bayer, J. M., H. Breuer, W. Nocke (1960): Vergleichende Untersuchungen über den Einfluß LH- und FSH-wirksamer Präparate sowie von ACTH auf die Nebennierenrindenfunktion, insbesondere auf die adrenalen Oestrogene bei ovariektomierten Frauen. Klin. Wschr. **38**, 1143–1146.

Bayer, J. M., H. Breuer, W. Nocke (1961): Beitrag zur Ausscheidung der Oestrogene im Urin bei ovariektomierten Frauen mit Mammacarcinom unter dem Einfluß von Cortison und seinen Derivaten. Endokrinologie **40**, 129–147.

Bomsel-Helmreich, O. (1983): The Preovulatory Human Oocyte and its Microenvironment. *In:* Beier, H. M., H. R. Lindner (eds.): Fertilization of the Human Egg In Vitro. Springer-Verlag, Berlin, Heidelberg, New York, Tokyo; pp. 19–34.

Borth, R., E. Diczfalusy, H. D. Heinrichs (1957): Grundlagen der statistischen Auswertung biologischer Bestimmungen. Arch. Gynäk. **188**, 497–538.

Borth, R. (1960): Simplified Mathematics for Multiple Bioassays. Acta endocr. (Kbh.) **35**, 454–468.

Breuer, H. (1969): Oestrogene und Mammacarcinom. *In:* Kracht, J. (Hrsg.): Oestrogene-Hypophysentumoren. 15. Symposion der Deutschen Gesellschaft für Endokrinologie, Köln, 6.–8. 3. 1969. Springer-Verlag, Berlin, Heidelberg, New York; pp. 81–93.

Brown, J. B., R. D. Bulbrook, F. C. Greenwood (1957): An Additional Purification Step for a Method for Estimating Oestriol, Oestrone, and Oestradiol-17β in Human Urine. J. Endocrinol. **16**, 49–56.

Brown, J. B., R. Kellar, G. D. Matthew (1959): Preliminary Observations on Urinary Oestrogen Excretion in Certain Gynaecological Disorders. J. Obstetr. Gynaec. Brit. Emp. **66**, 177–211.

Brown, J.B., H.A.F. Blair (1960): A Method for the Determination of Very Small Amounts of Oestrone in Human Urine. J. Endocrinol. **20**, 331–338.

Brown, J.B., G.D. Matthew (1962): The Application of Urinary Estrogen Measurements to Problems in Gynecology. Rec. Progr. Horm. Res. **18**, 337–385.

Bulbrook, R.D., F.C. Greenwood, G.J. Hadfield, E.F. Scowen (1958a): Oophorectomy in Breast Cancer; an Attempt to Correlate Clinical Results with Oestrogen Production. Brit. Med. J. **II**, 7–11.

Bulbrook, R.D., F.C. Greenwood, G.J. Hadfield, E.F. Scowen (1958b): Adrenalectomy in Breast Cancer. An Attempt to Correlate Clinical Results with Oestrogen Production. Brit. Med. J. **II**, 12–15.

Butcher, R.L, R.D. Page (1981): Role of the Aging Ovary in Cessation of Reproduction. *In:* Schwartz, N.B., M. Hunzicker-Dunn (eds.): Dynamics of Ovarian Function. Raven Press, New York; pp. 253-271.

Channing, C.P., L.D. Anderson, D.J. Hoover, J. Kolena, K.G. Osteen, S.H. Pomerantz, K. Tanabe (1982): The Role of Nonsteroidal Regulators in Control of Oocyte and Follicular Maturation. Rec. Progr. Horm. Res. **38**, 331–408.

Cooke, I.D. (1976): Endocrine Changes Associated with the Menopause and Postmenopausal Years. *In:* Campbell, St. (ed.): The Management of the Menopause & Post-Menopausal Years. MTP Press Ltd., Lancaster, England; pp. 49–62.

Dilman, V.M. (1971): Age-Associated Elevation of Hypothalamic Threshold to Feedback Control, and its Role in Development, Aging, and Disease. Lancet **I**, 1211–1219.

Edwards, R.G. (1980): Conception in the Human Female. Academic Press, London, New York, Toronto, Sydney, San Fracisco.

Franchi, L.L. (1970): The Ovary. *In:* Philipp, E.E., J. Barnes, M. Newton (eds.): Scientific Foundations of Obstetrics and Gynaecology. Heinemann, London; pp. 107–131.

Franchi, L.L., T.G. Baker (1973): Oogenesis and Follicular Growth. *In:* Hafez, E.S.E., T.N. Evans (eds.): Human Reproduction: Conception and Contraception. Harper & Row, Hagerstown, Md., New York, Evanston, San Francisco and London; pp. 53–83.

Forleo, R., W.P. Collins (1964): Some Aspects of Steroid Biosynthesis in Human Ovarian Tissue. Acta endocr. (Kbh.) **46**, 265–278.

Grodin, J.M., P.K. Siiteri, P.C. MacDonald (1973): Source of Estrogen Production in Postmenopausal Women. J. Clin. Endocrinol. Metab. **36**, 207–214.

Hammerstein, J. (1969): Oestrogene im biphasischen und im gestörten menstruellen Cyclus. *In:* Kracht, J. (Hrsg.): Oestrogene-Hypophysentumoren. 15. Symposion der Deutschen Gesellschaft für Endokrinologie, Köln, 6.–8.3.1969. Springer-Verlag, Berlin, Heidelberg, New York; pp. 57–80.

Hemsell, D.L., J.M. Grodin, P.F. Brenner, P.K. Siiteri, P.C. MacDonald (1974): Plasma Precursors of Estrogen. II. Correlation of the Extent of Conversion of Plasma Androstenedione to Estrone with Age. J. Clin. Endocrinol. Metab. **38**, 476–579.

Hodgen, G.D., A.L. Goodman, R.L. Stouffer, R.F. Williams, G.S. diZerega, O.L. Kreitmann, E.L. Marut, R.S. Schenken (1983): Selection and Maturation of the Dominant Follicle and its Ovum in the Menstrual Cycly. *In:* Beier, H.M., H.R. Lindner (eds.): Fertilization of the Human Egg In Vitro. Springer-Verlag, Berlin, Heidelberg, New York, Tokyo; pp. 57–69.

Johnson, S.G. (1958): A Clinical Routine Method for the Quantitative Determination of Gonadotrophins in 24-Hour Samples. Acta endocr. (Kbh.) **28**, 69–88.

Judd, H.L., W.E. Lucas, S.S.C. Yen (1974a): Effect of Oophorectomy on Circulating Testosterone and Androstenedione Levels in Patients with Endomedrial Cancer. Am. J. Obstetr. Gynecol. **118**, 793–798.

Judd, H.L., G.E. Judd, W.E. Lucas, S.S.C. Yen (1974b): Endocrine Function of the Postmenopausal Ovary: Concentration of Androgens and Estrogens in Ovarian and Peripheral Vein Blood. J. Clin. Endocrinol. Metab. **39**, 1020–1024.

Kaiser, R., E. Daume (1965): Über eine einheitliche Nomenklatur für das Klimakterium und seine Begleitsymptome. Geburtsh. u. Frauenheilk. **25**, 974–986.

Kellie, A.E., A.P. Wade (1957): The Analysis of Urinary 17-Oxosteroids by Gradient Elution. Biochem. J. **66**, 196–206.

Koering, M.J. (1969): Cyclic Changes in Ovarian Morphology during the Menstrual Cycle in *Macaca mulatta*. Amer. J. Anat. **126**, 73–101.

Knobil, E., L. Wildt (1983): Neuroendocrine Control of Ovarian Function in Higher Primates. *In:* Leyendecker, G., H. Stock, L. Wildt (eds.): Brain and Pituitary Peptides II: Pulsatile Administration of Gn-RH in

Hypothalamic Failure: Basic and Clinical Aspects. S. Karger, Basel, München, Paris, London, New York, Tokyo, Sidney; pp. 11–27.

Levin, L., H. H. Tyndale (1937): Quantitative Assay of "Follicle Stimulating" Substances. Endocrinology **21**, 619–628.

Leyendecker, G., S. Wardlaw, W. Nocke (1972): Experimental Studies on the Endocrine Regulations during the Periovulatory Phase of the Human Menstrual Cycle. Acta endocr. (Kbh.) **71**, 160–178.

Leyendecker, G., K. Hinckers, W. Nocke, E. J. Plotz (1975): Hypophysäre Gonadotropine und ovarielle Steroide im Serum während des normalen menstruellen Cyclus und bei Corpus-luteum-Insuffizienz. Arch. Gynäk. **218**, 47–64.

Leyendecker, G., L. Wildt, H. Gips, W. Nocke, E. J. Plotz (1976): Experimental Studies on the Positive Feedback Effect of Progesterone, 17α-Hydroxyprogesterone and 20α-Dihydroprogesterone on the Pituitary Release of LH and FSH in the Human Female. The Estrogen Priming of the Progesterone Feedback on Pituitary Gonadotropins in the Eugonadal Woman. Arch. Gyn. **221**, 29–45.

Leyendecker, G., L. Wildt, T. Struve, W. Nocke, E. J. Plotz (1977): Control of the Human Menstrual Cycle. *In:* James. V. H. T. (ed.): Proceedings of the V International Congress of Endocrinology, Hamburg, July, 18–24, 1976, Vol. I; Excerpta Medica International Congress Series No. 402 *Endocrinology*. Excerpta Medica Foundation, Amsterdam; pp. 199–204.

Leyendecker, G., L. Wildt (1983): Control of Gonadotropin Secretion in Women. *In:* Norman, R. L. (ed.): Neuroendocrine Aspects of Reproduction. Academic Press, New York; pp. 295–323.

Lindner, H. R., A. Tsafriri, M. E. Lieberman, U. Zor, Y. Koch, S. Bauminger, A. Barnea (1974): Gonadotropin Action on Cultured Graafian Follicles: Induction of Maturation Division of the Mammalian Oocyte and Differentiation of the Luteal Cell. Rec. Progr. Horm. Res. **30**, 79–138.

Longcope, C. (1971): Metabolic Clearance and Blood Production Rates of Estrogens in Postmenopausal Women. Am. J. Obstetr. Gynecol. **111**, 778–781.

MacDonald, P. C., R. P. Rombaut, P. K. Siiteri (1967): Plasma Precursors of Estrogen. I. Extent of Conversion of Plasma Δ^4-Androstenedione to Estrone in Normal Males and Nonpregnant Normal, Castrate and Adrenalectomized Females. J. Clin. Endocrinol. Metabl. **27**, 1103–1111.

Mattingly, R. F., W. Y. Huang (1969): Steroidogenesis of the Menopausal and Postmenopausal Ovary. Am J. Obstetr. Gynecol. **103**, 679-693.

Mauléon, P. (1969): Oogenesis and Folliculogenesis. *In:* Cole, H. H., P. T. Cupps (eds.): Reproduction in Domestic Animals, 2nd ed. Academic Press, New York; pp. 187–225.

Nimrod, A., K. J. Ryan (1975): Aromatization of Androgens by Human Abdominal and Breast Fat Tissue. J. Clin. Endocrinol. Metab. **40**, 367–372.

Nocke, L. (1970): Methode zur gleichzeitigen Bestimmung von Pregnandiol und Pregnantriol aus einer Urinprobe. Z. Anal. Chem. **252**, 322–327.

Nocke, W. (1961): A Study of the Colorimetric Estimation of Oestradiol-17β, Oestradiol-17α, Oestrone, Oestriol and 16-*epi*Oestriol by the Kober Reaction. Biochem. J. **78**, 593–602.

Nocke, W. (1969): In Vivo Studies on the Endocrine Activity of Normal and Tumorous Ovaries in Postmenopausal Women. *In:* Raspé, G. (ed.): Schering Workshop on Steroid Metabolism "In Vitro Versus In Vivo", Berlin 1968. Pergamon Press-Vieweg, Advances in the Biosciences 3, Oxford, London, Edinburgh, New York, Toronto, Sidney, Paris, Braunschweig; pp. 129–149.

Nocke, W., G. Leyendecker (1970): Die endokrinen Funktionen von Hypothalamus, Hypophysenvorderlappen und Ovar während der Prae- und Postmenopause. Gynäkologe **2**, 113–122.

Nocke, W., G. Leyendecker (1972a): Neue Erkenntnisse über die endokrine Physiologie des menstruellen Cyclus. Gynäkologe **5**, 39–72.

Nocke, W., G. Leyendecker (1972b): Neue Erkenntnisse über die endokrine Regulation der Ovarialfunktion. Gynäk. Rundschau **12**, 58–85.

Norymberski, J. K., R. D. Stubbs, H. F. West (1953): Assessment of Adrenocortical Activity by Assay of 17-Ketogenic Steroids in Urine. Lancet **I**, 1276–1281.

Pincus, G., R. I. Dorfman, L. P. Romanoff, B. L. Rubin, E. Bloch, J. Carlo, H. Freeman (1955): Steroid Metabolism in Aging Men and Women. Rec. Progr. Horm. Res. **11**, 307–341.

Plotz, E. J., M. Wiener, A. A. Stein (1966): Steroid Synthesis in Cystadenocarcinoma of the Ovaries. Am. J. Obstetr. Gynecol. **94**, 189–194.

Plotz, E.J., M. Wiener, A. A. Stein, B. D. Hahn (1967): Enzymatic Activities Related to Steroidogenesis in Postmenopausal Ovaries with and without Endometrial Carcinoma. Am. J. Obstetr. Gynecol. **99**, 182–197.

Procopé, B.-J. (1968): Studies on the Urinary Excretion, Biological Effects and Origin of Oestrogens in Post-Menopausal Women. Acta endocr. (Kbh.) **60**, Suppl. 135.

Procopé, B.-J., H. Adlercreutz (1969): Studies on the Influence of Age on Oestrogens in Postmenopausal Women with Atrophic Endometrium and Normal Liver Function. Acta endocr. (Kbh.) **62**, 461–467.

Reyes, F. I., J. S. D. Winter, C. Faiman (1977): Pituitary Ovarian Relationships Preceding the Menopause. – I. A Cross-Sectional Study of Serum Follicle-Stimulating Hormone, Luteinizing Hormone, Prolactin, Estradiol, and Progesterone Levels. Am. J. Obstetr. Gynecol. **129**, 557–564.

Rössle, R., F. Roulet (1941): Maß und Zahl in der Pathologie. Springer-Verlag, Berlin.

Schindler, A. E., A. Ebert, E. Friedrich (1972): Conversion of Androstenedione to Estrone by Human Fat Tissue. J. Clin. Endocrinol. Metab. **35**, 627–630.

Sherman, B. M., S. G. Korenman (1975): Hormonal Charcteristics of the Human Menstrual Cycle throughout Reproductive Life. J. Clin. Invest. **55**, 699–706.

Sherman B. M., J. H. West, S. G. Korenman (1976): The Menopausal Transition: Analysis of LH, FSH, Estradiol, and Progesterone Concentrations During Menstrual Cycles of Older Women. J. Clin. Endocrinol. Metab. **42**, 629–636.

Shettles, L. B. (1960): Ovum Humanum. Wachstum, Reifung, Ernährung, Befruchtung und frühe Entwicklung. Urban & Schwarzenberg, München, Berlin.

Siiteri, P. K., P. C. MacDonald (1973): Role of Extraglandular Estrogen in Human Endocrinology. *In:* Geiger, S. R., E. Astwood, R. O. Greep (eds.): Handbook of Physiology, Section 7.2, Endocrinology, Vol. II, Part I. The American Physiologic Society, Washington, D.C.; pp. 615–629.

Szöllösi, D., M. Gerard (1983): Cytoplasmatic Changes in Mammalian Oocytes During the Preovulatory Period. *In:* Beier, H. M., H. R. Lindner (eds.): Fertilization of the Human Egg in Vitro. Springer-Verlag, Berlin, Heidelberg, New York, Tokyo; pp. 35–55.

Tsafriri, A., S. Bar-Ami, H. R. Lindner (1983): Control of the Development of Meiotic Competence and of Oocyte Meturation in Mammals. *In:* Beier, H. M., H. R. Lindner (eds.): Fertilization of the Human Egg in Vitro. Springer-Verlag, Berlin, Heidelberg, New York, Tokyo; pp. 3–17.

Vermeulen, A. (1976): THe Hormonal Activity of the Postmenopausal Ovary. J. Clin. Endocrinol. Metab. **42**, 247–253.

Weir, B. J., I. W. Rowlands (1977): Ovulation and Atresia. *In:* Zuckerman, S., B. J. Weir (eds.): The Ovary, 2nd ed., Vol. I. Academic Press, New York, San Francisco, London; pp. 265–301.

Wildt, L., G. Leyendecker (1981): Die endokrine Kontrolle des menstruellen Zyklus. Gynäkologe **14**, 64–83.

Wildt, L., H. Schwilden, G. Wesner, C. Roll, K.-A. Brensing, J. Luckhaus, M. Bähr, G. Leyendecker (1983): The Pulsatile Pattern of Gonadotropin-Secretion and Follicular Development during the Menstrual Cycle and in Women with Hypothalamic and Hyperandrogenemic Amenorrhea. *In:* Leyendecker, G., H. Stock, L. Wildt (eds.): Brian and Pituitary Peptides II: Pulsatile Administration of Gn-RH in Hypothalamic Failure: Basic and Clinical Aspects. S. Karger, Basel, München, Paris, London, New York, Tokyo, Sydney; pp. 28–57.

Zuckerman, S., T. G. Baker (1977): The Development of the Ovary and the Process of Oogenesis. *In:* Zuckerman, S., B. J. Weit (eds.): The Ovary, 2nd ed., Vol. I. Academic Press, New York, San Francisco, London; pp. 41–67.

The climacteric syndrome

H. P. G. Schneider

Introduction

Until about 30 years ago, the climacteric was regarded as a period of undesirable physiologic changes from which menopausal women could not escape. Such views have changed. Although the menopause is still considered to be primarily an ageing event, we now look at it to be an anthropological process providing genetic protection at the expense of potential organic defects.

During the past 100 years, both the reproductive and total life span of women have increased gradually. In the Roman Empire the average life expectancy of women was 23 years. From the Middle Ages until the late 19th century, fewer than 30% of females reached the menopausal age of 51 years. Today, nearly 90% of women in western industrialized countries experience menopause; almost 60% live to age 75. In fact, recent census figures indicate that the average woman can expect to spend approximately one third of her life, some 30 years, in the post-menopausal state. With a life expectancy of 78 years, there are now a just under 10 million post-menopausal women in the United Kingdom and in West-Germany compared to 40 mill. in the United States. This is, in each case, about 17% of the total population. The average age of menopause has not changed since medieval times. The expanding reproductive years are due primarily to the earlier experience of menarche which is correlated with a critical body weight and percentage of body fat. The earlier reaching of the critical body weight can be attributed to improved nutrition and general health as well as better sociooeconomic conditions. The age of menopause does not appear to be related to the age of menarche, sociooeconomic factors, race, parity, weight, or height. The only factor that may influence the earlier onset of menopause is cigarette smoking [1].

Menopausal symptoms

Until the early 1970's, it was extremely difficult to discern which symptoms are truly associated with the climacteric. Symptoms of any type were usually divided on a empirical basis into "autonomic", "psychologic", and "metabolic", or simply itemized grocery-list style without any attempt at explanation [2]. The problem was a lack of established scientific data relating to the human climacteric. With the advent of serious menopause research, the institution of menopause clinics and the founding of the International Menopause Society, considerable progress has been achieved in defining menopausal symptomatology. According to international classification, the varied symptom profile after menopause is caused by an interaction between three components:

1. Decreased ovarian activity with altered hormone profiles
2. Sociocultural or environmental factors, and
3. Psychologic factors.

With respect to ovarian activity, the rate at which tissue levels of estrogen decline appears to be the most important factor. The second component involves the inherited or aquired propensity to withstand or succumb to the aging process. Finally, the third component refers to the woman's ability to cope with major alterations in her interpersonal relationships, especially with family members. Severe emotional distress may occur with the loss of one or both parents, or the "loss" of children to college or marriage. Women at menopausal age may have to cope with a husband who has become severely ill or who is seeking a younger woman. She is bombarded constantly by reminders that she is growing older in a youth-oriented culture. Her ability to cope with these stresses successfully will depend, in large part, upon her educational, sociooeconomic, racial, and cultural background.

In the literature there is little information concerning the number of women who have sufficient symptoms at the time of the menopause to seek medical advice. A statistical study of 1000 women in England indicated that 15.8% had no symptoms at the time of the menopause, 62.3% had only hot flushes for an average duration of 2 years, and 89.7% carried on their daily activities without interruption [3]. It is generally agreed that 10 to 15% of women will present themselves for medical advice for symptoms attributed to the climacteric [4].

The common menopause complaints are listed in a table from Neugarten and Kraines (1965) (Tab. 1) [46]. True milestones in the study of the climacteric were the prospective placebo trials of Utian (1972) [6] and of Campbell and Whitehead (1977) [5]. The former was an extensive single-blind study; the latter a double-blind investigation, in which 64 patients participated in a 2-month cross-over and 61 patients in a 6-month cross-over study using conjugated equine estrogens (Premarin) and a placebo (Tab. 2). A convincing placebo response was demonstrated with symptoms of vaginal dryness, coital satisfaction, urinary frequency and such elusive qualities as an improvement in memory and youthful skin appearance. This placebo effect on vaginal dryness and urinary frequency disappeared in the longer study, but the significant placebo effect on the youthful skin appearance was maintained. The clearly demonstrated benefits of estrogen therapy in the short study were related to hot flushes, insomnia, vaginal dryness, irritability, poor memory, anxiety, "worry about age", headaches, "worry about self", urinary frequency and good spirits.

Table 1 Frequency of Complaints in Menopausal Women, Ages 45–54 Years.

Complaint	%
Irritability	92
Lethargy/Fatigue	88
Depression	78
Headaches	71
Hot flushes	68
Forgetfulness	64
Weight gain	61
Insomnia	51
Joint pain/backache	48
Palpitations	44
Crying spells	42
Constipation	37
Dysuria	20
Decreased libido	20

Data from Neugarten BL, Kraines RJ. "Menopausal symptoms" in women of various ages. Psychosom Med. 1965; 27:270.

Table 2 Symptoms significantly improved by estrogen therapy when compared with placebo (Campbell and Whitehead, 1977)

2-months crossover study (64 patients)	6-months crossover study (61 patients)
1. Hot flushes	1. Hot flushes
2. Insomnia	2. Vaginal dryness
3. Vaginal dryness	3. Insomnia
4. Irritability	4. Urinary frequency
5. Poor memory	5. Poor memory
6. Anxiety	
7. Worry about age	
8. Headaches	
9. Worry about self	
10. Urinary frequency	
11. Optimism	
12. Good spirits	

Many of these beneficial effects were maintained and enhanced by prolonged therapy, and a significant improvement by estrogen therapy compared with placebo in the 6-month cross-over study was found in hot-flushes, vaginal dryness, insomnia and poor memory.

A potential criticism of this convincing classical study is that there was no "washout period" between the medication and the placebo courses. In order to refute this criticism Campbell showed that even using only the symptoms present in the last 2 months of the 6-months-periods in the cross-over study, the results were still valid and, furthermore, that a beneficial effect upon libido and a surprisingly beneficial effect upon backache were shown for the first time.

Vasomotor symptoms

There is international agreement that the two most common acute problems during the climacteric are vasomotor instability (flushing and sweating episodes) and symptoms due to atrophy of the lower genital tract (vulva and vagina). Vasomotor instability is characterized by a rise in skin temperature, peripheral vasodilatation, a transient increase in heart rate, and changes in skin impedance [7 + 8].

The hot flush is described as a sudden onset of warmth in the face and neck that progresses to the chest. Recent thermographic studies have shown peripheral skin temperature changes of up to 5° C during flushing attacks. These occur all over the body but are often felt by the woman only in the face and upper thorax. This sensation generally lasts several minutes and is often accompanied by a visible red flush. The hands become warm and the skin of the face and neck become moist. These episodes may last for several minutes, be exceedingly uncomfortable, and are frequently associated with dizziness, nausea, headaches, palpitations, diaphoresis, and "night sweats". These unpleasant symptoms can also be triggered by emotional stress, excitement, fear, or anxiety and disappear just as quickly as they appear. 80% of women who experience hot flushes have symptoms for more than one year, but less than 25% symptoms for more than 5 years.

Physiology of the vasomotor flush

Flushing attacks are associated with a reduction in central body temperature and with an increase in heart rate of up to 13 beats per minute. In general, there is no correlation between the absolute levels of estrogen concentrations and the occurence of vasomotor symptoms. Flushes frequently occur during clomiphene citrate therapy or danazol administration. Not all postmenopausal women experience vasomotor symptoms, perhaps because alterations in metabolism of catecholamine or catecholestrogen within the brain or extraglandular formation of estrone was sufficient in these women to suppress the symptoms. Thus, it appears that hot flushes are triggered by "estrogen withdrawal" rather than by a lack of estrogen.

The simultaneous changes of skin temperature and resistance can be used as an objective marker of the occurrence of menopausal hot flushes during sleep [9]. Simultaneous changes of finger temperature and skin resistance over the sternum were found to be the most specific marker of a hot flush (Fig. 1). A significant association was found between the occurrence of hot flushes and waking episodes in

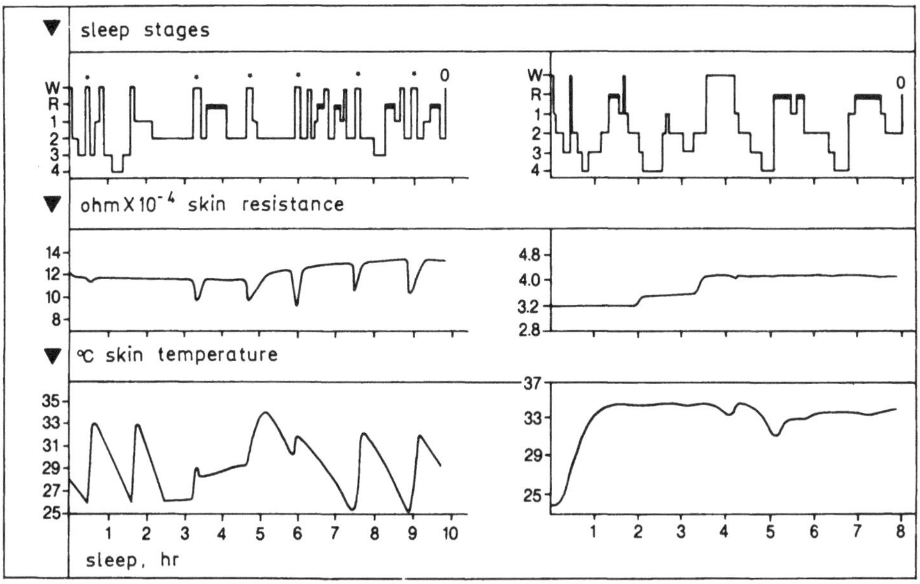

Fig. 1 Sleepgram and recordings of skin resistance and temperature in a postmenopausal (left panel) and a premenopausal (right panel) woman. Each asterisk marks occurrence of an objectively measured hot flush. Open circle indicate arousal of patient by investigator at end of study (based on Erlik et al., 1981)

8 of 9 postmenopausal patients examined. A rise of skin temperature with sleep onset has been described previously and is believed to reflect changes of the set-point of temperature-regulating centers of the hypothalamus [10].

With most flushes the onset of waking preceded any pleythysmograhic change in skin resistance (perspiration) or temperature (vasodilatation). The mean intervals from waking onset to any measurable change of skin resistance and temperature were 0.59 and 0.81 min, respectively, while the intervals from wake onset to maximal proliferal changes were 3.96 and 8.21 min, respectively. These temporal relationships were remarkably similar to the relationship of the onset of a subjective hot flush and the occurrence of the same peripheral changes in symptomatic patients studied while awake. Judd and co-workers therefore concluded that the onset of waking and the commencement of cortical awareness of a subjective hot flush are due to a central disturbance rather than to the discomfort associated with cutaneous perspiration and flushing.

Thermoregulatory control of the vasomotor flush

What is our current understanding of the mechanism responsible for the vasomotor flush? Although the flush is synchronous with a pulsatile release of LH from the pituitary, LH-levels per se do not activate the vasomotor centers. After pituitary

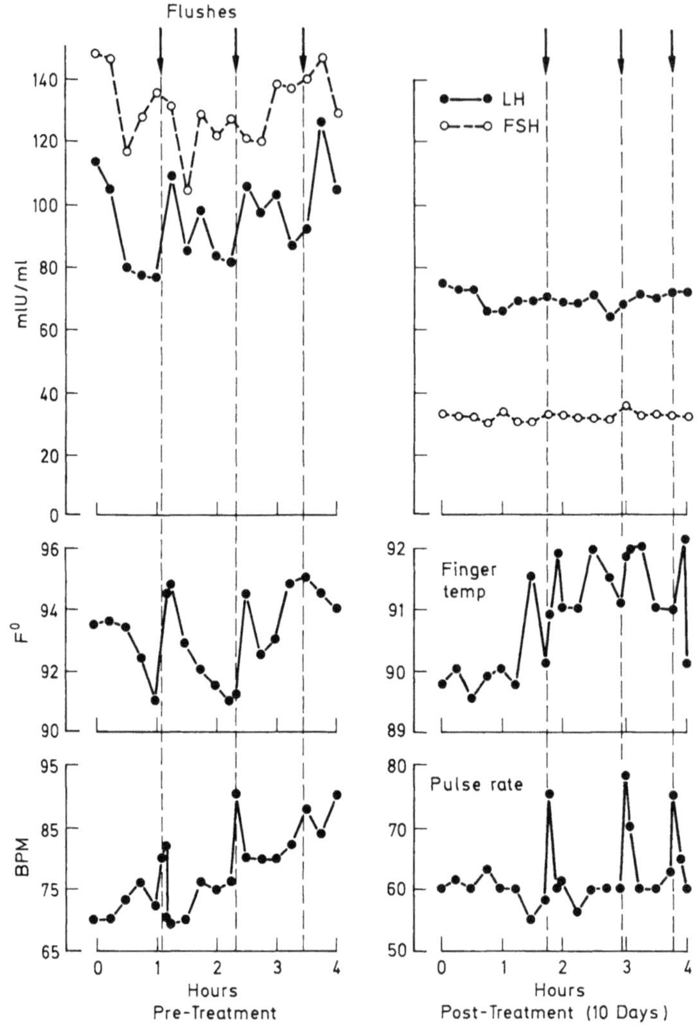

Fig. 2 Changes in finger temperature (degree Fahrenheit) and pulse rate (beats per min) in association with flush episodes (arrows and serum concentrations of LH (•--•) and FSH (o--o) in a representative study of one hypogonadal subject before and after 10 days of daily LRF-Agonist administration (50 μg s.c.) (based on Casper and Yen, 1981)

gonadotropin desensitization by an LH-RH agonist, LH and FSH pulses were equalized, and serum gonadotropin levels were decreased. Flush episodes, however, were unaltered (Fig. 2) [11]. These findings demonstrate that pulsatile LH release by the pituitary is not causally related to menopausal flushes, and support the contention that flush episodes are initiated by a hypothalamic mechanism.

According to present concepts of thermoregulatory control in men, a central hypothalamic thermostat compares the core temperature of the body with a set-point temperature [12]. This set-point temperature can be altered by a variety of agents, such as a pyrogen. When the hypothalamus is exposed to a pyrogen, the central set-point is reset at a new level which is then higher than the actual core temperature, and the person feels cold. Through increased heat production (shivering) and decreased heat loss (cutaneous vasoconstriction), the core temperature rises to the new, high set-point [13, 14, 15].

According to this concept it seems that the menopausal flush is triggered by a sudden, downward setting of the central thermostat. To adjust the core temperature to this new set-point, effector heat-loss mechanisms (cutaneous vasodilatation and perspiration) are activated. The lines of support for this hypothesis are as follows: As mentioned above, there is an actual fall in core temperature during a flush episode; furthermore, the clear association of pulsatile LH release and the occurrence of vasomotor changes both point to the rostral hypothalamic centers that trigger menopausal flushes as well as pulsatile secretion of LH. In fact, hypothalamic LH-RH neurons and the preoptic-anterior hypothalamic nuclei that regulate body temperature are in close anatomic relationship, and neurotransmitter signals associated with release of LH-RH may modify thermoregulatory neurons [16, 17, 18]. The initiation of a waking episode before any measurable change of cutaneous vasodilatation and perspiration may reflect this downward setting of hypothalamic thermostats.

Estrogen deficiency and psychological function

There is disagreement as to whether ovarian failure causes psychological changes. Much of this controversy has arisen because studies of varying scientific merit have reported conflicting results. The observations of a well-designed study of the King's College Group [5], in which men were also included and in which the word "Menopause" did not appear, were the following: As expected, flushing and sweating increased in incidence only in women and reached peak prevalence in the late 40's and early 50's. Interestingly, a variety of psychological symptoms, such as difficulty in making decisions, loss of confidence, anxiety and irritability also achieved peak prevalence at this time (Fig. 3). Thus, these results support the hypothesis that estrogen deficiency increases the incidence of minor psychological dysfunction. It is doubtful whether endogenous depression results from lack of estrogen.

Role of catecholamines and prostaglandins

The close association between vasomotor instability and hypothalamic dysfunction suggested that alterations in the metabolism of catecholamines coupled with decreased estrogen production are causally involved. Catecholamines, particularly

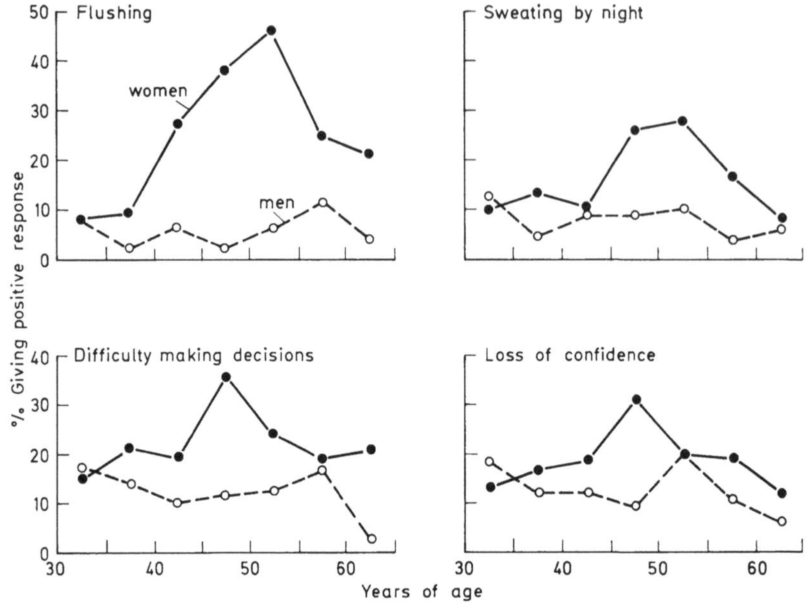

Fig. 3 Vasomotor symptoms (flushing and sweating at night) and pschological factors (difficulty in making decisions and loss of confidence) in women and men in their late 40's and early 50's. Scores as percent giving positive response (n=64) (courtesy of Dr. M. Whitehead).

dopamine and norepinephrine, act as rostral hypothalamic neurotransmitters. These agents appear to play a significant role in modulating mood, behaviour, motor activity and hypothalamic-pituitary function.

Monoaminoxydase (MAO) and catechol-o-methyl transferase (COMT) activities increase, and neuronal uptake of catecholamines decreases, as a function of aging [19]. The concentrations of dopamine in the hypothalamus fall and those of norepinephrine increase following castration [20]. Moreover, the activity of tyrosine hydroxylase and the turnover rate of norepinephrine in the hypothalamus increase following castration [21]. These changes are reversed by estrogen treatment. Thus, aging and decreased estrogen levels may alter dopamine-norepinephrine metabolism in the brain sufficiently to result in an instability of the autonomic nervous system (Table 3).

Prostaglandins are also present in high concentrations in the hypothalamus. Many cerebral vessels, in particular those in the hypothalamus, are innervated by noradrenergic neurons. These neurons may be stimulated by either norepinephrine or prostaglandin to produce central vasospasm which results in nervousness, anxiety, irritability, depression, and loss of memory [22].

Norepinephrine is the predominant neurotransmitter in the nuclei of the upper pons, which controls REM sleep. Serotonin is the predominant neurotransmitter in the

Table 3 Interplay of central nervous system neurotransmitters and sleep in the menopause; the effect of estrogen.

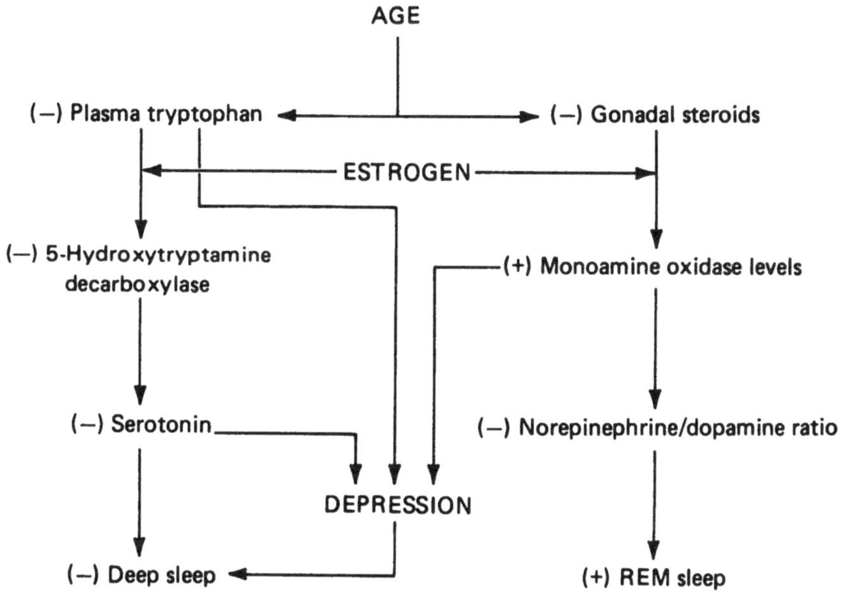

midline brain stem nuclei, which control deep sleep. When these biogenic amines are depleted, a patient is more likely to become depressed. Menopausal patients do sleep less, possibly as a result of the same biogenic amine depletion.

Norepinephrine was the first biogenic amine implicated in regulating the sleep-wake cycle. Evidence has been presented that the ratio of norepinephrine to serotonin in the brain is related to proportions of REM and non-REM sleep; higher ratios are associated with more REM sleep [27].

Hormonal effects on menopausal symptoms

When double-blind studies of the effects of estrogens or progesterone on vasomotor flushes are conducted, the placebo effect observed is significant. There is a marked therapeutic effect when placebo is given initially, but further improvement occurs when the active drug is then given. In contrast, when estrogen is first introduced, symptoms significantly worsen at the cross-over from drug to placebo. Albrecht et al. [23] (1981) demonstrated a significant decrease in the amount of objectively recorded vasomotor flushes when placebo and medroxyprogesterone acetate were studied, the latter causing greater suppression.

The fact that placebo had such a large effect in menopausal studies needs additional discussion in regard to recent literature on endorphins. Opiates interfere with dopaminergic systems in the brain; they decrease both the storage and turnover of brain dopamine in the median eminence [24]. Thus they may modulate LH and prolactin secretion [25]. Since endorphins seem to affect behavior and mental illness, many authors tried to relate endorphins to the placebo effect. However, De Fazio et al. (1984) [26] recently demonstrated that naloxone did not change the rate of objectively measured hot flushes (continuous recordings of finger temperature and skin resistance in 16 postmenopausal women on naloxone infusion (22 μg/min) vs. saline during 8 h). These data suggest that there is a very low input of endogenous opiates on gonadotropin secretion in postmenopausal women and that opioid peptides do not play a role in the initiation of the postmenopausal hot flush.

There is growing knowledge concerning the effects of age and estrogen deficiency on tyrosine hydroxylase, monoamine oxydase and catechol-o-methyl transferase (COMT) levels (Table 3).

Monoamine oxydase (MAO) (which inactivates norephinephrine, tryptophan, and serotonin) levels are elevated and plasma tryptophane levels are lowered with increasing age [28], depressive syndromes (Nies et al., 1971), amenorrheic disorders, and menopause (Klaiber et al., 1971). Aging also decreases levels of the biosynthetic enzymes tyrosine hydroxylase and dopa-decarboxylase (McGeer & McGeer, 1976). Estrogens may have a MAO inhibitor effect (Klaiber et al., 1972). During the menstrual cycle, when estrogens reach peak levels, and during therapy with oral contraceptives, higher estrogen doses are associated with a lowering of MAO activity (Holzbauer & Yondin, 1973; Luhby et al., 1970).

Estrogens interfere with certain vitamin B_6 enzyme systems in tryptophane metabolism and dopamine metabolism. Via induction of 5-hydroxytryptophane decarboxylase and dopa-decarboxylase, they affect the ratio of norepinephrine to dopamine in the brain. Catecholestrogens, metabolic products of estrogens, are responsible for buffering the effects of estrogen on the hypothalamic-pituitary system, thereby controlling gonadotropin release via the CNS (Ball & Knuppen, 1980). According to these authors, 2-hydroxyestradiol-17β is the key agent in the regulation of gonadotropin release. They speculate that this compound – by competing for COMT – inhibits the metabolism of catecholamines which results in either prolongation and/or potentiation of the action of catecholamines.

Attempts to correlate peripheral plasma norepinephrine, epinephrine, and dopamine levels with LH spikes in objectively recorded hot flushes have failed so far (Casper et al., 1980). However, peripheral concentrations of these amines may not reflect central changes.

Kronenberg et al. (1984) monitored thermoregulatory, cardiovascular and endocrine changes in 11 post-menopausal women with frequent hot flushes. These authors measured catecholamine and LH levels in peripheral plasma obtained at 1- and 5-min-intervals (Fig. 4). Hot flushes were accompanied by abrupt increases in plasma epinephrine (about 150%) and concomitant decreases in norepinephrine

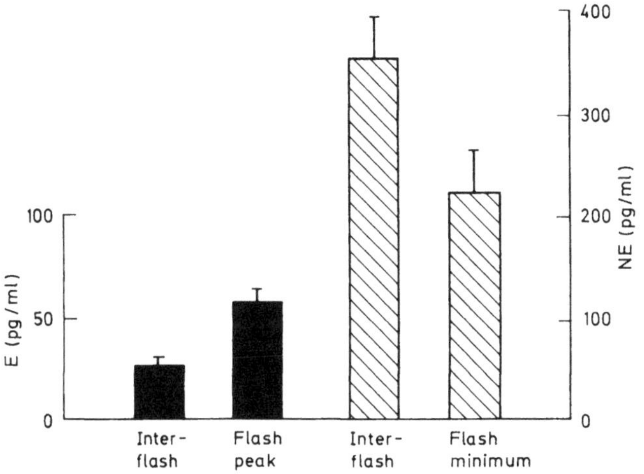

Fig. 4 Mean (± SEM) levels of plasma epinephrine (E) and norepinephrine (NE) for 5 subjects between and during hot flushes for NE. (according to Kronenberg et al., 1984)

(about 40%). These observations are consistent with the hypothesis that hot flushes are due to a change in the thermoregulatory set-point. Furthermore, the changes in catecholamine levels are consistent with the cardiovascular changes accompanying hot flushes, since Hartman's experiments demonstrated that central noradrenergic neurons innervate cerebral and hypothalamic blood vessels (1973).

In summary, the presence of estrogens increases nervous system levels of those transmitters which regulate both sleep and mood.

There is a high rate of anxiety and mood depression during the menopause, and suicide and mental illness peak at this time [33]. Klaiber (1972) treated ambulatory depressed patients with pharmacologic doses of estrogens which lowered MAO levels and had some effect on psychiatric symptoms. Aylward (1975), in double-blind cross-over study, demonstrated that estrogens increased plasma free tryptophane and thereby decreased mental illness. Campbell and Whitehead (1977), who compared 1,25 mg Premarin with placebo, found a significant improvement in well-being, both psychologic and symptomatic, in patients with moderate or severe menopause symptoms.

Therapeutic aspects of menopausal symptoms

The thick, well-stratified vaginal epithelium of the reproductive area becomes thin and atrophic following loss of ovarian function. Resultant symptoms include vaginal dryness and dyspareunia and an increase in the incidence of bacterial infections. Since the urethra has the same embryological origin as the vagina,

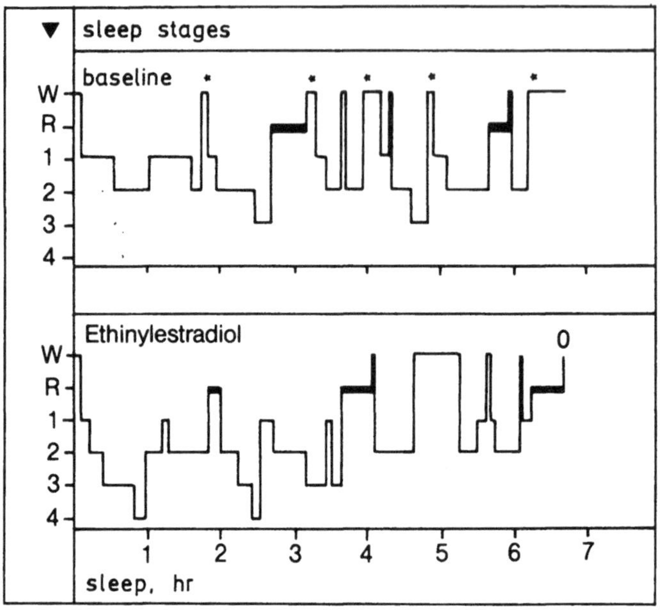

Fig. 5 Sleepgrams measured in symptomatic patient before and after 30 day administration of ethinyl-estradiol, 50 μg four times daily. (based on Erlik et al., 1981)

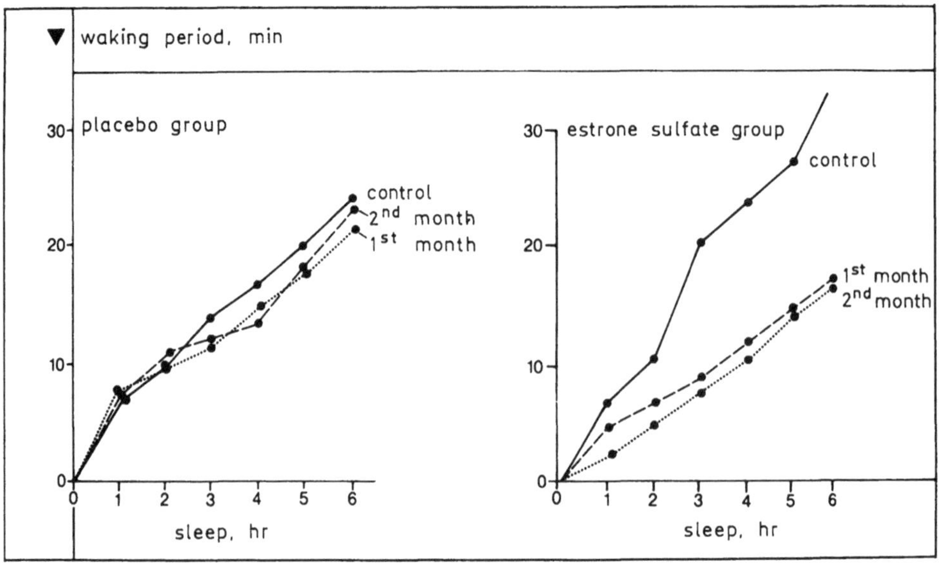

Fig. 6 Cumulative waking episodes during the first 6 hours of sleep before and following placebo (left) or estrone-sulfate (right) (based on Thomson & Oswald, 1977)

atrophic urethritis can develop in a small percentage of women. This may increase the risk of recurrent urinary infections. Resulting dysuria and stress incontinence will significantly improve following estrogen replacement.

With the use of randomized, prospective, double-blind studies, the administration of estrogen to postmenopausal women has been shown to significantly reduce the occurrence of hot flushes and improve the quality of sleep (Fig. 5). The beneficial effects on sleep include decreases in insomnia, sleep, latency, and the number and duration of episodes of wakefulness and increases in the length of sleep and the amount of rapid eye movement sleep (Fig. 6) [38, 9, 39].

These actions differ from those observed with most sleeping pills, which reduce both sleep latency and the time of rapid eye movement sleep [40].

Current research demonstrates the close relationships among the abatement of vasomotor symptoms via estrogen therapy, the improvement of sleep, the stabilization of thermoregulation, and LH releasing hormone pulses. Thus estrogens may definitely have a "central tonic effect". This effect may be mediated through catecholamines or endogenous opioids. The lessening of depression with estrogens also supports this hypothesis. Finally, it is difficult to separate the effects of aging and the effects of hormonal deprivation (Table 4).

Our current knowledge of psychoneuroendocrinology suggests additional *Pharmacological Approaches* to menopausal symptoms. Of these, two interesting lines of therapeutic investigation should be mentioned. Several investigators applied veralipride to symptomatic postmenopausal women; this compound is a benzamide derivative with a central anti-dopaminergic action. De Cecco et al. (1981) [41] gave a daily dose of 100 mg veralipride for 20 days to 21 women with menopausal disorders. The treatment improved the climacteric syndrome, particularly the sudden hot flushes. FSH plasma levels remained unchanged, LH levels were reduced, although they remained high, and PRL levels increased. Clayden et al. (1974) were the first to try clonidine in a double-blind cross-over fashion; they demonstrated a significant reduction of hot flushes. Many authors tried this nonhormonal treatment at varying doses (0.05–0.15 mg orally). At these dose levels, clonidine has less effect on blood pressure and no serious side effects. Other authors failed to demonstrate a response of menopausal vasomotor symptoms to clonidine [43]. Finnish authors found that clonidine was highly effective in young, ovariectomized women (Ylikorkala, 1975) [44].

In a randomized, multicentric, double-blind study of 83 out-patient women with climacteric symptoms, a combined treatment with clonidine (.05 mg b.i.d.) and low-dose conjugated estrogens (.6 mg s.i.d.) was compared to the oral administration of estrogens at a higher dose (1.25 mg s.i.d.). Over a period of 12 weeks, frequency and intensity of hot flushes, sweating, intensity of migraine attacks and a modified Kupperman index were recorded and statistically evaluated. A clear improvement in

Table 4 Therapeutic Strategies to Menopausal Symptoms

	compound	mechanism of action	clinical effects	metabolic effects
	estrogen[1]	↓ MAO ↓ COMT	anxiety and mood-depression alleviated	BP ↔ HDL/LDL ↑
		↑ tryptophane	mental illness decreased	Hemostasis ↔
		↑ NE / 5-HT	rem-non rem proportion of sleep	
		↑ NE / DA	VMF vaginal dryness urinary frequency memory	
Hormonal	progesterone[2]	? opiates ? NE / DA	VMF – insomnia – mental – relief	Ca[3] balance restored plasma lipids ↔ serum androgen ↔
	estrogen –[4] progestagen	continuous	VMF – paraesthesia – insomnia irritability vertigo atrophic endometrium rare & slight bleeding	$\frac{\text{HDL}}{\text{LDL}}$ cholesterol ↔

1 Schiff et al., 1979
2 Albrecht et al., 1981; F. A. Aleem, 1984
3 F. A. Aleem, 1984
4 Mattson, Cullberg, Samsioe, 1982 & 1984

all parameters was observed in both groups. Differences in the groups were not significant, nor was there any difference between the groups with respect to other complaints (pain in the lower back, pain in the joints, libido loss, reduced sexual arousability, vaginal dryness). No serious side-effects were observed. In both groups heart-rate, blood-pressure and body-weight remained fairly constant. In their final assessment of efficacy and tolerance the investigators and patients judged the combination to be somewhat more favourable than the higher dose estrogen treatment. According to these findings the combination treatment is of at least equal value as the higher dose estrogen monotherapy [45].

Clonidine, by acting as a central α-2-receptor agonist, may inhibit central adrenergic neurons and possibly also the release of peripheral vasoactive compounds. It is

Table 5 Therapeutic Strategies to Menopausal Symptoms

	compound	mechanism of action	clinical effects	metabolic effects
Pharmacological	clonidine[1]	α-adrenergic agonist ↓ NE ↓ DA	VMF	–
Pharmacological	veralipride[2]	central anti-dopaminer-gic ↔ FSH ↓ LH ↑ PRL	VMF	–
Pharmacological	lofexidine[3]	α-adrenergic agonist	VMF (74%) $p < .001$	–
Combination	clonidine[4] & estrogen	α-adrenergic 1.25 mg E_1-S ≅ 0.6 mg E_1-S & 0.05 mg clonidine b. i. d.	Kupperman-index all parameters BP	BWt ↔

1 Clayden et al., 1974
2 De Cecco, 1981
3 Parker, Jones, Ravnikar, Schiff, 1985
4 Schindler et al., 1984

unclear whether clonidine also acts on diaphoresis via the cholinergic postsynaptic receptor.

For patients unable or unwilling to take estrogens alternative treatments may prove beneficial in some cases. Alternative treatment includes placebo, tranquilizers and sedatives in addition to veralipride and clonidine (Table 5).

The occurrence of waking episodes with hot flushes contributes to insomnia in older women. This chronic sleep disturbance can alter psychological function and provides a plausible explanation for the improvement of affective and cognitive functions observed with substitution of hormones in postmenopausal women experiencing severe flushes.

References

[1] Frie, J.F. (1980) Ageing, natural death, and the compression of morbidity. N. Engl. J. Med. 303:130–135

[2] Utian, W.H. (1980) Menopause in modern perspective. Appleton-Century-Crofts, New York

[3] Subcommittee of Council of Medical Women's Federation of England: Investigation of menopause in 1000 women. Lancet 1:106 (1933)

[4] For Ref. see 2. Utian, W.H. (1980)

[5] Campbell, S. & Whitehead, M. (1977) Oestrogen therapy and the menopausal syndrome. In: Greenblatt, R.G. & Studd, J.W.W. (eds.) Clinics in Obstetrics and Gynecology. Vol. 4, pp. 31–48 (London: W.B. Saunders)

[6] Utian, W.H. (1972) The true clinical features of postmenopause and oophorectomy and their response to estrogen therapy. S. Afr. Med. J. 46:732

[7] Tataryn, I.V., Meldrum, D.R., Lu, K.H., et al. (1979) LH, FSH and skin temperature during the menopausal hot flushes. J. Clin. Endocrinol. Metab. 49:152–154

[8] Meldrum, D.R., Shamonki, I.M., Frumar, A.M., et al. (1979) Elevations of skin temperature of the finger as an objective index of postmenopausal hot flushes: Standardization of the technique. Am. J. Obstet. Gynecol. 135:713–717

[9] Erlik, Y., Tataryn, I.V., Meldrum, D.R., Lomax, P., Bajorek, J.G., and Judd. L. (1981) Association of waking episodes with menopausal hot flushes. Jama 245:1741–1744

[10] Hayward, J.N. (1972) The anatomy of heat exchange. In: Schonbaum, E. & Lomax, P. (eds.) Proceedings of the Vth International Congress of Pharmacology: The pharmacology of thermoregulation. Basel, Switzerland, S. Karger, pp. 26–27

[11] Casper, R.F. & Yen, S.S.C. (1981) Menopausal flushes: Effect of pituitary gonadotropin desensitization by a potent luteinizing hormone-releasing factor agonist. J. Clin. Endocrinol. Metab. 53:1056–1058

[12] Cooper, K.E. (1972) The body temperature "setpoint" in fever. In: Blight, J., Moore, R. (eds.) Essays on temperature regulation. New York, Elsevier/North Holland, pp. 149–162

[13] Cooper, K.E., Cranston, W.I., Snell, E.S. (1964a) Temperature regulation during fever in man. Clin. Sci. 27:345–356

[14] Cooper, K.E., Johnson, R.H., Spalding, J.M.K. (1964b) Thermoregulatory reactions following intravenous pyrogen in a subject with complete transaction of the cervical cord. J. Physiol. 171:55–56

[15] Cooper, K.E., Veale, W.L., Pittman, Q.L. (1976) Pathogenesis of fever, brain dysfunction and infantile febrile convulsions. New York, Raven Press, pp. 107–115

[16] Lomax, P., Bajorek, J.G., Chesarek, W., et al. (1979) Thermoregulatory effects of luteinizing hormone releasing hormone in the rat. In: Cox, B., Lomax, P. (eds.) Thermoregulatory mechanisms and their therapeutic implications. Basel, Switzerland, S. Karger, pp. 208–211

[17] Reaves, T.A., Hayward, J.N. (1979) Hypothalamic and extra-trypothalamic thermoregulatory centers. In: Lomax, P. & Schonbaum, E. (eds.) Body temperature: Regulation, drugs effects and therapeutic implications. New York, Marcel Dekker Inc. pp. 39–70

[18] Kobayashi, R.M., Lu, K.H., Moore, R.Y., et al. (1978) Regional distribution of hypothalamic luteinizing hormone releasing hormone in proesterus rats – effects of ovariectomy and estrogen replacement. Endocrinology 102:98–105

[19] Yen, S.S.C. (1977) The biology of menopause. J. Reprod. Med. 18:287–296

[20] Donoso, A.L., Stefano, I.J.E., Biscardi, A.M., et al. (1967) Effects of castration on hypothalamic catecholamines. Am. J. Physiol. 212:737–739

[21] Fuxe, K., Höckfelt, T., Nilsson, O. (1969) Castration, sex hormones, and tuberoinfundibular dopamine neurons. Neuroendocrinology 5:107–120

[22] Finch, C.E. (1975) Neuroendocrinology of ageing: A view of an emerging area. Biol. Sci. 25:645–647

[23] Albrecht, B., Schiff, I., Tulchinsky, D., et al. (1981) Objective evidence that placebo and oral medroxyprogesterone acetate diminishes menopausal hot flushes. Am. J. Obstet. Gynecol. 139:631–636

[24] Meites, J., Bruni, J.F., van Vugt, A., et al. (1979) Relation of endogenous opioid

peptides and morphine to neuroendocrine function. Life sci. 24:1325–1336
[25] Van Loon, G. R., Ho, D., Kim, C. (1980) Beta-endorphin-induced decrease in hypothalamic turnover. Endocrinology 106:76–80
[26] De Fazio, J., Verheugen, C., Chetkowski, R., et al. (1984) The effects of naloxone on hot flashes and gonadotropin secretion in postmenopausal women. J. Clin. Endocrinol. Metab. 58:578–581
[27] Webb, W. B. (1969) Partial and differential sleep deprivation. In: Kayes, A. (ed.) Sleep physiology and pathology. Philadelphia: Lippincott, pp. 221–244
[28] Tryding, N., Tufeessom, G., Nilsson, S., et al. (1972) Aging, monoamins and monoamine oxidase levels. Lancet 1:489
[28a] Nies, A., Robinson, A. S., Rovares, C. L., et al. (1971) Amine and monoamine oxidase levels in relation to aging and depression in man. Psychosom. Med. 33:470
[28b] McGeer, E., McGeer, P. L. (1976) Neurotransmitter metabolism in the aging brain. In: Terry, R. D., Gerkson, S. (eds.) Neurobiology of aging. Raven Press, New York, 389–403
[29] Klaiber, E. I., Broverman, D. M., Vogel, W., et al. (1972) Effects of estrogen therapy on plasma MAO activity and EEG during responses in depressed women. Am. J. Psychiatr. 28:1492–1498
[30] Holzbauer, M., Yondin, M. B. H. (1973) The estrous cycle and monoamine oxydase levels. Br. J. Pharmacol. 48:600–608
[31] Luhby, A. L., Dawis, P., Murphy, M., et al. (1970) Pyridoxine and oral contraceptives. Lancet 2:1083
[32] Ball, P., Knuppen, R. (1980) Catecholestrogens (2- and 4-hydroxy-estrogens): Chemistry, biogenesis, metabolism, occurrence and physiological significance. Acta Endocrinol. (Suppl.) 93:232
[33] Hagnell, O. (1970) The incidence and duration of episodes of mental illness in a total population. In: Hare, F. H. & Wing, J. K. (eds.) Psychiatric epidemiology. London: Oxford University Press, 213–224
[34] Aylward, M. (1975) Estrogens, plasma tryptophan levels in perimenopausal patients. Chapter 12, in: Campbell, S. (ed.) The management of the menopausal and post-menopausal years. London, University Part Press, pp. 135–147
[35] Campbell, S. & Whitehead, M. (1977) Oestrogen withdrawal therapy and the menopausal syndrome. Clin. Obstet. Gynecol. 31–47
[36] Kronenberg, F., Cote, L. J., Linkie, D. M., Dyrenfurth, I., and Downey, J. A. (1984) Menopausal hot flashes: Thermoregulatory, cardiovascular, and circulating catecholamine and LH changes. Maturitas 6:31–43
[37] Hartman, B. K. (1973) The innervation of cerebral blood vessels by central noradrenergic neurons. In: Ustin, E. & Snyder, S. H. (eds.) Frontiers in catecholamine research. New York, Pergamon Press, p. 91
[38] Schiff, I., Regestein, W., Tulchinsky, D., et al. (1979) Effects of estrogens on sleep and psychological state of hypogonadal women. JAMA 242:2405–2407
[39] Thompson, J. & Oswald, I. (1978) Effect of estrogen on the sleep, mood and anxiety of postmenopausal women. Br. Med. J. 2:1317–1319
[40] Kales, A., Kales, J. D., Bixler, E. O., et al. (1975) Effectiveness of hypnotic drugs with prolonged use: Flurozepan and pentobarbital. Clin. Pharmacol. Ther. 18:356–363
[41] De Cecco, L., Venturini, P. L., Alibrandi, M. P., et al. (1981) Effét du veralipride sur les taux de LH, FSH et PRL et sur le syndrome climaterique. Rev. F. R. Gynecol. Obstet. 76/10:691–694
[42] Clayden, J. R., Bell, J. W., Pollard, P. (1974) Menopausal flushing: Double-blind trial of a non-hormonal medication. Br. J. Med. 1:409
[43] Lindsay, R., Hart, D. M. (1978) Failure of response of menopausal vasomotor symptoms to clonidine. Maturitas 1:21
[44] Ylikorkala, O. (1975) Clonidine in the treatment of menopausal symptoms. Ann. Chir. Gynaecol Finn. 64:242
[45] Schindler, A. E., Heners, D., Pater, T. H., Wendel, U., and Donath, E. M. (1984) Behandlung des klimakterischen Syndroms. Fortschr. Med. 102/47–48:1213–1216
[46] Neugarten, B. L., Kraines, R. J. (1965) "Menopausal symptoms" in women of various ages. Psychosom. Med. 27:270

Skin and the menopause

M. Brincat

Introduction

The skin, one of the largest organs in the body, undergoes changes after the menopause in women. Many of these changes have previously been described simply as part of the 'ageing' process. This explanation, however fails to explain how the skin of women who are maintained on hormone therapy looks healthier than the skin of women of similar age who are not. After the menopause women start to complain of generalised dry flaky skin and of easy bruising. These symptoms are almost always reversible with appropriate sex hormone replacement, within a very short space of time, usually within the first six months. It is evident, therefore, that the sex hormones and, in particular, estrogens play an important part in the maintenance of skin quality in women. This chapter discusses how the sex hormones effect skin. The possible similarities between the relationship of the connective tissue in the skin and sex hormones and the connective tissue in the bone and sex hormones will be discussed.

Fig. 1 shows a cross-section of human skin. The dermis is largely composed of collagen; elastin fibres (2.5%) make up the rest.

The effects of estrogen on animal and human skin

Little work has been done on the effect of estrogen on the skin. Estradiol is concentraded in the basal cell layers of the epidermis (Shahrad & Marks 1977). Both estrogen and androgen receptors have been identified on fibroblasts in the skin (Back et al. 1970, Stumpf et al. 1976).

In animals, estrogens appear to alter the vascularisation of the skin (Goodrich 1966) and affect changes in the connective tissue of the dermis as reflected by increased mucopolysaccharide incorporation, hydroxyproline turnover and alterations in ground substance (Goodrich 1966). In addition to an increase in dermal turnover of hyaluronic acid, the dermal water content is enhanced with estradiol therapy (Grosman 1971, 1973). Atrophy of the epidermis disappeared after treatment lasting six weeks with the number of capillaries increasing and collagenous fibres

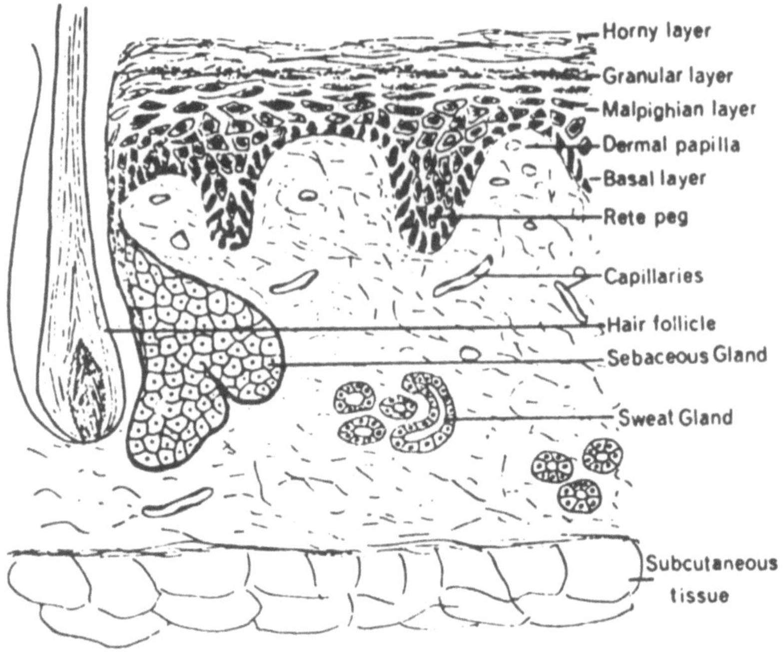

Fig. 1 Diagram shows a cross-section of the human skin demonstrating its normal structure.

appearing less fragmented. Both testosterone and estrogen ointments had similar effects on the skin of both sexes (Goldzieher 1946, 1949, 1952). Rauramo (1969) observed that oral estrogen therapy in castrated women caused thickening of the epidermis for three months which persisted for six.

Punnonen (1973) used two different strengths of estrogens in castrated women, estriol succinate and the stronger estradiol valerate. Both caused statistically significant thickening of the epidermis after three months but, whereas this thickness persisted with the estradiol succinate, 34% of the patients on estradiol valerate started to get significant thinning of their epidermis. It was postulated that this was happening because the dosage and treatment was too strong.

Mitotic activity in the epidermis

The descriptions of effects of estrogens on mitotic activity in the epidermis are conflicting. Punnonen (1973) claimed significantly higher mitotic activity in the epidermis in studies carried out using 3H-Thymidine labelling in-vitro, while Shahrad (1977), who used the same labelling agent in his in-vitro studies, claimed a depressor effect of estrogen on thymidine incorporation in the human epidermis. However, since Shahrad used pharmacologically high concentrations of estrone, there might be an optimum dose of estrogen which gives the maximum beneficial results.

Collagen in the Dermis: (This will be discussed more fully below). Collagenous fibrils were less fragmented in the dermis of women treated with estrogens (Goldzieher 1952). An increase in the number of capillaries in the dermis of these women was also noted.

Estrogens, and amorphous ground substance

The production of mucopolysaccharades is another fibroblast function. Estrogen could increase the rate of collagen production (Boueck 1959) by altering the polymerization of mucopolysaccharides. Estrogens increase the hydroscopic qualities and reduce the adhesion of collagen fibres in connective tissues (Danforth et al. 1974). The dermis is one such site where estrogens work in this way. As has been seen above, due to enhanced synthesis of dermal hyaluronic acid, the dermal water content increases (Grosman 1971, 1973).

In mice, hyaluronic acid content was shown to increase dramatically with estrogens; a close linear relationship exists between the in increase in high molecular weight hyaluronic acid and the increase in tissue water (Grossman 1971, 1973). Uzuka, who also worked with mice and whose findings were similar to Grossman's suggested that the stimulation of hyaluronic acid synthesis in mouse skin in response to estrogens is mediated through estrogen receptors and involves the induction of the enzyme, hyaluronic acid synthetase (Uzuka et al. 1980, 1981).

Skin thickness, collagen content and disease – Relationship between skin thickness and skin collagen

The skin is known to be affected by various systemic and endocrine disorders. Studies have been carried out on skin changes in various connective tissue and endocrine disorders. A brief review is presented below.

Black et al. (1970a, 1970b) and Shuster et al. (1970) looked at the relationship between skin thickness and skin collagen in systemic sclerosis, osteoporosis of mixed aetiology and hirsutes and found a good correlation between the two. In a small study, Black et al. (1970b) demonstrated changes in the collagen content and thickness of the skin in osteoporotics (mixed aetiology) treated with androgens, when compared to osteoporotics who had not been on this treatment. Shuster et al. (1970) found an increase in skin collagen in women with hirsutes, but the increase was not statistically significant. In scleroderma, Black (1970a) demonstrated a decrease in total collagen content and skin thickness in affected areas. In clinically normal areas, the skin thickness was decreased but the collagen content was not significantly altered. Arho (1972) did not show any difference between skin thickness and collagen content in patients with scleroderma when compared to normal patients. He did find a good correlation between skin thickness and collagen content in a number of patients with a variety of endocrine and collagen disorders. The conditions looked at by Arho, apart from normal skin, were acromegaly, rheumatoid arthritis, lupus erythematosus, scleroderma, prurigo Besnier, psoriasis and Cushing's syndrome. Patients with prurigo Besnier and scleroderma had normal skin collagen contents. Acromegaly produced both thicker skin and higher skin collagen content. Patients with Cushing's syndrome and those who had been treated with costicosteroids had thinner skin and lower skin collagen content than normals (Arho 1972).

Fibroblasts

The fibroblast (fibra = fiber and blastos = germ) is the most numerous cell encountered in loose connective tissue. Fibroblasts are responsible for the production of fibers and for most of the amorphous components of the intercellular substance (ground substance, glycosaminoglycans). The loose connective tissue of the dermis develops from mesenchyme with the mesenchymal cells differentiating into various cell types including the fibroblast.

Fibroblasts and sex hormones

As has already been mentioned, both estrogen and testosterone receptors have been identified on fibroblasts in the skin (Black et al. 1970, Stumpf et al. 1976).

Estrogens affect connective tissue by increasing the intercellular fluid content and rendering the ground substance more metachromatic and the fibroblasts more 'succulent' in appearance (Barnwood 1963a). Testosterone causes fibroblastic proliferation; the cells are larger than in control experiments with abundant, strongly basophilic and pyroninophilic cytoplasm (Barnwood 1963a).

The effect of sex hormones has been shown by examining the histological changes of ground substance and collagen. Estrogen administration although showing little morphological effect on fibroblasts, resulted in the formation of metachromatic ground substance rich in hyaluronic acid (HA) and containing, due to the increased HA, an increased intercellular fluid content. Testosterone causes more definite morphological changes with increased metachromatic ground substance which is also rich in hyaluronic acid (Boas 1949).

That sex hormones can influence fibroblast function has been shown by studying collagen formation and degradation by the sponge – implant – biopsy technique. Using this method Boucek et al. 1959 showed fundamental sex difference in collagen turnover. Collagen synthesis and accumulation proceed at comparable rates in male and female rat tissues up to a certain time (approximately 40 days in this study). Thereafter, in males, although the rate of collagen accumulation slows, the total amount of collagen persists. In females, however, after this particular time, the amount of collagen formed is reduced. This suggests that once a certain collagen level is achieved in the female, the collagen degradation exceeds collagen synthesis. This finding is associated with morphological changes in the related fibroblasts which become narrower and show decreased cytoplasmic content and nuclear thinning during this period.

The sponge – implant – biopsy technique is used for the assessment of fibroblast activity as determined by their healing activities (invasion of implanted sponge by fibroblasts and subsequent collagen formation). Boucek (1959) also looked at the difference between intact and oophorectomised female rats and observed that the oophorectomised rats had depressed fibroblast activity.

Collagen

Collagen is the most abundant protein in mammals, constituting 25% of their total protein (Alberts et al. 1983). In the dermis, as has been indicated, collagen accounts for 97.5%, by weight, of the fibrous protein present. Studies on collagen from various sites have indicated the presence of two basic alpha-chains, alpha-1 and alpha-2. These alpha chains consist of just over 1000 amino acid residues arranged in groups of three in the basic collagen triple helix configuration. This very stable structure forms the basic building unit of collagenous structures. Proline and hydroxproline constitute 20 to 25% of the total number of amino acids in collagen.

Skin and bone share a common collagen, Type I. Skin also contains some of Type III collagen. Type I, which constitutes 90% of the total collagen in the body, (Alberts et al. 1983) is the most important.

The effects of growth, development and ageing on collagen

Growth, development and ageing involve major changes in collagen biosynthesis and metabolism. For example, the amount of Type III collagen, frequently measured as the ratio of Type III to Type I collagen, is greater in the skin of young animals than in the skin of old animals (Miller 1976). The basis for this observation is not fully understood, but it indicates "gene switching" similar to, although less complete than the switch from embryonic and fetal haemoglobins to haemoglobin A. Growth of connective tissues involves an increased rate of collagen biosynthesis, and the increased rates of the pro-alpha chain translation are generally accompanied by increased tissue levels of intracellular post-translational enzymes. Conversely, both the rates of translation and the levels of these enzymes decrease with age (Prockop et al. 1976, Cardinale et al. 1974, Tuderman et al. 1977, Risteli et al. 1976, Anttinen et al. 1973, Anttinen et al. 1977). The hydroxylysyl glycosyltransferases (Risteli et al. 1976, Anttinen H. et al. 1977) tend to decrease less with age than do prolyl (Tuderman 1977) and lysyl (Risteli 1976, Anttinen H. 1973) hydroylases, but levels of these enzymes generally change in a parallel manner. In addition, collagen degradation parallels the decrease in collagen synthesis which, according to some authors, occurs with age (Kivirriko 1973).

Although the bulk of body collagen in adults is remarkably stable, a fraction of the collagen in all tissues is continuously degraded and replaced, even in old age. Such changes in overall collagen metabolism can be (roughly) followed by assaying excretion of peptide-bound hydroxyproline or hydroylysine in urine (Kivirriko 1973, Krane et al. 1977) since excretion of these substances is largely caused by collagen degradation (Kivirriko 1973).

In addition to changes in the genetic type and the amount of collagen, changes in the quality of collagen accompany growth and ageing. The amounts of hydroylysine (Barnes et al. 1974, Royce et al. 1977) and glycosylated hydrosylysine (Royce et al. 1977, Murai et al. 1975) in Type I collagen and the amount of immature and reducible crosslinks tend to decrease with age (Risteli et al. 1976). These observations indicate that the chemical characteristics and perhaps the function of collagen change with age. To what extent these changes are fundamental to the ageing process is still unknown. The role of sex hormones which change dramatically with age is likewise unknown (Prockop 1979a, b).

Studies on postmenopausal women

Brincat et al. (1983) looked at the skin collagen content of a number of postmenopausal women who had been on the same estrogen and testosterone implant combinations as hormone replacement for at least two years and not more than ten years, and compared this to that of an untreated age-matched group of postmenopausal women. The treated group had a highly significant greater skin collagen content than the untreated group (Fig. 2). In later studies (Brincat et al. 1984b, c, 1985a), it was shown that in the treated group of women, no correlation existed between the skin collagen content and the duration of therapy, suggesting that after a certain period (less than two years) the skin collagen content equilibrated and did not continue to increase indefinitely (Fig. 3). These same authors (Brincat 1984b, c, 1985) showed highly significant correlations between years since menopause, and skin collagen content in the untreated group of women with the skin collagen content declining in an exponential manner. (Fig. 3).

Using a radiological method for measuring skin thickness, skin was also shown to be significantly thicker in postmenopausal women who had been on hormone treatment than those age-matched women who had not (Brincat et al. 1984b). (Fig. 4).

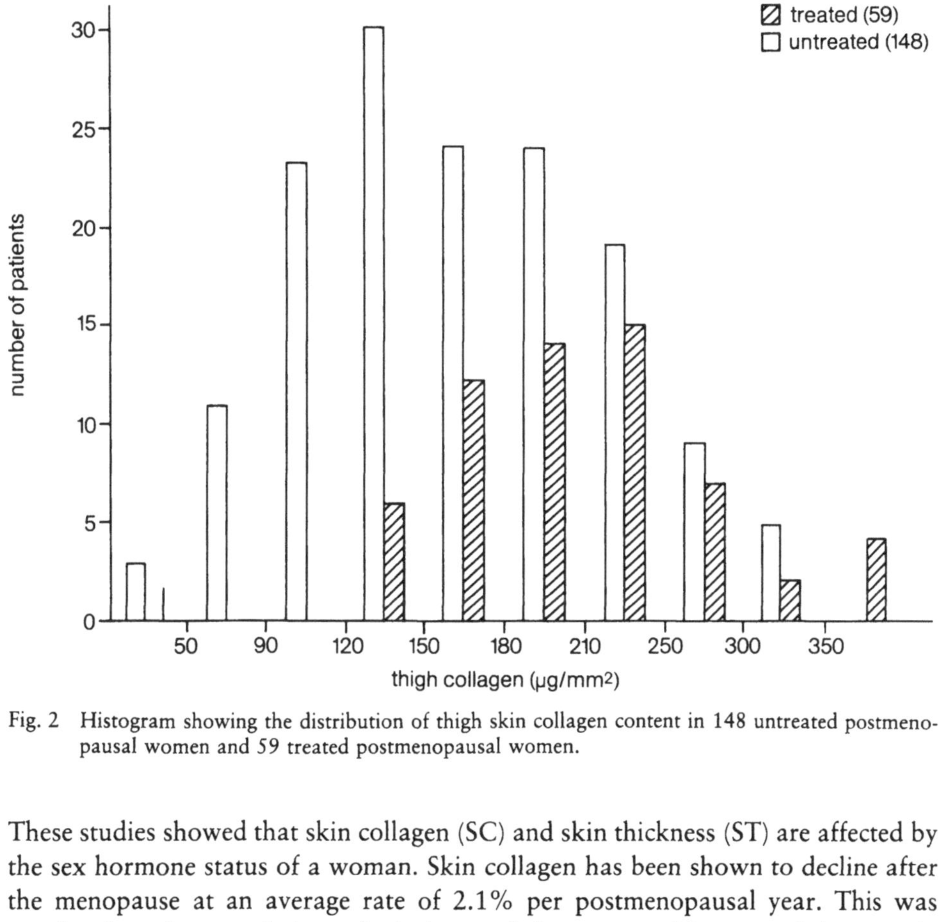

Fig. 2 Histogram showing the distribution of thigh skin collagen content in 148 untreated postmenopausal women and 59 treated postmenopausal women.

These studies showed that skin collagen (SC) and skin thickness (ST) are affected by the sex hormone status of a woman. Skin collagen has been shown to decline after the menopause at an average rate of 2.1% per postmenopausal year. This was unrelated to the actual chronological age of the woman. The rate of decrease in collagen content was higher in the initial postmenopausal years than in the latter ones, the decline being exponential in nature.

In prospective studies carried out on postmenopausal women (Brincat 1985b), it has also been shown that skin collagen content can actually be improved with estrogen or estrogen and testosterone hormone replacement. This improvement is self-limiting. There seems to be an optimum collagen content that a woman achieves, beyond which no further collagen increase occurs. This is shown as the '0' collagen value in Fig. 5. A very strong correlation exists between the original collagen content that the woman has at the start of her treatment and the change in collagen that occurs after six months of treatment (Brincat 1985b). In those women with a low skin collagen content who are several years postmenopausal estrogens are therapeutic and later of prophylactic value, while in those who have a high skin collagen content, and who are in their early postmenopausal years, estrogens are of prophylactic value only. Thus a deficiency in skin collagen can be corrected but not over-

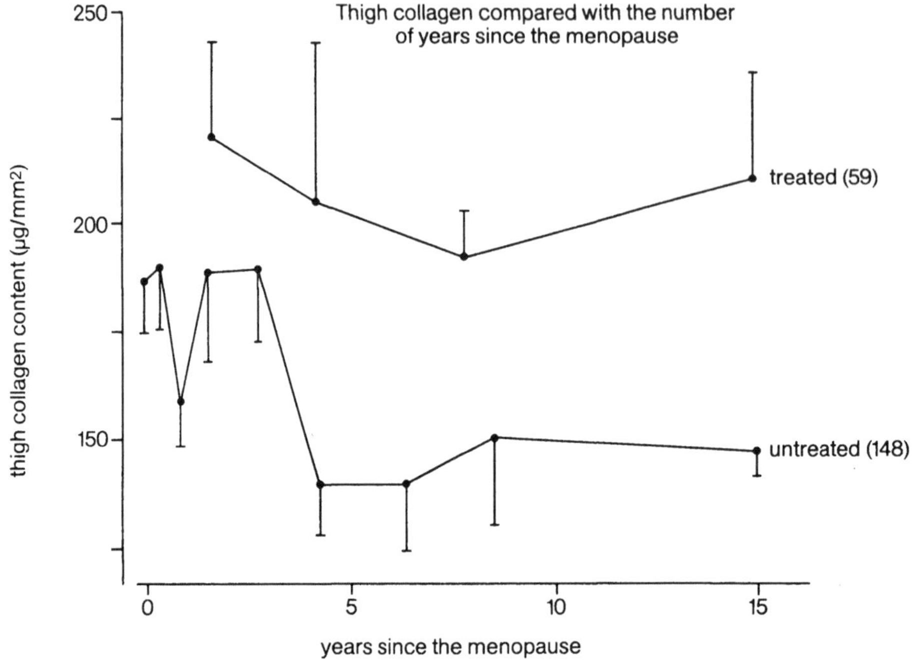

Fig. 3 Thigh skin collage content (M±SE) with years since menopause in 148 untreated postmenopausal women and in 59 postmenopausal women who had been on sex hormone treatment for between two to ten years.

corrected. Similarly, as has been noted above, there seems to be an optimum physiological estrogen dose for the epidermis also beyond which thinning rather than thickening of the epidermis occurs (Punnonen 1973, Shahrad 1977).

After six months of therapy with various physiological regimens of estrogens and one regimen which included a small dose of testosterone, skin collagen levels were restored to levels similar to those in the treated group of postmenopausal women discussed above, and to those in premenopausal women (Brincat 1985b).

Skin thickness, measured radiologically represents dermal connective tissue as a whole, rather than collagen only (i.e. it also represents the amorphous ground substance). This has, however, been shown to have a highly significant correlation with skin collagen content in both the treated and the untreated group of postmenopausal women (Brincat 1975a). Skin thickness has been shown to become thinner after the menopause (Brincat et al. 1984b, c). It has been shown to decline at an average rate of fall in the initial postmenopausal years which is not as high as with the skin collagen content.

In summary, from the retrospective studies quoted above, it can be said that there is evidence that skin collagen content and skin thickness can be restored and/or be

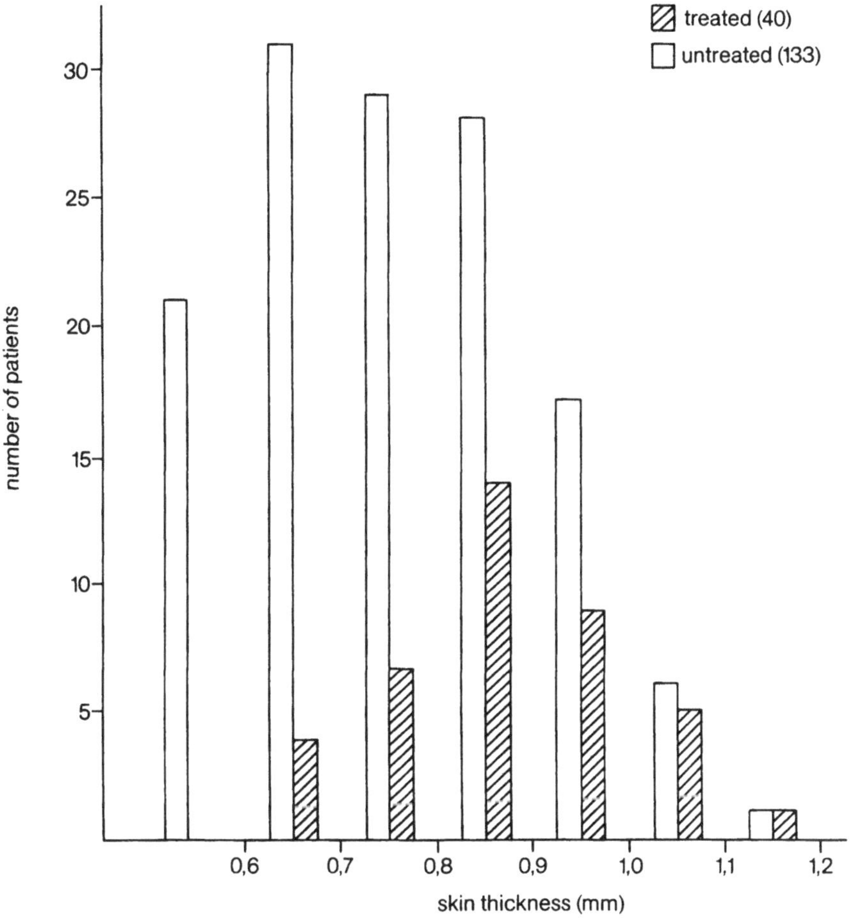

Fig. 4 Histogram showing the distribution of forearm skin thickness in 133 untreated postmenopausal women and 40 treated postmenopausal women.

prevented from falling in a period of under two years of sex hormone treatment. From the prospective studies described, the skin collagen content has been shown to be restituted after six months of physiological sex hormone replacement.

Finally, no correlation was found between skin thickness and skin collagen content and the actual chronological age of a woman, which suggests that actual age is not as important a factor in determining these parameters as the years since menopause. (Brincat et al. 1985a).

Sex hormones, skin and bone

Apart from indicating the relationship of skin with the sex hormones, studies on the dermis and the menopause suggest the possible behavior of connective tissue in

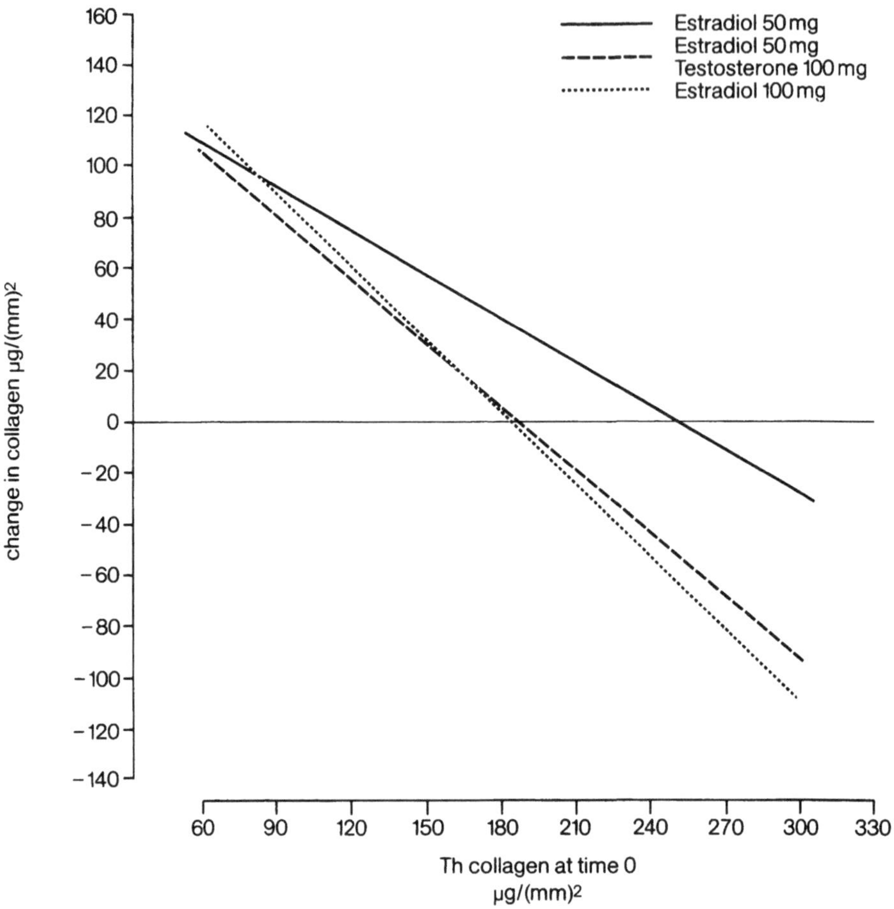

Fig. 5 Diagram shows the relationship between the change in thigh skin collagen content that occurred in postmenopausal women after 6 months of receiving an estradiol 50 mgs, an estradiol 50 mgs and testosterone 100 mgs and estradiol 100 mgs implant, and their original baseline thigh skin collagen content.

general with the sex hormones. The importance of this suggestion lies in the fact that it might be possible to predict the behavior of the connective tissue element, the organic matrix in bone mass in a particular individual, from the state of the skin and thus be able to predict who is most at risk of developing a bone mass that is sufficiently decreased so as to risk developing an osteoporotic fracture.

References

Alberts, B., Bray, D., Lewis, J., Raff, M., Roberts, K., Watson, J. D.: Cell-Cell Adhesion and the Extracellur Matrix. In: Molecular Biology of the Cell. (Alberts, B. et al. eds.). Garland Publishing Inc. New York & London 1983; 12:673–715.

Anttinen, H., Orava, S., Ryhanen, L. et al.: Assay of protocollagen Lysyl hydroxylase activity in the skin of human subjects and changes in the activities with age. Clin. Chim. Acta 1973; 47:289–94.

Anttinen, H., Oikarinin, A., Kivviriko, K. I.: Age related changes in human skin collagen galactosyltransferase and collagen glucosyl transferase activity. Clin. Chim. Acta 1977; 76:95–101.

Arho, P.: Skin thickness and collagen content in some endocrine connective tissue and skin diseases. Acta Derm. Venerol. (Suppl.) Stockholm 1972; 69:1–48.

Barnwood, A. W.: The Fibroblast. Int. Rev. of Connective Tissue Research 1963; 1:1–28.

Black, M. M., Bottoms, E., Shuster, S.: Skin Collagen Content and Thickness in systemic sclerosis. Br. J. Dermatol. 1970a; 83:552–555.

Black, M. M., Shuster, Bottoms, E.: Osteoporosis, Skin Collagen and Androgen. Br. Med. J. 1970b; 4:773–4.

Boucek, R. J., Noble, N. L., Woessner, J. F. Jnr.: Properties of Fibroblasts. In: Connective Tissue Thrombosis and Atherosclerosis. (IH Page ed). Academic Press, New York 1959; 193–211.

Brincat, M., Moniz, C. F., Studd, J. W. W., Darby, A. J., Magos, A. L., Cooper, D.: Sex Hormones and skin collagen content in postmenopausal women. Br. Med. J. 1983; 287:1337–8.

Brincat, M., Moniz, C. F., Studd, J. W. W., Darby, A. J., Magos, A. L., Eumbery, G., Versi, E.: The Long Term Effects of the Menopause and of Administration of sex hormones on skin collagen and skin thickness. Br. J. Obstet. Gynaecol. 1985; 92:256–59.

Brincat, M., Studd, J. W. W., Moniz, C. J., Parsons, V., Darby, A. F.: Skin thickness and skin collagen mimic an index of osteoporosis in the postmenopausal woman. In: Osteoporosis (Christiansen, C. et al., eds.). Proceedings of the Copenhagen International Symposium on Osteoporosis 1984b, 353–355.

Brincat, M., Studd, J. W. W., Moniz, C. F., Parsons, V., Darby, A. J.: Skin thickness measurement. A simple screening method for determining patients at risk of developing postmenopausal osteoporosis. In: Osteoporosis (Christiansen, C. et al., eds.). Proceedings of the Copenhagen International Symposium on Osteoporosis 1984c; 1:323–326.

Brincat, M.: Skin collagen, skin thickness and Metacarpal Index in the diagnosis of women at risk of developing postmenopausal osteoporosis. Drug therapy 1985; In press.

Cardinale, G. J., Udenfriend, S. B.: Prolyl hydroxylase Adv Emzymol 1974; 41:245–300.

Danforth, D. N., Veis, A., Breen, M., Weinstein, H. G., Buckingham, J. C., Manalo, P.: The Effect of Pregnancy and Labour on the Human Cervix: Changes in collagen, glycoproteins and glycosaminoglycans. Am. J. Obstet. Gynaecol. 1974; 120:641–651.

Goldzieher, M. A.: The effects of Oestrogens on the senile skin. J. Gerontol. 1946; 1:196.

Goldzieher, J. W.: The direct effect of steroids on the senile human skin. J. Gerontol. 1949; 4:104.

Goldzieher, J. W., Roberts, I. S., Rasols W. B., Goldzieher, M. A.: Local action of steroids on senile human skin. Arch. Derm. 1952; 66:304.

Goodrich, S. M., Wood, J. E.: The effect of Oestradiol-17β on peripheral venous distensibility and velocity of venous blood flow. Am. J. Obstet. Gynaecol. 1966; 96:407–41.

Grosman, N., Hirdberg, E., Schon, J.: The effect of Oestrogenic Treatment on the Acid Mucopolysaccharide Pattern in Skin of Mice. Acta Pharmacol. et Toxicol. (1971); 30:458–64.

Grosman, N.: Studies on the hyaluronic acid protein complex, the molecular size of hyaluronic acid and the exchangeability of chloride in skin of mice before and after oestrogen treatment. Acta Pharmacol. et Toxicol. 1973; 33:201–208.

Kivirikko, K. I.: Urinary excretion of hydroxyproline in health and disease. Int. Rev. Connect. Tissue Res. 1973; 5:93–163.

Krane, S. M., Kantrowitz, F. G., Byrne, M. et al.: Urinary excretion of hydroxylysine and its glycosides as an index of collagen degradation. J. Clin. Invest. 1977; 59:819–27.

Murai, A., Miyahara, T., Shiozawa, S.: Age related variations in glycosylation of hydroxylysine in human and rat skin collagens. Biochem. Biophys. Acta 1975; 404:345–48.

Prockop, D. J., Kivirikko, K. L., Tuderman, L., Guzman, N.: The Biosynthesis of Collagen and its disorders. NEJM 1979; 301 (2); 77–85.

Punnonen, R.: Effect of castration and peroral therapy on skin. Acta Obstet. Gynaecol. Scand. (Suppl.) 1973; 21:1–44.

Rauramo, L., Punnonen, R.: Wirkung einer oralen Oestrogentherapie mit oestriolsuccinat auf die Haut kastrierter Frauen. Z. Haut Geschlechts-Kr. 1969; 44, 13:463–470.

Risteli, J., Kivirikko, K. I.: Intracellular enzymes of collagen biosynthesis in rat liver as a function of age and in hepatic injury induced by dimethylnitrosamine: changes in prolyl hydroxylase, lysyl hydroxylase, collagen galactosyltransferase and collagen glucosyltransferase activities. Biochem. J. 1976; 158:361–67.

Royce, P. M., Barnes. M. J.: Comparative studies on collagen glycosylation in chick skin and bone. biochem. Biophys. Acta 1977; 498:132–142.

Shahrad, P., Marks, R.: A Pharmacological effect of oestrone on human epidermis. Br. J. Dermat. 1977; 97:383–386.

Shuster, S., Black, M. H., Bottoms, E.: Skin collagen and thickness in women with hirsutes. Br. Med. J. 1970; 4:772.

Stumpf, W. E., Sur, M., Joshi, S. E.: Estrogen target cells in the skin. Experientia 1976; 30:196.

Tuderman, L., Kivirikko, K. I.: Immunoreactive prolyl hydroxylase in human skin, serum and synovial fluid: changes in the content and components with age. Eur. J. Clin. Invest. 1977; 7:295–299.

Uzuka, M., Nakamiza, K., Ohta, S., Mori, Y.: The mechanism of oestrogen-induced increase in hyaluronic acid biosynthesis with special reference to oestrogen receptors in the mouse skin. Biochem. Biophys. Acta 1980; 627:199–206.

Uzuka, M., Nakamiza, K., Ohta, S., Mori, Y.: Induction of Hyaluronic acid Synthetase by Oestrogen in the mouse skin. Biochem. Biophys. Acta 1981; 673:387–393.

Osteoporosis: occurrence and diagnosis

R. Lindsay

Osteoporosis is a major public health problem of the 1980's. The postmenopausal variety of the disorder is, by far, the most common. It is estimated that in the U.S.A. there may be as many as 15 million women who have evidence of osteoporosis. Because of the size of the problem, in terms of morbidity, mortality and cost, increasing attention is being addressed to the problems remaining in diagnosis, prevention and treatment of the disorder.

Osteoporosis can be defined as reduction in bone mass per unit volume such that there is a significantly increased risk of fracture. This definition requires a premorbid period of bone loss but not the presence of fracture since the occurrence of fracture does not change the underlying pathology. Also, the availability of techniques for bone mass measurement allows diagnosis prior to fracture which, until recently, was the prime method of presentation. Thus osteoporosis is undergoing a change, similar to that observed for hyperparathyroidism or hypertension, where a previously fairly less common symptomatic disorder is now being diagnosed commonly in its relatively asymptomatic period, with consequent problems in determining appropriate management.

It has been known for many years that fracture frequency changes with age [1]. After the peak in traumatic fractures in the teenage years and early twenties, there is a relatively stable fracture rate in both sexes until the fifth decade when fracture incidence begins to increase among women, doubling approximately every eight years thereafter. A similar increase in fractures among men is evident, but not until the seventh decade, that is, at least twenty years later than among women. The commonest fractures are those of the wrist (colles fractures), vertebrae (crush fractures) and of the hip, but fracture of any bone can occur.

Recent evidence suggests that fractures consequent upon osteoporosis are an increasing clinical problem [2]. Our own data (Fig. 1) suggests that between 1970 and 1980 there was an overall increase of about 40% in the annual frequency of fractures of the hip in the U.S.A. Similar data have been reported from the U.K. [3, 4]. This year more than 300,000 hip fractures are expected in the U.S.A., and if the present trend continues to the end of the century, this figure may climb to almost 1/2 million annually. With considerable morbidity and a 10–15% mortality within six months of the fracture, hip fracture clearly is a major concern in many health care

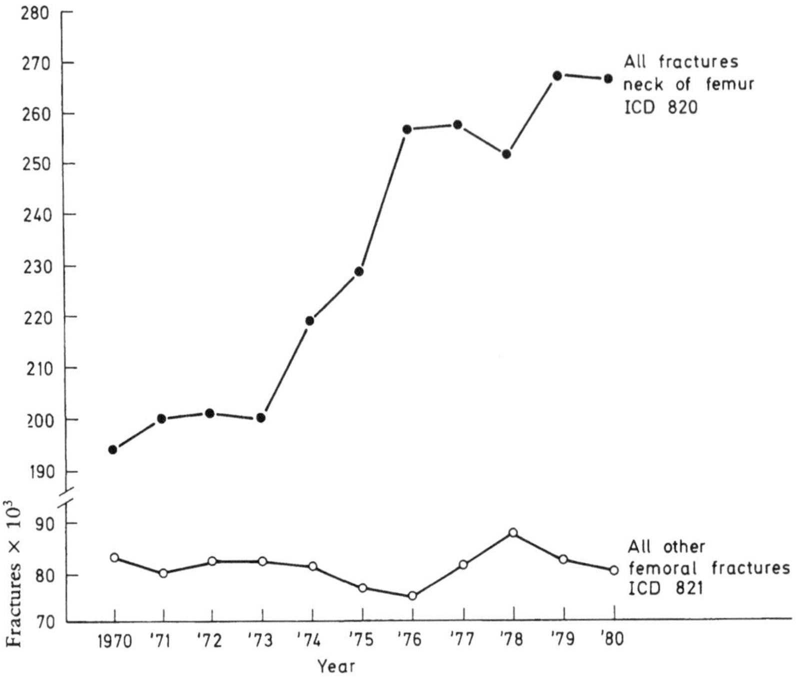

Fig. 1 Increase in the annual frequency of hip fractures in the U.S.A.

systems. Indeed the overall annual health care cost of osteoporosis in the U.S.A. was estimated to be nearly $4 billion in 1983 [5].

Realization of the health care costs involved has renewed interest in the early diagnosis of patients with osteoporosis, and recognition of those who are liable to develop the disorder. This is not a simple problem. Because those factors considered to contribute significantly to this risk for osteoporosis yield such a protean group, (Table 1) they fail to define adequately 'high-risk' status. No prospective studies of sufficient magnitude have examined the risk hypothesis, and the majority of data has been accumulated either using retrospective analyses of patients with established fracture syndromes or relatively short-term studies of younger peri- and postmenopausal groups. Despite these limitations there is some value in examining those risk factors currently thought to be of importance, since they provide the only measure of risk available presently.

Assessment of risk

Clearly osteoporosis tends to occur within families. This may be due to a genetic influence exerted on bone mass at maturity or a sharing of environmental influences within family groups. The relative importance of these two factors is undecided and more defined evaluation of this familial trait is required. Genetic influences on bone mass may also explain the racial differences in expression of the fracture syndromes which are considerably more common in Caucasian and Oriental races. The protective effect of obesity may again be a genetic issue, but may also represent an effect of increased stress upon the skeleton, as well as an effect of higher endogenous estrogens in the postmenopausal years since peripheral conversion of adrenal androgens to estrogen occurs mainly in fatty tissue [6].

Table 1 Risk Factors for Osteoporosis

Female sex	
Caucasian or Oriental ethnic origin	
Positive family history for osteoporosis	
Reduced weight for height	
Poor diet:	Calcium
	Caffeine
	Alcohol
	Protein
	Phosphate
Sedentary life-style	
Cigarette smoking	
Nulliparity	
Other disorders affecting mineral metabolism	

Since Albright's classical clinical description [7] of the disorder, an early menopause or prememopausal oophorectomy has been recognized as a risk factor. However, its relative importance has been questioned repeatedly. Review of all data available currently, however, leads to the conclusion that this is a very significant risk factor, especially when compounded by the presence of others. Cross-sectional and prospective studies have demonstrated an increase in bone remodeling [8] across the menopause, and the kinetic data obtained for calcium homeostasis correlates well with much of the prospective data on bone mass changes obtained using the newer techniques of bone mass measurement (Table 2). Long-term data suggest that bone loss accelerates following menopause for perhaps 3–6 years [9] and that this loss contributes 30–50% of the total age-dependent loss of bone among women. This accelerated phase of bone loss currently appears to be sensitive only to ovarian steroids [10–13], being inhibited in a dose-dependent fashion by low doses of estrogen [14]. However, when the mechanism of the estrogen effect is uncovered,it is entirely possible that an effective therapy may be obtained which may not be an estrogen.

Loss of bone mass, in addition to loss of the organic matrix, clearly also results in loss of mineral content. Since dietary calcium supplementation has significant effects

Table 2 Non-invasive Techniques for Measurement of Bone Mass

Technique	Site	Cortical/ Trabecular Ratio	Accuracy	Precision	Radiation
Radiogrammetry	Metacarpal	99:1	?	+2%	5–8mrem
Radiodensitometry	Metacarpal	99:1	?	2–15%	5–8 mrem
Single-Photon Absorptiometry	Mid-Radius	95:5	4%	2–4%	5 mrem
	Distal Radius	75:25	5%	2–4%	5 mrem
Dual-Photon Absorptiometry	LV 2–4	40:60	5–7%	2–5%	5–15 mrem
	Femur Neck	75:25	?	?	5–15 mrem
	Total Skeleton	80:20	2–4%	2–4%	10–40 mrem
Computerized Tomography	Vertebral Body	5:95	?*	?*	>200 mrem
Neutron Activation Analysis	Total Body	80:20	3–5%	2–3%	>1 rem
	Trunk	30:70	+10%	5%	400 mrem

* Precision and accuracy of CT vary depending on methodology; dual energy scanning improves accuracy (by providing some correction for marrow fat), but precision does not appear to change. Radiation dosage doubles, however.

on skeletal turnover in a wide variety of models, it is not surprising that dietary calcium deficiency has been postulated to be a cause of osteoporosis. From the elegant studies of Heaney, it is clear that the female population of the U.S.A. consumes less than the optimum amount of calcium in the daily diet [15]. However, it is a significantly large jump from that observation to the hypothesis that calcium supplementation can provide and maintain positive skeletal balance. Additionally, it is pertinent to recognize that while many populations are relatively calcium deficient, the prevalence of osteoporosis does not mimic the population prevalence of calcium deficiency.

Of the other dietary factors suggested as risk factors, alcohol is clearly the most important, having significant negative effects on calcium and skeletal homeostasis in both females and males [16] as well as in model systems. The positive relationship between urinary sodium and calcium suggests that a high sodium intake will adversely affect calcium homeostasis. Caffeine appears to adversely affect calcium balance, and may increase bone resorption *in vitro*. The role of protein, within the normal range of intake, is not clear, although diets high in animal protein can induce urinary calcium loss [17–18] by virtue of their high sulphate content. It is also entirely possible that lifetime relative vitamin D malnutrition of insufficient magnitude to cause osteomalacia, can accelerate or exacerbate bone loss with aging, although this possibility still requires vigorous examination. The impact of phosphate, the final dietary factor thought to be incriminated in the pathogenesis of osteoporosis, is still uncertain, and further work is necessary. Cigarette consumption is a risk factor by itself [19, 20], since it is associated with reduced bone mass even when corrections are made for differences in factors such as weight which exist between smokers and non-smokers and may in themselves be a direct cause of reduced bone mass, rather than exerting purely a permissive effect as would be the case for calcium deprivation.

It has been generally assumed that activity is the most relevant of the so-called lifestyle risk factors. This assumption comes from observations on extreme activity patterns, in which inactivity (complete bed rest or spaceflight) is associated with hypercalciuria and loss of trabecular bone mass [21], while excessive activity (marathon running, professional tennis, etc) leads to at least local hypertrophy of skeletal tissue [22–23]. However, whether changing activity patterns within the confines that are acceptable to most individuals can influence skeletal mass both generally and significantly remains controversal. Among premenopausal women, activity of sufficient severity to produce amenorrhea is undoubtedly associated with *reduced* bone mass [24]. Indeed, it has been suggested that this may be exacerbated by dietary calcium insufficiency. This finding corroborates our own data suggesting that even in normal amenhorreic young women increased activity by itself is insufficient to obtain maximum skeletal mass unless there is adequate availability of calcium [25]. It appears, therefore, that a complex interaction of these three risk factors, dietary calcium, exercise and sex hormones, provides important control of skeletal status, probably in both males and females. *Clearly,* however, the menopause, with its catastrophic fall in ovarian steroid production becomes, in women, *probably* the single most important factor affecting the skeleton.

Bone mass measurement

With the increasing availability of bone mass measurements, interest has peaked in the possibility that such non-invasive techniques will provide further separation of those at risk from their peers. Currently, however, this is not possible. Firstly, it is not clear which is the most relevant measurement of mass, or if, indeed, estimates of single sites are representative of other skeletal sites. Secondly, no technique is of sufficient precision to allow calculation of rate of change of bone mass for individual patients within a reasonable time frame (Table 2). Currently, we use, for the younger asymptomatic women, a combination of dual and single photon absorptiometry, which gives an estimate both of the axial skeleton (mostly trabecular bone) and the peripheral skeleton. A relationship between measurements at these sites is observed, but it is not sufficiently close to allow estimation of one site from a measurement taken at the other (the standard error of estimation is about the same as the population standard deviation for the second site). When one wishes to examine rates of change, then there is almost no meaningful correlation between sites.

Notwithstanding these problems, bone mass measurements undoubtedly will become more generally available. Physicians are to be discouraged from basing clinical judgements on such results until a clearer definition of their meaning is evident. Single time point measurements provide no historical or prospective insight. Indeed calculation of rate using duplicate measures over a fixed time scale may provide a false impression of the real biological status. Nonetheless, such measurements will play an increasing role, and it is clear that those whose vertebral mass measurements are above the average of the maximum vertebral mass are fairly unlikely to suffer crush fractures in the near future. Equally, those whose bone mass is below the 5 percentile are clearly at greater risk. However, the magnitude of this risk and whether risk continues to increase as bone mass falls further is not understood.

In the future the combined use of risk factor assessment and bone mass measurements may define the population requiring preventive therapy. Currently we attempt to eliminate those risk factors which are amenable to such an approach and those that we feel, perhaps intuitively, may be of major importance. Thus, since 99% of the body's calcium is present in the skeleton, an adequate dietary supply of calcium seems prudent. According to kinetic data the median intake for the postmenopausal woman should be 1.5 g of elemental calcium per day [26]. Provision of this amount, preferably by dietary sources, should be an integral part of the general approach to osteoporosis. Calcium might best be regarded like iron; its deficiency causes a disorder, but not all osteoporoses are consequent upon calcium deficiency, just as not all anemias are resultant on iron deficiency. Likewise, because inactivity is deleterious to good health for a variety of reasons, a consistent, reasonable program of skeletal loading seems appropriate. The exact requirements are unknown, but those stated in the guidelines for prevention of cardiovascular disease, seems, at this time, to be appropriate. Avoidence of excessive alcohol, sodium and caffeine also seems sensible, as is cessation of cigarette consumption. Despite such measures, estrogen therapy remains the single most effective approach to the prevention of bone attrition. Long-term studies have shown efficacy in preventing both loss and fracture. However, the mechanism of the estrogen effect on

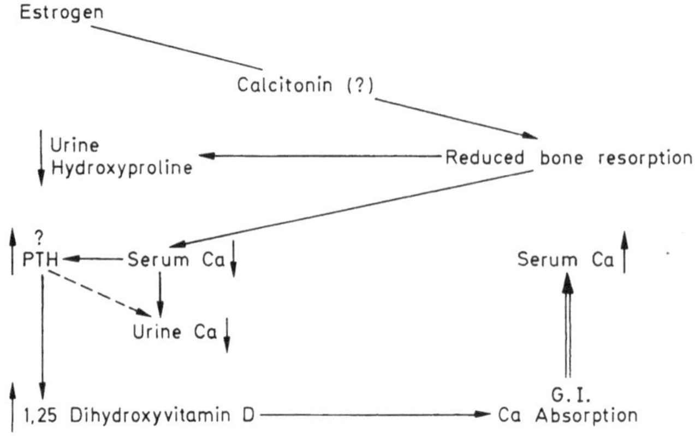

Fig. 2 Hypothesis for skeletal effects of estrogen.

the skeleton remains obscure. The hypothesis that estrogens act through calcitonin as an intermediary (Fig. 2), although the most popular of the current hypotheses, remains unproven [27], and other modes of action for sex steroid effects on the skeleton cannot be ruled out.

Recent advances in diagnosis of osteoporosis have stressed early diagnosis in the asymptomatic phase of bone loss. This has resulted, at least partially, from the difficulty in treatment of the fracture syndromes. Unfortunately, risk factor assessment and bone mass measurement have yet to become sufficiently refined in clinical use to allow accurate definition of the individual at high risk of fracture. Future developments will require clearer definition of high risk individuals to allow programs of prevention to be instituted at a time point when maximum efficacy can be expected.

References

[1] Gordan, G. S., Vaughan, C. (1976): Clinical management of the osteoporosis. Publishing Sciences, Inc., Acton, MA.

[2] Lindsay, R., Herrington, B. S. (1983): Estrogens and osteoporosis. Seminars in Reproductive Endocrinology, **1**, 55–67.

[3] Fenton-Lewis, A. (1981): Fracture of neck of the femur in changing incidence. Brit. Med. J., **283**, 1217–1220.

[4] Wallace, W. A. (1983): The increasing incidence of fractures of the proximal femur: an orthopedic epidemic. Lancet i, 1413–1414.

[5] National Institute of Health Consensus Development Conference. (1984) Osteoporosis. American Journal of Medicine.

[6] Siiteri, P. C. (1975): Postmenopausal estrogen production. Frontiers of Hormone Res, **3**, 40–44.

[7] Albright, F., Bloomberg, E., Smith, P. H. (1940): Postmenopausal osteoporosis. Trans. Assoc. Amer. Phys., **55**, 298–305.

[8] Heaney, R. P., Recker, R. R., Saville, P. D. (1978): Menopausal changes in bone remodeling. J. Lab. Clin. Med., **92**, 964–970.

[9] Lindsay, R., Hart, D. M., MacLean, A., Clark, A. C., Kraszewski, A., Garwood, J. (1978): Bone response to termination of estrogen treatment. Lancet i, 1325–1327.

[10] Lindsay, R., Hart, D. M., Aitken, J. M., MacDonald, E. B., Anderson, J. B., Clark, A. (1976): Long term prevention of postmenopausal osteoporosis by estrogen. Lancet i, 1038–1041.

[11] Lindsay, R., Hart, D. M., Forrest, C., Baird, C. (1980): Prevention of spinal osteoporosis in oophorectomised women. Lancet ii, 1151–1154.

[12] Recker, R. R., Saville, P., Heaney, R. P. (1977): Effects of estrogen and calcium carbonate on bone loss in postmenopausal women. Ann. Intern. Med. **87**, 649–655.

[13] Horsman, A., Gallagher, J. C., Simpson, M., Nordin, B. E. C. (1977): Prospective trial of estrogen and calcium in postmenopausal bone loss. B. Med. J. **2**, 789–792.

[14] Lindsay, R., Hart, D. M., Clark, D. M. (1984): The minimum effective dose of estrogen for prevention of postmenopausal bone loss. Obstetrics and Gynecology **63**, 750–763.

[15] Heaney, R. P., Gallagher, J. C., Johnston, C. C., Neer, R., Parfitt, A. M., Whedon, G. D. (1982): Calcium nutrition and bone health in the elderly. Amer. J. Clin. Nutrition **36**, 986–1103.

[16] Seeman, E., Melton, L. J., III, O'Fallon, W. M., Riggs, B. L. (1983): Risk factors for spinal osteoporosis in men. Amer. J. Med. **75**, 977–983.

[17] Heaney, R., Recker, R. R. (1982): Effects of nitrogen, phosphorus and caffeine on calcium balance in women. J. Lab. Clin. Med. **99,** 46–55.

[18] Lemann, J., Adams, N. D., Grow, R. W. (1979): Urinary calcium excretion in human beings. N. Eng. J. Med. **301,** 535.

[19] Daniell, H. W. (1976): Osteoporosis and the slender smoker. Arch. Int. Med. **136,** 298–304.

[20] Lindsay, R. (1981): The influence of cigarette smoking on bone mass and bone loss. In Osteoporosis: Recent Advances in Pathogenesis and Treatment. Eds. DeLuca H. F. et al., University Park Press, Baltimore, p. 477.

[21] Schneider, U. S., McDonald, J. (1981): Prevention of disuse osteoporosis: clodronate therapy. In Osteoporosis: Recent Advances in Pathogenesis and Treatment. Eds. DeLuca H. F. et al., University Park Press, Baltimore, p. 491.

[22] Aloia, J. F., Cohen, F. H., Tabu, T., Abesamis, C., Kalici, N., Ellis, I. (1978): Skeletal mass and body composition in marathon runners. Metabolism **27,** 1793–1796.

[23] Huddleston, A. L., Rockwell, D., Kulund, D. M., Harrison, R. B. (1980): Bone mass in lifetime tennis athletes. JAMA **244,** 1107–1109.

[24] Drinkwater, B. L., Nilson, K., Chestnut, C. H., Brenner, W. T., Shamholtz, S., Southworth, M. B. (1984): Bone mineral content of amenorrheic and eumenorrheic athletes. NEJM **311,** 277–281.

[25] Kanders, B., Lindsay, R., Dempster, D., Markhard, L., Valiquette, G. (1984): Determinants of bone mass in young healthy women. In Osteoporosis. Eds. Christiansen, C., et al. Aalborg Stiftsbogtrykkeri, pp. 337–340.

[26] Heaney, R. P., Recker, R. R., Saville, P. D. (1977): Calcium balance and calcium requirements in middle-aged women, Amer. J. Clin. Nutrition **30,** 1603–1611.

[27] Stevenson, J. C., Abeyasekeva, G., Hillyard, C. J., Phang, K., MacIntyre, I., Campbell, S., Lane, G., Townsend, P. T., Young, O., Whitehead, M. I. (1983): Regulation of calcium regulating hormones by exogenous sex steroids in early postmenopause. European J. Clin. Invest. **13,** 481–487.

Lipids, hormonal status and the cardiovascular system in the postmenopause

M. J. Tikkanen, E. A. Nikkilä, T. Kuusi

Introduction

One of the most puzzling questions is why women are relatively more immune to coronary heart disease (CHD) than men. Among most populations CHD is much more prevalent in men than in women. Even in familial hypercholesterolemia, in which premature CHD is due to a single-gene defect, females affected develop coronary heart disease at a later age than their male relatives with the same genetic defect [1]. This demonstrates that factors other than genetics ones influence the rate of atherogenesis which can ultimately result in CHD.

In this paper, serum lipid and lipoprotein risk factors are discussed in relation to sex and hormonal status. It will be argued that at all ages the female serum lipid pattern is more advantageous than the male, and that this may be the major female protective factor. The sex difference in serum lipids seems to be maintained by endogenous sex hormones; estrogens may therefore have an important role in the protection of women against CHD. The argument implies that in estrogen-deficient conditions, administration of exogenous hormone could be beneficial in the restoration of the serum lipid pattern, which, in turn, might reduce the risk of CHD.

Serum lipids as risk factors for coronary heart disease

Lipids (including cholesterol and triglycerides) are transported in the circulation as combinations of protein and fat called lipoproteins. Three major classes of serum lipoproteins are related to coronary heart disease (CHD). Two of them transport lipids from the liver to the peripheral cells for utilization or storage: Very low density lipoproteins (VLDL) are the major carriers of triglycerides, and low density lipoproteins (LDL) are carriers for cholesterol. High density lipoproteins (HDL) also transport cholesterol, but it is likely that they carry it in the opposite direction, from the peripheral tissues to the liver.

There is convincing evidence that elevated LDL cholesterol levels (also reflected as high total cholesterol) cause an increased risk of coronary heart disease [2]. There are studies suggesting that elevated VLDL levels have a similar, but probably weaker, effect on the risk. In contrast, the CHD risk is inversely related to HDL cholesterol level [3]. Thus, low HDL cholesterol increases risk but a high HDL cholesterol level provides protection against CHD. The HDL/LDL cholesterol ratio combines the two major lipid risk factors and is therefore a particularly powerful predictor of coronary risk.

Serum lipid risk factors: comparisons by hormonal status

Low density lipoprotein cholesterol. Until the age of fifty, the serum levels of LDL cholesterol (and therefore serum total cholesterol) are lower in women than in men [4]. This is illustrated in Fig. 1 which also shows that at the time of menopause this pattern is reversed. A progressive rise in the average LDL cholesterol level in women after the age of fifty results in higher LDL cholesterol than is present in men of similar age. The fact that the cessation of ovarian hormone production occurs at the same time as the surge in LDL cholesterol has led to the assumption that endogenous estrogen somehow reduces LDL cholesterol levels during the fertile years, whereas estrogen deficiency results in postmenopausal elevation of LDL cholesterol. This view is supported by evidence derived from studies using exogenous estrogens. During replacement therapy with estradiol valerate, which is metabolized to the natural human estrogen, estradiol, we originally observed a marked reduction in serum LDL cholesterol levels of hypercholesterolemic postmenopausal women [5]. The magnitude of the reduction in LDL cholesterol was directly proportional to the

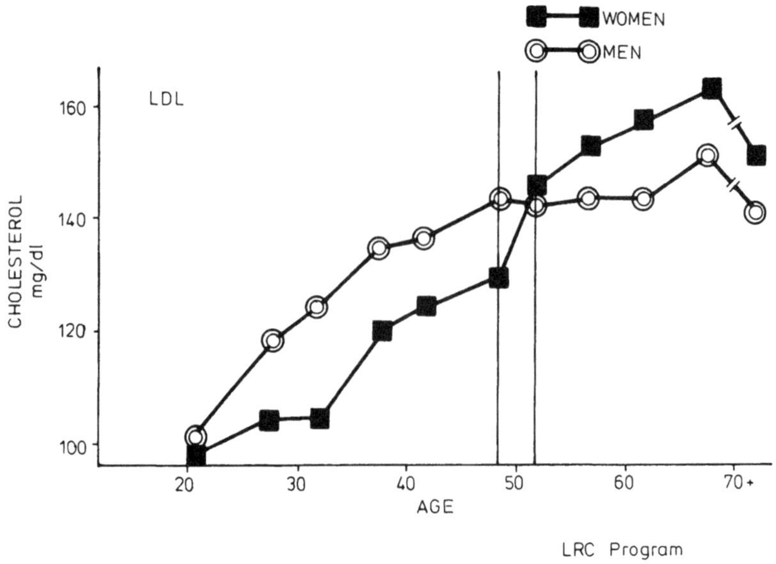

Fig. 1 Average LDL cholesterol levels at various ages [4]

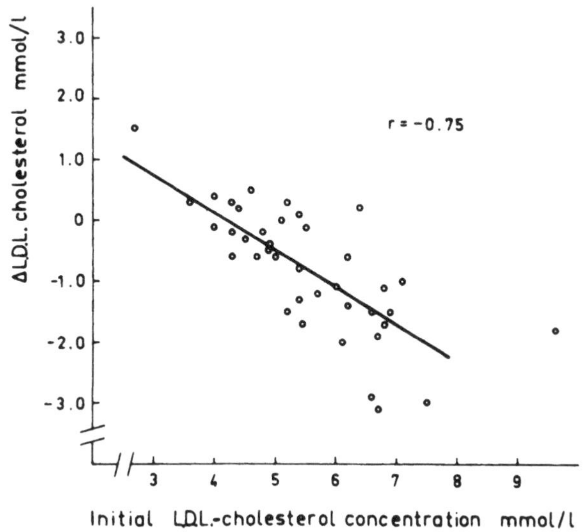

Fig. 2 Reduction of LDL cholesterol (LDL) during therapy with estradiol valerate 2 mg/day [5]

initial LDL cholesterol level (Fig. 2). Accordingly, women with initially high LDL cholesterol levels responded best to estrogen therapy but little change was observed in women with normal or low pretreatment levels. Cross-sectional studies at population level confirmed that postmenopausal women on estrogen have lower LDL cholesterol levels than women not taking any hormones (Fig. 3) [6]. Thus epidemiological and clinical observations suggest that endogenous estrogens participate, at least to some extent, in the regulation of serum and LDL cholesterol levels and hence contribute to the sex differences in the serum lipid pattern.

High density lipoprotein cholesterol. In all age groups the HDL cholesterol concentrations in women exceed those of men (Fig. 4) [4]. It is possible that ovarian estrogens contribute to this difference during the fertile years of the female. Synthetic alkylated estrogens and estradiol (Fig. 5) [5] probably increase HDL cholesterol levels by a dual mechanism involving both enhanced synthesis [7] and decreased catabolism [8] of the lipoprotein. Population studies have also demonstrated that estrogen-treated postmenopausal women have uniformly higher HDL cholesterol levels than women not on estrogen (Fig. 6). However, estrogens are not the only hormonal factors influencing the lipoprotein pattern. The male sex hormones have effects opposite to those of estrogens [9]. Thus the sex difference in HDL cholesterol persists when women become estrogen deficient after the menopause, possibly because of the HDL-lowering effects of male sex hormones. The metabolic basis of the sex hormone mediated regulation of high density lipoprotein concentrations is now slowly being clarified. At least partly, the hormonal up- and down-regulation of the HDL cholesterol level is determined by stimulation and

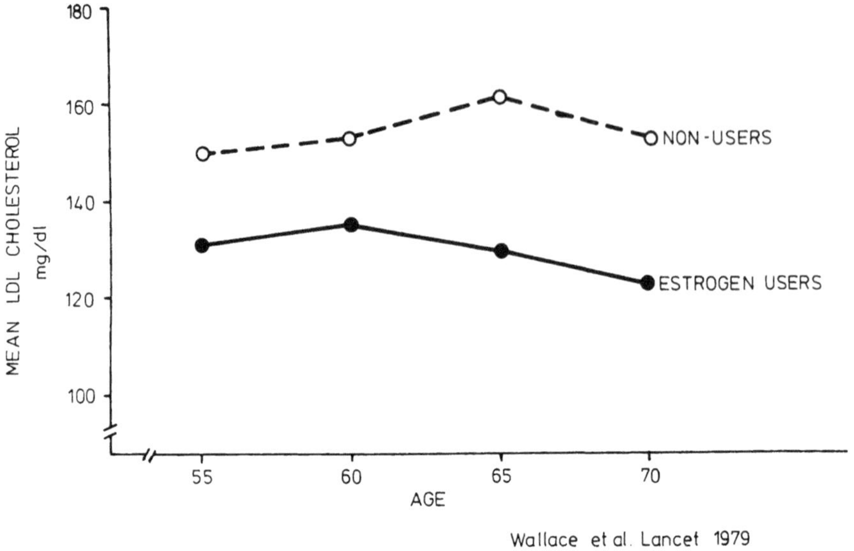

Fig. 3 Average LDL cholesterol levels in users and non-users of postmenopausal estrogen replacement therapy [6]

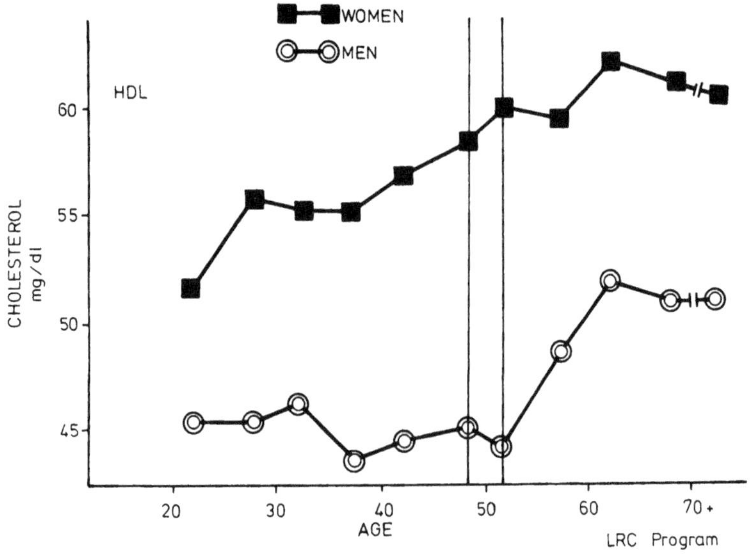

Fig. 4 Average HDL cholesterol levels at various ages [4]

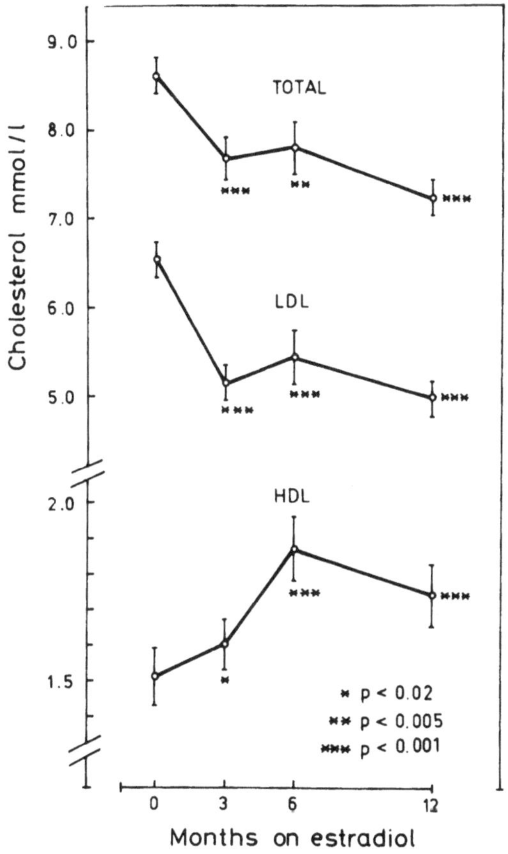

Fig. 5 Effect of estradiol valerate 2 mg/day on serum lipoprotein lipids in postmenopausal women (Mean ± SD, n = 30).

inhibition of hepatic lipase [8]. Androgens enhance, and estrogens suppress, the activity of this lipolytic enzyme which degrades HDL [8, 10–14]. Changes in the synthesis rate of HDL proteins which are presumably due to sex hormone effects, may also contribute to this regulation [7, 15].

The LDL/HDL cholesterol ratio. As shown in Fig. 7, which depicts data from the Lipid Research Clinics Prevalence Survey [4], the LDL/HDL cholesterol ratio remains favorable in women at all ages.

VLDL triglycerides. With regard to triglyceride metabolism an important distinction must be made between natural human estrogens (e.g. estradiol) and all other estrogens, including alkylated synthetic and conjugated equine estrogens. Alkylated steroids like ethinyl estradiol and mestranol [16, 17] but also equine estrogens [18] may elevate serum and VLDL triglyceride levels. In contrast, estradiol valerate does not influence serum or VLDL triglyceride concentrations in postmenopausal women

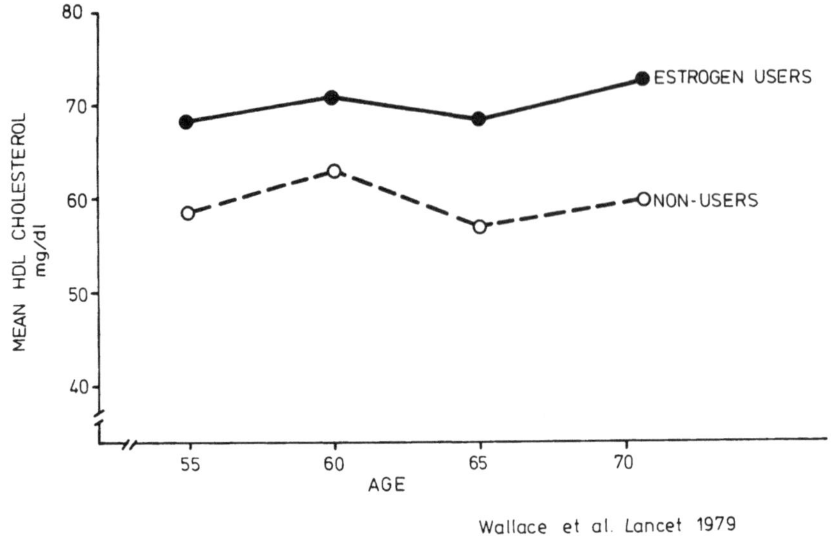

Fig. 6 Average HDL cholesterol levels in users and non-users of postmenopausal estrogen replacement therapy [6]

[17, 19, 20]. Kinetic studies have confirmed this by showing that slight increments occurring in VLDL triglyceride production rates are compensated for by accelerations in fractional catabolic rates [21] and thus result in only insignificant changes in serum VLDL triglyceride levels.

Estrogen replacement therapy and prevention of coronary heart disease

There are many indications that hormonal factors play an important role in the modification of the serum lipid pattern. In the female, ovarian estrogens probably have a beneficial effect on both LDL and HDL cholesterol levels, and even more so on the HDL/LDL cholesterol ratio. Postmenopausal estrogen deficiency results in the loss of this benefit when LDL cholesterol levels increase and surpass those of men, but the advantage in HDL cholesterol persists. Studies carried out in Goteborg [22] and Framingham [23] have reported that postmenopausal women have an increased risk of CHD in comparison to premenopausal women of the same age.

Replacement therapy with natural estrogen can be used to normalize elevated postmenopausal LDL cholesterol levels [5]. Although there is no unequivocal proof that estrogen substitution in the postmenopause lessens or delays the development of CHD, the balance of evidence favors this possibility. Population studies have demonstrated either a significant protective effect [24, 25] or no effect at all [26, 27]

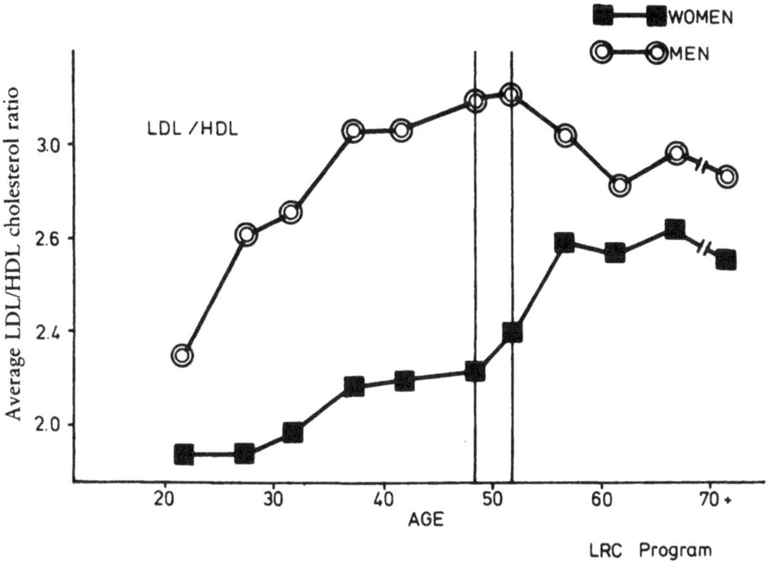

Fig. 7 Average LDL/HDL cholesterol ratios at various ages [4]

of estrogen replacement. The Lipid Research Clinic's Primary Prevention Trial established that the lowering of LDL cholesterol in middle-aged men by cholestyramine therapy was associated with a significant reduction in coronary risk [28]. Accordingly, a reduction in LDL cholesterol due to estrogen treatment with an accompanying increase in HDL cholesterol could probably have a similar risk lowering effect. However, many other factors, which are beyond the scope of the present paper, contribute to the sex differential in susceptibility to disease and longevity (for extensive review, see ref. [29]).

It has been suggested that postmenopausal estrogen substitution therapy increases the risk of various thromboembolic complications. This suspicion is based on the increase of thromboembolic phenomena observed in males with coronary heart disease who were treated with large doses of conjugated equine estrogens [30], and in women taking oral contraceptives [31]. No such association between postmenopausal estrogen replacement and thromboembolic or other cardiovascular complications has been observed [32–36]. It is not known whether addition of sequential progestin to cyclic estrogen regimens will cause any problems with regard to thromboembolic phenomena, but this addition should not have any major effect on HDL cholesterol levels, especially if non-androgenic progestins are used [37].

It is unlikely that large-scale prospective studies comparable to the Lipid Research Clinic's Primary Prevention Trial [28] will soon be carried out in postmenopausal women receiving estrogen replacement therapy. Because of the overwhelming importance of CHD in the postmenopausal age group, primary prevention by means of estrogen substitution should be considered. Based on indirect evidence from studies using exogenous estrogen administration, and on results from epidemiological surveys, one can conclude that the probable beneficial effects of estrogen replacement therapy on the cardiovascular system outweigh its possible adverse effects.

Acknowledgements: The authors have received support from the Sigrid Juselius Foundation, Paavo Nurmi Foundation, Nordisk Insulin Fond and the Academy of Finland.

References

[1] Goldstein, J. L., Fredrickson, D. S., Brown, J. S.: Familial hyperlipoproteinemia. In: The metabolic basis if inherited disease (Eds. Stanbury, J. B., Wyngaarden, J. B., Fredrickson, D. S.) McGraw-Hill Book Co., New York, 1977.

[2] Castelli, W. B., Doyle, J. T., Gordon, T., Humes, C. G., Hjortland, M. C., Halley, S. B., Kagan, A., Zukel, W. J.: HDL cholesterol and other lipids in coronary heart disease: The cooperative lipoprotein phenotyping study. Circulation 1977; 55:767–772.

[3] Gordon, T., Castelli, W. P., Hjortland, M. C., Kannel, W. B., Dawber, T. R.: High density lipoprotein as a protective factor against coronary heart disease: The Framingham study. Am. J. Med. 1977; 62:707–714.

[4] Heiss, G., Tamir, I., Davis, C. E., Tyroler, H. A., Rifkind, B. M., Schonfeld, G., Jacobs, D., Frantz, I. D.: Lipoprotein-cholesterol distributions in selected North American populations: The Lipid Research Clinics Program prevalence study. Circulation 61:302–315, 1980.

[5] Tikkanen, M. J., Nikkilä, E. A., Vartiainen, E.: Natural oestrogen as an effective treatment for type-II hyperlipoproteinaemia in postmenopausal women. Lancet 1978; 2:490–492.

[6] Wallace, R. B., Hoover, J., Barrett-Connor, E., Rifkind, B. M., Hunninghake, D. B., Mackenthun, A., Heiss, G.: Altered plasma lipid and lipoprotein levels associated with oral contraceptive and oestrogen use. Lancet 2:111–115, 1979.

[7] Schaefer, E. J., Foster, D. M., Zech, L. A., Lindgren, F. T., Brewer, H. B. Jr., Levy, R. I.: The effects of estrogen administration on plasma lipoprotein metabolism in premenopausal females. J. Clin. Endocrinol. Metab. 1983; 57:262–267.

[8] Tikkanen, M. J., Nikkilä, E. A., Kuusi, T., Sipinen, S.: High density lipoprotein-2 and hepatic lipase: reciprocal changes produced by estrogen and norgestrel. J. Clin. Endocr. Metab. 1982; 54:1113–1117.

[9] Furman, R. H., Alaupovic, P., Howard, R. P.: Effects of androgens and estrogens on serum lipids and the composition and concentration of serum lipoproteins in normolipemic and hyperlipidemic states. Progr. Biochem. Pharmacol. 1967; 2:215–249.

[10] Ehnholm, C., Huttunen, J. K., Kinnunen, P. J., Miettinen, T. A., Nikkilä, E. A.: Effect of oxandrolone treatment on the activity of lipoprotein lipase, hepatic lipase and phospholipase A1 of human postheparin plasma. N. Engl. J. Med. 1975; 292:1314–1317.

[11] Taggart, H. M., Applebaum-Bowden, D., Haffner, S., Warnick, G. R., Cheung, M. C., Albers, J. J., Chestnut, III, C. H., Hazzard, W. R.: Reduction in high density lipoproteins by anabolic steroid (stanozolol) therapy for postmenopausal osteoporosis. Metabolism 1982; 31:1147–1152.

[12] Tikkanen, M. J., Nikkilä, E. A., Kuusi, T., Sipinen, S.: Different effects of two progestins on plasma high density lipoprotein (HDL2) and postheparin plasma hepatic lipase activity. Atherosclerosis 1981; 40:365–369.

[13] Applebaum, D. M., Goldberg, A. P., Py-

kälistö, O. J., Brunzell, J. D., Hazzard, W. R.: Effect of estrogen on post-heparin lipolytic activity. Selective decline in hepatic triglyceride lipase. J. Clin. Invest. 1977; 59:601–608.
[14] Tikkanen, M. J., Kuusi, T., Vartiainen, E., Nikkilä, E. A.: Treatment of post-menopausal hypercholesterolaemia with estradiol. Acta Obstet, Gynecol. Scand. 1979; Suppl. 88:83–88.
[15] Solyom, A.: Effect of androgens on serum lipids and lipoproteins. Lipids 1972; 7:100–105.
[16] Aitken, J. M., Lorimer, A. R., McKay, Hart, D., Lawrie, T. D., Smith, D. A.: The effects of oophorectomy and long term mestranol therapy on the serum lipids of middle-aged women. Clin. Sci. 1971; 41:597–603.
[17] Wallentin, L., Larsson-Cohn, U.: Metabolic and hormonal effects of post-menopausal oestrogen replacement treatment. II Plasma lipids. Acta Endocrinol. 1977; 86:597–607.
[18] Robinson, R. W., Lebeau, R. J.: Effect of conjugated equine estrogens on serum lipids and the clotting mechanism. J. Atheroscler. Res. 1965; 5:120–124.
[19] Tikkanen, M. J., Nikkilä, E. A., Kuusi, T., Sipinen, S.: Effects of oestradiol and levonorgestrel on lipoprotein lipids and postheparin plasma lipase activities in normolipoproteinaemic women. Acta Endocrinol. 1982; 99:630–635.
[20] Pyörälä, T.: The effect of synthetic and natural estrogens on glucose tolerance, plasma insulin and lipid metabolism in postmenopausal women. In: The management of the menopause and postmenopausal years (ed. Campbell, S.). Lancaster: MTP Press Limited 1976; 195–210.
[21] Tikkanen, M. J., Kuusi, T., Nikkilä, E. A., Sane, T.: Very low density lipoprotein triglyceride kinetics during hepatic lipase suppression by estrogen. FEBS Lett. 181:160–164, 1985.
[22] Bengtsson, C.: Ischemic heart disease in women. Acta Med. Scand. 1973; 549:75–81.
[23] Kannel, W. B., Hjortland, M. C., McNamara, P. M., Gordon, T.: Menopause and risk of cardiovascular disease. The Framingham study. Ann. Int. Med. 1976; 85:447–452.
[24] Ross, R. K., Paganini-Hill, A., Mack, T. M., Arthur, M., Henderson, B. E.: Menopausal oestrogen therapy and protection from death from ischaemic heart disease. Lancet 1981; 1:858–860.
[25] Bain, C., Willett, W., Hennekens, C. H., Rosner, B., Belanger, C., Speizer, F. E.: Use of postmenopausal hormones and risk of myocardial infarction. Circulation 1981; 64:42–46.
[26] Rosenberg, L., Armstrong, B., Hershel, J.: Myocardial infarction and estrogen therapy in post-menopausal women. N. Engl. J. Med. 1976; 294:1256–1259.
[27] Pfeffer, R. I., Whipple, G. A., Kurosak, T. T., Chapman, J. M.; Coronary risk and estrogen use in postmenopausal women. Am. J. Epidemiol. 1978; 107:479–487.
[28] Lipid Research Clinics program. The lipid research clinics coronary primary prevention trial results II. The relationship of reduction in incidence of coronary heart disease to cholesterol lowering. J. Amer. Med. Ass. 1984; 251:365–374.
[29] Hazzard, W. R.: The sex differential in longevity (Chap. 7). In: Principles of geriatric medicine (eds. Andres, R. A., Bierman, E. L., Hazzard, W. R.) McGraw-Hill Book Co. New York, 1984.
[30] Coronary Drug Project. Findings leading to discontinuation of the 2.5 mg/day estrogen group. J. Amer. Med. Ass. 1973; 226:652.
[31] Vessey, M. P.: Female hormones and vascular disease: epidemiologic overview. Br. J. Fam. Plann. 1980; 6:1–12.
[32] Burch, J. C., Byrd, B. V., Vaughn, W. K.: Results of estrogen treatment in one thousand hysterectomized women for 14,318 years. In: Consensus on menopause research (Eds. van Keep, P. A., Greenblatt, R. B., Albeaus-Fernet, M.) MTP Press, Lancaster, England, 1976.
[33] Hammond, C. B., Jelovsek, F. R., Lee, K. L., Creasman, W. T., Parker, R. T.: Effects of long-term estrogen replacement therapy I. Metabolic. Am. J. Obstet. Gynecol. 1979; 133:525.
[34] Nachtigall, L. E., Nachtigall, R. H., Nachtigall, R. B., Beckmann, E. M.: Estrogen replacement II. A prospective study in the relationship to carcinoma and cardiovascular and metabolic problems. Obstet. Gynecol. 1979; 54:74.
[35] Boston Collaborative Drug Surveillance Program. Surgically confirmed gallblad-

der disease, venous thromboembolism, and breast tumors in relation to postmenopausal estrogen therapy. N. Engl. J. Med. 1974; 290:15–19.

[36] Gambrell, R. D., Jr.: The menopause: benefits and risks of estrogen-progestogen replacement therapy. Fertil Steril. 1982; 37:457–474.

[37] Tikkanen, M. J., Kuusi, T., Nikkilä, E. A., Sipinen, S.: Postmenopausal hormone replacement therapy: effects of progestins on serum lipids and lipoproteins. Maturitas 8:7–17, 1986.

Psychosocial aspects in the perimenopause

J. M. Wenderlein

Gerontological research warns us against making generalised statements about people in any one age group. That growing old is a highly individual process is particularly apparent in perimenopausal women. Despite similar physiological changes secondary to the cessation of ovarian function, effects at the experience and behavioural levels are highly diverse.

Associating psychosocial changes in the perimenopausal years with the loss of a role is of little use in counselling. For women, there are no distinct age limits for the role of mother, housewife or job holder. It is just as difficult to make generalised statements about these roles as about how the loss of fertility occurring with the perimenopause is experienced by the individual.

The perimenopause is often still associated with a reduced feeling of selfe-steem and completeness as a woman, particularly in those of low social status and low educational level. Quite often, these women also have a negative picture of ageing. If this is based on a one-sided traditional understanding of the role, then general satisfaction with life can rarely be achieved by a change of attitude since negative cliché attitudes or stereotypes are usually acquired in early childhood.

This is not to suggest that doctors should take a negative attitude towards counselling. However, counselling success resulting in a greater ability to make social contacts and to create a wider scope of interests is not the rule in psychosocially dissatisfied women. The same applies to perimenopausal women with long-standing partner conflicts.

If partner conflicts, stress problems in occupation and household and reactive dissatisfaction with the role first occur with the onset of climacteric complaints, then prompt gynaecological assistance is possible. The following descriptions of climacteric symptoms with some psychosocial sequelae have been deliberately greatly simplified. There are still too few women who know about these interactions, and it should be realised that such knowledge is of greater assistance in coming to terms with reality than psychiatric treatment, which is only of use in neurotic conflicts. It has not been demonstrated, nor is it likely, that neuroses have a higher incidence in the perimenopause than in other phases of life.

It is also known that mental diseases which became manifest for the first time with the cessation of ovarian function are rare in perimenopausal women requiring assistance.

This, among other things, suggests that psychotherapeutic or psychiatric help is only indicated in exceptional cases.

It is hoped that the following will illustrate just how the gynaecologist can provide psychosocial assistance.

Estrogens and the psyche

Research into the effects of natural and synthetic estrogens on the brain is far from complete. How do the central nervous effects of estrogens affect psychic functions and, in particular, behavior? It will be a long time before this question is answered since too many social and psychic factors are involved.

The menstrual cycle can be mentioned as an example. Positive effects such as well-being, assurance and self-confidence are said to be promoted in the first half of the cycle under the influence of estrogens. In the final analysis, however, mood is decided by situational factors and individual experience.

In the premenstrual syndrome, too, the hormonal imbalance is nothing more than one explanatory influence in a multifactorial etiology.

The attempts to explain psychosocial changes in the perimenopause with the falling production of endogenous estrogens are just as unsatisfactory. Whether, and to what extent, vegetative disorders are involved is determined essentially by the individual biographical factors of the woman, e.g., her experience of the menarche, menstruation and other gynaecological events.

In comparison to this, the influences of verifiable changes in gonadotropin secretion, hypothalamic hormones and the limbic system are still too uncertain to permit a prediction or quantification of perimenopausal symptoms.

Although, at present, it is very difficult to place the relatively nonspecific disorders of experience and behaviour during the perimenopause into the framework of our endocrinological knowledge, the positive psychotropic effects of estrogen replacement can be exploited therapeutically with great success.

Antidepressant and anxiolytic effects of estrogens

How estradiol exerts central nervous effects through biotransformation into, for example, 2-hydroxyestrone is of interest.

It is an established fact that estrogen replacement in the perimenopause results in excellent antidepressant and anxiolytic effects.

My own psychometric studies support this. Before the start of therapy, pronounced anxiety was demonstrated by means of test procedures in 20% of cases. This number fell to 7% after 3 months of estrogen therapy and to 1% after 6 months.

122 post-menopausal women received 2 × 2 mg estriol succinate and 1.25 mg conjugated estrogens for half a year alternately by year of birth (even – odd).

Using an anxiety scale, it was shown over the same period that the number of women without any anxiety at all increased from 15% before the estrogen treatment to 50% after 3 months of estrogen therapy. This percentage did not change any further in the following 3 months of estrogen therapy.

Antidepressive effects were also reliably verified by psychometric methods in the same study. Before the start of therapy, 3 of the 10 women in the group who were a few years after the menopause were suffering from depressive moods. After 6 months of estrogen therapy, this applied to only 1 of the 10 women. The antidepressive effects of the estrogens were therefore sufficient in two thirds of the women. Psychotropic drugs or specific antidepressants and counselling were helpful in the other third.

Critics might justifiably argue that psychosocially orientated exploration and counselling were primarily called for here.

Depression and anxiety which occur for the first time in the perimenopause are usually the result of an estrogen deficit. It ist very difficult to say whether the depression is of central-nervous origin or whether it occurs as a reaction to climacteric deficiency symptoms. Whatever the answer is, it would make little difference in practice. The object is, after all, to provide practical help to a relatively large group of perimenopausal women, estimated to number several million. The reduction of depression and anxiety by counselling aimed at modifying behavior is often not only an unrealistic target, but also a stressful process with uncertain success at the end.

For a woman who suffers from depression and anxiety for the first time with the perimenopause, it can be distressing when the doctor looks for psychosocial conflicts as the cause.

The object of what I have just said is to warn against applying too much psychology in the climacteric. What most perimenopausal women expect from the gynaecologist ist prompt help against estrogen deficiency symptoms, almost all of which lead to psychosocial impairment, as the following example shows.

Disorders of bladder function and some psychosocial consequences

How often do atrophic changes in the urethra and bladder lead via frequent inflammation to pollakiuria and dysuria? According to my own statistics, every 4th climacteric woman complains about this. Depressive women were affected three times more frequently by these problems than non-depressives. After urinary tract infections had been ruled out, estrogen therapy proviced the anticipated help for both problems. I shall mention just one aspect of the well-known interactions between disturbed micturition and depressive tendencies. If antidepressants are prescribed instead of estrogens, the disorder of micturition can be exacerbated as a result of the concomitant anticholinergic effects.

In women with a feeling of prolapse and "downward pressure" in the genital region without an anatomical substrate, depressive moods were three times more frequent than in non-depressive climacteric women. Here again, much thought was given to the interactions. In our own survey of a total of 122 women, this ratio could no longer be found after 3 months of estrogen therapy. The complaints were reported less frequently, which meant an improved quality of life for most of the women.

It is impossible to say how often surgery has been attempted as the first measure instead of several months of estrogen therapy in urinary incontinence or prolapse complaints occurring for the first time in the perimenopause and without a convincing anatomical substrate.

Sexual-medical aspects

Women expect changes in the sexual sphere during the perimenopause just about as often as they experience them. Almost half of the women expect a reduced desire for sex, and just as many expect reduced sexual enjoyment.

These perimenopausal problems correlate hightly significantly with a negative experience of gynaecological events in the fertile phase of life, such as menstruation and giving birth.

As was expected, negative expectations and experience of sexuality were less frequent among women with a high level of education and of at least average intelligence.

Lively and sociable, that is, more extroverted women suffer less frequently from perimenopausal impairment of sexuality than introverted women of the same age. The latter group is not only almost inaccessible to counselling, but also rejects estrogen therapy more often, for example even for atropic changes in the vulvovaginal region.

Relatively few women complain to the gynaecologist about sexual disorders occurring for the first time after the menopause and resulting from vaginal involution and dryness. On the other hand, quite a few complain about a greater tendency towards inflammation in the years after the menopause. This should prompt the doctor to inquire about the sexual-medical history.

In our own survey, every fifth post-menopausal woman complained about unpleasant discharge before therapy, but only every tenth after 3 months of estrogen therapy.

The number of women with pain during sexual intercourse decreases analogously. No direct influence on sexual interest can, of course, be expected from the administration of estrogens in the perimenopause.

The ways in which sexual interest can be influenced indirectly by estrogen therapy are, unfortunately, still experienced by too few perimenopausal women. In our survey, every second woman in the non-depressive group complained of rapid fatigability. After 6 months of estrogen therapy, this symptom was reported by only 1 in 6 of the women. The effects on their sex life require no discussion.

Not infrequently, women who had experienced therapy with psychotropic drugs for subjective perimenopausal complaints, including depression, complained about sedative side effects. In cases in which this increased previously existing rapid fatigability, complaints were also made about tension in the partner relationship including the sexual sphere. Here again, there is no point discussing the question of what is cause and what is effect.

Estrogen therapy instead of counselling?

The appropriate use of estrogens – that is, the lowest possible but still effective dosage administered cyclically with the addition of a progestogen – could provide a better quality of life for even more perimenopausal women.

Reducing psychometrically verified incidence of reduced well-being in climacteric women from 25% to 6% after 3 months of oral treatment with estrogens then allows a highly specific search for psychosocial conflicts and their usually difficult counselling.

The same procedure should be used in climacteric psychovegetative disorders. As documented by a list of complaints, these occurred in 32% of women before the start of therapy and in only 8% after a few months of estrogen therapy. It is not known how often psychosocially oriented counselling results in a better quality of life in these remaining women who require assistance and who usually suffer from a feeling of reduced self-esteem and self-assurance secondary to vegetative disorders.

Will more women suffering from agitation brought on by the climacteric, which makes a normal life in marriage, family and occupation difficult, ask for the help of estrogen therapy in the future? This is to be expected if women are informed about the climacteric more objectively and at an earlier stage, preferably while they are still at school as part of health and sex education. Very few women know about the positive psychotropic effects of estrogen therapy in the perimenopause. Such information is more likely to be accepted by women who have had many years' positive experience with the use of hormones in the form of hormonal contraceptives.

But it will also very much depend on the gynaecologist whether more climacteric women will have the courage to improve their quality of life through estrogen-progestogen therapy. My own experience at post-graduate training events suggests that there are still quite a few doctors who are biased by their own negative attitudes towards sex hormones. One need only mention the now pointless discussion about the risk of carcinoma, which can be regarded as long-concluded in regard to combined estrogen-progestogen therapy. The physician's slightest doubt about this question is sensed by most women, not only the anxious ones, even when it is not verbalized.

A colleague cited the following example at a medical post-graduate training event. A perimenopausal patient with depressive moods presented at the practice with simultaneous unpleasant tachycardia and palpitations. In response to the antidepressant prescribed, the functional heart complaints worsened and became even more unpleasant. These well-known concomitant cardiovascular effects of antidepressants led to termination of the therapy and to a dissatisfied, dissapointed patient. The doctor in question sumarily rejected the suggestion that he should try therapy with estrogens, which not only reduce the depression, but also eliminate the functional heart complaints in more than half of the cases. In support of his attitude, he listed a number of contraindications which apply to synthetic steroids for hormonal contraception, but not to optimal hormone therapy in the perimenopause.

It was impossible to clarify the interactions here – whether more rational information would mean less emotional defence against such treatment, or whether rational reasons were being sought for the emotional rejection of estrogen therapy.

The following solution to this dilemma is suggested: in all cases of subjectively functional and objectively organic consequences of a protracted estrogen deficit in the perimenopause, all psychosocial consequences should be considered including, for example, osteoporosis.

Doctors who take the trouble to think deeply about this subject will be able to provide convincing help to any climacteric woman seeking assistance.

The bladder in the menopausal woman

E. Versi

Introduction

In developed countries with increased life expectancy, the geriatric population will continue to grow. In this population one of the most distressing and debilitating problems is urinary incontinence. Since these lower urinary tract symptoms are generally considered to be a part of the menopause syndrome, it has been assumed that the problem is sex hormone dependent.

Both the urethra and the vagina develop from the urogenital sinus and their anatomical proximity results in a frequent association between gynaecological and urological pathology. Both the vaginal epithelium and the urethral epithelium are subject to estrogenic action (Everett, 1941). The submucosal vascular plexuses of the urethra contribute to sphincteric function and these too are estrogen dependent (Versi & Cardozo, 1985) as may be the collagenous matrix of the urethral submucosal connective tissue (Versi et al., 1986). Estrogen receptors have been detected in the human female urethra (Iosif et al., 1981) suggesting a direct action of the hormone. It would therefore appear that both the genital and lower urinary tract are influenced by estrogens.

Symptomatology

The common urological complaints that confront the practising gynaecologist are:

1. Incontinence
2. Frequency, urgency and dysuria
3. Voiding difficulties

The presentation of these complaints are by no means exclusive in that any given patient will usually have more than one urinary complaint and often a gynaecological one as well. Therefore it is appropriate for the gynaecologist to investigate and treat both urological and gynaecological symptoms.

1. Incontinence

Iosif and Bekassy (1984) reported a survey on 902 Swedish women aged 61 and found that 29.2% complained of urinary incontinence. The majority of these women related the onset of their symptoms to the menopause. However Osborne (1976) in an earlier survey of 600 women aged beeween 35 and 60 was unable to show an increased prevalence at the time of the menopause. Similarly, the data from Thomas et al. (1980) of a postal survey of incontinence in nearly 10,000 women could not specifically incriminate the menopause.

2. Urgency, frequency and dysuria

These are symptoms of urinary tract infection, but when present in the absence of an infective pathogen, they are collectively known as the urethral syndrome. The incidence of urinary tract infections does not increase at the menopause, remaining about 3% from the age of 20 to 65 (Sussman, 1969; Brocklehurst, 1972), but is markedly increased in the aged population (Brocklehurst, 1968). Smith (1976) studied women with the urethral syndrome and correlated symptoms with changes in urethral cytology. However, the prevalence of the urethral syndrome does not increase after the menopause. It may be that symptoms due to atrophic urethritis and those encountered in sexually active women have a different aetiology. The prevalence of 'frequency and urgency' in 1120 women aged between 30 to 64 was not found to be raised following the menopause (Bungay et al., 1980).

3. Voiding diffuculties

These symptoms are less common in women but the usual complaint is that of poor stream, straining to void, incomplete emptying and postmicturition dribbling. Patients often have a concomitant cystocele. Voiding difficulties can be caused by either outflow obstruction or inadequate detrusor activity during voiding. Roberts and Smith (1968) suggested that estrogen deficiency results in distal urethral stenosis and therefore advocated estrogen replacement therapy for this condition. However, in the majority of cases of voiding difficulty in women, the problem is due to an inefficient detrusor muscle (Blaivas and de la Rocha, 1985). Nonetheless, Hilton and Stanton (1983b) reported an improvement in these symptoms following hormone replacement therapy.

Investigations

The bladder is, unfortunately, an unreliable witness: solely from an analysis of the symptoms, it is not possible to accurately predict the diagnosis (Cardozo & Stanton,

1980; Jarvis et al., 1980; Shepherd et al., 1982). Urodynamic investigation is therefore an essential part of the management of lower urinary tract dysfunction. Prior to embarking on any such investigation, it is important to ensure that no infection is present as this will be exacerbated and will lead to unreliable results (Bergman & Bhatia, 1985).

The function of the urinary system is to collect and store urine and then to expel it efficiently when it is appropriate to do so. Urodynamic investigations are designed to test various functional aspects of this system. Tests concerned with upper urinary tract function are probably not relevant to the menopause and so shall not be considered here. Numerous tests exist for the evaluation of lower urinary tract activity, but some are clinically more useful than others. In this article only pad tests, uroflowmetry, videocystourethrography and urethral presure profilometry will be discussed. Given the spectrum of urinary symptoms encountered during the climacteric, these are the tests that are likely to yield a definitive diagnosis.

Pad testing (Versi & Cardozo, 1986) is a very simple method for the quantification of urine loss. The patient is asked to wear a pre-weighed perineal pad and is given a fluid load to drink. She then carries out a series of exercises including walking and coughing. At the end of the test the pad is reweighed to determine the weight gain which is interpreted as being the quantity of urine lost. This test can therefore be used to objectively detect incontinence even when it is quite subtle.

Uroflowmetry is the measurement of the flow rate of urine. When it is found to be normal, it implies that the bladder and the urethra are working efficiently as a functional unit (Arbuckle & Paquini, 1963). However, when the peak flow rate is reduced, it may be due either to outflow obstruction or to poor detrusor (bladder) contractibility. The underlying cause can be determined by making concomitant voiding intravesical pressure measurements (Backman et al., 1966). The most common cause of this complaint in women is inadequate detrusor activity. A poor flow rate combined with high residual urine is urodynamic proof of voiding difficulty.

Videocystourethrography (Bates et al., 1970) is the most comprehensive and useful technique and so could be called the "Rolls Royce" of urodynamic tests. It involves filling and voiding cystometry with simultaneous radiological screening of the bladder and urethra. Cystometry (Cardozo, 1981) is the assessment of detrusor activity. During the filling phase it will detect aberrant detrusor contractions (detrusor instability), and during the voiding phase it will help diagnose outflow obstruction (high voiding pressure). When a patient with a full bladder (containing radiological contrast medium) is asked to cough, the integrity of her urethral sphincter can be assessed. Continence is maintained by the internal (bladder neck) and external (urethral) sphincters. If there is "beaking" of the bladder neck but no passage of contrast medium past the mid-urethral point when the patient coughs, then continence is being maintained by the external sphincter even though the internal sphincter is incompetent. If the cough results in streaking of contrast medium down the urethra and past its midpoint, then the internal and external sphincters are both incompetent. This is known as genuine stress incontinence if it occurs in the absence of a detrusor contraction (simultaneous cystometry). It will be appreciated that this is an important condition when it is understood that just prior to, and during, a detrusor contraction, the urethra usually relaxes. So a sphincter cannot be said to be incompetent if it is relaxed or relaxing at the time of the cough. With videocystourethrography it is also possible to detect morphological abnormalities such as bladder and urethral divericula, trabeculation, vesico-uretric reflux and mobility of the bladder neck and urethra giving an indication of fibrosis that may be present consequent to previous surgery.

Urethral pressure profilometry has become more reliable and reproducible since the advent of solid state microtransducers mounted on flexible catheters (Asmussen & Ulmsten, 1975), which allow simultaneous pressure measurements of the urethra and bladder. The catheter is inserted into the bladder and is then withdrawn at a steady speed. This yields a pressure profile of the urethra at rest. If this is done while the patient is coughing, then a stress provile can be obtained. This latter profile is of course, the relevent one when stress incontinence is being investigated. Whereas videocystourethrography can determine the absolute competence of the urethral sphincter, urethral pressure profilometry enables more subtle changes to be documented and so can possibly detect weakness of the sphincter before it fails completely.

Climacteric survey

At the Dulwich Menopause Clinic, patients presenting with climacteric symptoms were assessed for urological symptoms and then subjected to urodynamic investigations. These consisted of a pad test, uroflowmetry, videocystourethrography and urethral pressure profilometry. If the menopause had an effect on lower urinary tract symptomatology and the incidence of pathology, then it might be supposed that postmenopausal women would present with greater morbidity then perimenopausal women. In the Dulwich study women were deemed to be postmenopausal only if they had experienced climacteric symptoms and had been amenorrhoeic for more than 6 months. Furthermore they had to have serum LH levels of greater than 25 ng/ml, FSH greater than 40 ng/ml and estradiol of less than 220 pmol/ml. If only some of these criteria were satisfied, the patients were classed as perimenopausal. In the postmenopausal group, the menopausal age, that is, the time from the last menstrual period or, in the case of those who had previously had a hysterectomy (30%), from the onset of typical climacteric symptoms, was 4.2 ± 0.5 years.

Symptoms

Table 1 shows that the prevalence of stress incontinence, frequency, nocturia and urgency is quite high. However, pain on micturition is a less common climacteric complaint than are the symptoms of voiding difficulties. The latter is in contrast to the findings of Stanton et al. (1983) who found a prevalence of 30%. There is no statistically significant difference between the peri- and postmenopausal women for the prevalence of any of the symptoms listed in Table 1. This suggests either that the menopause has no effect on lower urinary tract symptomatology or that whatever effect estrogen deficiency has, it has already been manifested by the time the women presented to the menopause clinic. This would suggest that the urological changes occur as an early event in the climacteric process. At present there is no comparable data for younger (pre-climacteric) and older (late postmenopausal) women. We hope to further address this issue by carrying out a more precise menopausal age related analysis of climacteric women. It is also possible that, as the menopause is a relatively gradual process and hormone profiles are only representative of the menopausal status at a specific point in time (estrogen levels fluctuate during the climacteric), analyses relying upon a sharp definition of the menopause may be confounded.

Table 1 A Comparison of Lower Urinary Symptomatology in Peri- and Postmenopausal Women

	Perimenopausal	Postmenopausal
N	54	89
Age	46.5 ± 0.6	52.2 ± 0.5
Stress Incontinence (Occasional)	33.3%	40.4%
Stress Incontinence (Frequent)	9.3%	10.1%
Frequency (> 8 per day)	31.5%	28.2%
Nocturia (> once per night)	29.6%	29.2%
Urgency (occasional)	16.7%	33.7%
Urgency (frequent)	31.5%	21.3%
Painful Micturition	13.0%	10.3%
Poor Stream	5.6%	10.1%
Incomplete bladder emptying	11.3%	13.0%

Urodynamic findings

Table 2 displays the results of urodynamic tests on these climacteric patients, again distinguishing between peri- and postmenopausal women. The first striking result is that only two thirds of climacteric women could be considered to be urodynamically normal. The most common pathology was genuine stress incontinence (15%), which is also the most common cause of incontinence seen in gynaecological practice. Detrusor instability was the next most common condition (10%); as the patients were neurologically normal, this was idiopathic detrusor instability. Only 5% of patients had voiding difficulties and only one had the urethral syndrome. This latter result is in sharp contrast to the report by Smith (1976) in which a much higher incidence was observed after the menopause. This discrepancy is explicable. Since Smith's results were retrospectively analysed from records of patients of a urological clinic, the sample cannot be said to be representative. Further it should be remembered that in the Dulwich study, stringent urodynamic criteria were used to diagnose the condition and that most of the patients were actually undergoing, or had only just undergone their menopause. It is possible that the urethral syndrome commonly occurs only after atrophic changes have been established for some time. There was no significant difference between peri- and postmenopausal patients in the prevalence of urodynamically diagnosed pathology. The same arguments apply to this data as to the symptomology data (see above). Work from other menopause clinics is expected to confirm these findings, and at present we are prospectively scrutinising the effect of HRT on these prevalence rates.

Urethral sphincter

In this series of climacteric women who were continent on pad testing (Versi and Cardozo, 1986) and videocystourethrography, 45 ± 9% of perimenopausal and 46 ± 6% of postmenopausal women had an incompetent bladder neck, thus demoting the role of this sphincter in the maintenance of continence. Because it is not known what the incidence of internal sphincter incompetence is in the normal population, it is not certain whether this is an age related phenomenon (Versi et al., 1986). The fact that there was no significant difference in the prevalence for peri- and postmenopausal women may suggest that the bladder neck is not estrogen dependent. The results of intervention studies (post HRT) are awaited.

Urethral pressure profilometry

The measurements taken from the urethral pressure profiles were carried out as described by Hilton and Stanton (1983a). The functional urethral length is the length of the urethra over which the intralumenal pressure exceeds bladder pressure at rest or under stress. The maximum closure pressure is the maximum pressure difference between the urethra and the bladder at rest or under stress. The transmission pressure ratio (TPR) of a cough is computed by dividing the magnitude of the cough pulse in the urethra by that in the bladder and multiplying by 100. The greater the TPR, the more competent the sphincter. Table 3 displays the results of these measurements; the data is again divided to distinguish between peri- and postmemopausal women. No difference was found between the groups, in the resting profile but under stress (during coughing), perimenopausal women were found to have a more efficient sphincter. Parametric tests were used for the statistical comparison except when the data was not normally distributed. The finding that postmenopausal women have a weaker urethral spincter suggests that estrogen withdrawal does have an effect on sphincteric action. This subtle change is demonstrable using urethral pressure profilometry, though it is not shown in the prevalence rates of genuine stress incontience based on videocystourethrography (Table 2). It has been shown that maximum urethral pressure and urethral length decrease with age (Rud 1980a) and so the results in Table 3 may merely reflect an

Table 2 The Prevalence of Urodynamically Diagnosed Pathology in Women undergoing the Climacteric

	Perimenopausal	Postmenopausal
Total	54	89
Normals	33 (61%)	62 (70%)
Genuine Stress Incontinence	10 (19%)	12 (13%)
Detrusor Instability	5 (10%)	10 (11%)
Voiding Difficulty	3 (6%)	4 (4%)
Urethral Syndrome	0 (0%)	1 (1%)

Table 3 Urethral Pressure Profile Measurements in Peri- and Postmenopausal Women

Parameter	Perimenopausal	Postmenopausal	Significance
Resting Profile			
Functional Length (mm)	28.5 ± 0	28.4 ± 0.6	NS
Maximum Closure Pressure (cm water)	49.6 ± 2.2	50.4 ± 3.7	NS
Stress Profile			
Functional Length (mm)	21.4 ± 1.5	17.1 ± 1.0	$p < 0.05$
Maximum Closure Pressure (cm water)	70.0 ± 18.7	46.2 ± 11.3	NS
Response to a Single Cough			
Instantaneous closure pressure (cm water)	35 ± 4	33 ± 3	NS
Substained closure pressure (cm water)	44 + 2	36 ± 3	$p < 0.05$
Recovery time (secs)	6.1 ± 0.8	9.5 ± 1.5	$p < 0.05$*
Transmission Pressure Ratios (TRP)			
First quartile	94.4 ± 3.9	83.8 ± 2.7	$p < 0.05$
Maximum TPR	118 ± 20	105 ± 2	$p < 0.05$*

* Nonparametric Test

age dependent difference. However it should be borne in mind that the mean age difference between peri- and postmenopausal women was only 5.7 years and Rud's work reports trends observed in women aged between 25 and 71+ years. This area requires further exploration and new data is needed to clarify this point. Although it has been reported that estrogen replacement therapy increases sphincteric function at rest (Faber & Heidenreich, 1977; Beisland, 1984) and under stress (Rud, 1980b; Hilton & Stanton, 1983 b), these studies were on relatively small series of patients and there is no universal agreement on the actual effects.

At the Dulwich Menopause Clinic it has been noted that urethral pressure profile parameters correlate with skin collagen content: the greater the collagen content, the better the sphincteric action (Versi et al., 1986). Hormone replacement therapy increases skin collagen content (Brincat et al., 1985) and those patients whose pretreatment levels were low, accrued greater benefit. This may explain why the effects of estrogens on the urethral sphincter are not uniform. Skin collagen could perhaps be used as a prognostic index for the selection of patients whose urethral sphincters are likely to improve with replacement therapy.

Conclusion

Since lower urinary tract symptomatology is a part of the menopause syndrome, it has been assumed that the bladder is estrogen dependent. Epidemiological surveys have revealed a high prevalence of symptoms but the data do not consistently support the thesis that the menopause, *per se*, is responsible for this morbidity. Even if a causal relationship exists, it would be difficult to demonstrate since the process of estrogen deprivation occurs over a number of years. Also, because urinary symptoms do not faithfully reflect the underlying urological pathologies that give rise to them, surveys of symptoms without urodynamic studies are difficult to interpret.

To elucidate this problem, women presenting to the Dulwich Menopause Clinic were investigated from a urological view point. Assessment consisted of history, examination, urine culture, pad testing, uroflowmetry, videocystourethrography and urethral pressure profilometry. Patients were regarded as postmenopausal if they had had symptoms and been amenorrhoeic for more than 6 months, had serum LH $>$ 25 ng/ml, FSH $>$ 40 ng/ml and estradiol $<$ 220 pmol/ml. If only some of these criteria were satisfied, they were regarded as perimenopausal.

There was a high prevalence of urinary symptoms (about 30%), but there was no significant difference between peri-and postmenopausal rates. Similarly the prevalence of urodynamically recognised pathology was high (30%), but here again there was no statistically significant difference between the peri- and postmenopausal groups. The most common pathology was genuine stress incontinence with detrusor instability, being the second most common. Surprisingly, the urethral syndrome was a rare diagnosis.

Urethral pressure profilometry revealed that postmenopausal women had weaker urethral sphincters under stress than the perimenopausal group. This technique allows a more sensitive measurement of urethral function so that degress of weakness can be monitored whereas videocystourethrography can only differentiate a competent from an incompetent sphincter.

It is therefore possible that estrogen withdrawal does have an effect on the urethral sphincter but more intervention studies are needed to confirm this. Lower urinary tract problems are very much a part of the menopause, but, as yet, it is not known whether they are just age-related or are specifically estrogen dependent.

References

[1] Arbuckle, L. D., Paquin, A. J. (1963): Urinary outflow resistance in normal human females. Invest. Urol. **1**, 216–228.

[2] Asmussen, M., Ulmsten, U. (1975): Simultaneous urethrocystometry and urethral pressure profiles measurement with a new technique. Acta Obstet. Gynecol. Scand. **54**, 385–386.

[3] Backman, K. A., Garrelts, B. von and Sundblad, R. (1966): Micturition in normal women. Studies of flow pressure Acta Chir. Scand. **132**, 403–413.

[4] Bates, C. P., Whiteside, C. G., Turner-Warwick, M. (1970): Synchronous cine/pressure/flow cystourethrography with special reference to stress and urge incontinence. Br. J. Urol. **42**, 714–723.

[5] Bent, A. E., Richardson, D. A.; Ostergard, D. R. (1983): Diagnosis of lower urinary tract disorders in postmenopausal patients. Am J. Obstet. Gynecol **145**, 218–222.

[6] Bergman, A. and Bhatia, N. N. (1985): Urodynamics: effect of urinary tract infection on urethral and bladder function. Obstet. Gynecol. **66**, 366–371.

[7] Blaivais, J. G., de la Rocha, R. E. (1985): Impaired urinary flow rate. The distinction between bladder and outlet obstruction and poor detrusor contractibility. Proc. Int. Cont. Soc., pp. 51–52 London.

[8] Brincat, M., Moniz, C. J., Studd, J. W. W., Darby, A., Magos, A., Embrey, G. and Versi, E. (1985): Long-term effects of the menopause and sex hormones on skin thickness. Br. J. Obstet. Gynaecol. **92**, 256–259.

[9] Brocklehurst, J. C., Fry, J., Griffiths, L. L. and Kalton, G. (1972): Urinary infection and symptoms of dysuria in women aged 45–64 years: their relevence to similar findings in the elderly. Age and Aging **1**, 41–47.

[10] Bungay, G. T., Vessey, M. P, and McPherson (1980): Study of symptoms in middle life with special reference to the menopause. Br. Med. J. **281**, 181–183.

[11] Cardozo, L. D. (1981): The use of cystometry in the understanding of urinary incontinence. In: Progress in Obstetrics and gynaecology, J. W. W. Studd (Ed.) pp. 151–166. Churchill Livingstone.

[12] Cardozo, L. D., Stanton, S. L. (1980): Genuine Stress Incontinence and detrusor instability, a review of 200 patients. Br. J. Obstet. Gynaecol. **87**, 184–190.

[13] Everett, H. S. (1941): Urology in the female. Am. J. Surg. **52**, 521.

[14] Hilton, P., Stanton, S. L. (1983a): Urethral pressure measurement by microtransducer: the results in symptom-free women and in those with genuine stress incontinence. Br. J. Obstet. Gynaecol. **90**, 919–933.

[15] Hilton, P., Stanton, S. L. (1983b): The use of intravaginal estrogen cream in genuine stress incontinence. Br. J. Obstet. Gynaecol. **90**, 940–944.

[16] Iosif, C. S., Batra, S., Ek, A. and Astedt, B. (1981): Estrogen receptors in the hu-

man female lower urinary tract. Am. J. Obstet. Gynecol. **141**, 817–820.

[17] Iosif, C. S. and Bekassy, Z. (1984): Prevalence of genito-urinary symptoms in the late menopause. Acta Obstet. Gynecol. Scand. **63**, 257–260.

[18] Jarvis, G. J., Hall, S., Stamp, S., Millar, D. R. and Johnson, A. (1980): An assessment of urodynamic examination in incontinent women. Br. J. Obstet. Gynaecol. **87**,893–896.

[19] Osborne, J. L. (1976): Postmenopausal changes in micturition habits and in urine flow and urethral pressure studies. In Campbell, S. (ed.) The Management of the Menopause and Post Menopausal Years, pp. 285–289. MTP Publications.

[20] Roberts, M., Smith, P. (1968): Non-malignant obstruction of the female urethra. Br. J. Urol. **40**, 694–702.

[21] Rud, T. (1980a): Urethral pressure profile in continent women from childhood to old age. Acta OBstet. Gynaecol. Scand. **59**, 331–335.

[22] Rud, T. (1980b): The effect of estrogens and gestagens on the urethral pressure profile in urinary continent and stress incontinent women. Acta Obstet. Gynecol. Scand. **59**, 265–270.

[23] Shepherd, A. M., Powell, P. H., Ball, A. J. (1982): The place of urodynamic studies in the investigation and treatment of female urinary tract symptoms. J. Obstet. Gynaecol. **3**, 123–125.

[24] Smith, P. J. B. (1976): The effect of estrogens on bladder function in the female. In Campbell S. (Ed.) The Management of the Menopause and Post Menopausal Years, pp. 291–198 MTP press.

[25] Sussman, M., Asscher, A. W., Water, W. E., Evans, J. A. S., Campbell, H., Evans, K. T. and Williams, J. E. (1969): Asymptomatic significant bacteriuria in the non-pregnant women. I. Description of a population. Brit. Med. J. **1**, 799–803.

[26] Thomas, T. M., Plymat, K. R., Blanin, J. and Meade, T. W. (1980): Prevalence of urinary incontinence, Br. Med. J. **281**, 1243–1245.

[27] Versi, E., Cardozo, L. D. (1985): Urethral Vascular Pulsations. pp. 503–594, Proc. Int. Cont. Soc., London.

[28] Versi, E., Cardozo, L. D., Studd, J. W. W., Brincat, M., O'Dowd, T. M. and Cooper, D. J. (1986): The internal urinary sphincter in the maintenance of female continence. Br. Med. J. **292**, 166–7.

[29] Versi, E. and Cardozo, L. D. (1986): Perineal pad weighing versus videographic analysis in genuine stress incontinence. Br. J. Obstet. Gynaecol. **93**, In Press.

[30] Versi, E., Brincat, M., Cardozo, L. D., Cooper, D. and Studd, J. W. W. (1986): Correlation of urethral physiology and skinn collagen in postmenopausal women. Br. J. Obstet. Gynaecol. Submitted.

[31] Zuckerman, S. (1940): Histogenesis of tissue sensitive to estrogens. Biol. Rev. Cambridge Philosoph. Soc. **15**, 231–271.

Discussion

Editor's note: The following questions and answers have been selected from the transcript of the discussion. They form a representative cross-section of the discussion but are not a complete record. This applies for all other discussions.

Hammerstein: Dr. Nocke, I wonder whether we have more than one type of menstrual cycle in the premenopause. There is the one which you have shown us, with a decrease in both progesterone and estrogens, but Sherman and Korenman* have described another type and given several examples – cycles with a decrease in estrogens, but not in progesterone. In one case – in the woman's very last menstrual cycle – I think they even demonstrated rather high progesterone values in the presence of low estrogens. Then, of course, there are anovulatory cycles as a third possibility. Two decades ago we described cycles in which you cannot find any progesterone activity whatsoever in the blood or urine with estrogens being low or even high. On this basis, I would say that there are at least 3 different types of the cycle which must take into account before the menopause.

Nocke: This was just one example within a wide scale of variations which might occur durig the perimenopausal phase – the phase immediately before and after the menopause. However, these cycles may start many years earlier – at about the age of 30 – and this scale includes the cycle which I showed you. At one end of the scale we have the very mild forms of luteal insufficiency, and at the other the abrupt cessation of bleeding. In between, we have the whole range of cyclical disturbances with and without ovulation. You are, of course, right that this is not the only type of cycle which we observe in the perimenopause.

Diczfalusy: I would certainly agree with Dr. Nocke – you do sometimes get cycles with no more progesterone, but then you also get follicular enlargement and very high estrogen levels. Because of this, it is extremely difficult to decide when postmenopausal levels are reached as far as ovarian estrogens are concerned. May I ask Dr. Nocke a question? You mentioned FSH and LH levels in the perimenopausal period. There have been at least two papers – one of them by Dr. Judd – indicating that there can be a major discrepancy between immunoreactive and bioactive LH in this period. Dr. Judd traced most of this activity – i.e. a very great rise in LH levels – to an increase in the alpha subunit. However, there was no biological activity. I wonder whether you have seen anything similar.

Nocke: We have no experience with these different kinds of research, but I would like to comment that we often find that LH is not increased as much as FSH in postmenopausal and perimenopausal women. Differentiating between the intact molecule and the subunits may, of course, produce different results. But, as most of you certainly know, in the era of the bioassay we obtained quite different figures

* Sherman, B. M., Korenman, page 6, J. Clin. Endocrinol. Metab. 39, 1: 145–149 (1974)

from animal experiments than from radioimmunoassays in blood. These figures are, of course, from urine.

Schwartz: We are unable to establish an FSH model to determine the time of cessation of ovarian follicular function, since there have been a number of case reports where pregnancies have occurred even after the demonstration of elevated FSH levels. I think this is very important from the clinical viewpoint.

Diczfalusy: I can certainly confirm that pathologically elevated FSH levels can be found in the presence of normal estradiol and progesterone levels in the perimenopause.

Question: I have two questions for Dr. Lindsay. His slide showed a really big increase in fractures starting after the age of 73. Can he give me an explanation for this phenomenon, since I cannot believe that aging is the only factor – a longer period of hypoestrogenic status in the menopause. The second question concerns the effect of estrogen. He pointed to young women who had had six months of oral contraceptives and claimed that there was an increase of bone and that this was an estrogen effect. I find this hard to believe.

Lindsay: I think the slide you are referring to was from the Mayo Clinic, which showed an increase of fracture frequency as a function of age. The increase of fracture frequency in women is clearly at least 20 years in advance of that in the male, starting somewhere between the ages of 40 and 50. I don't think you can attribute all the fractures that occur in the aging female or aging male to either the menopause or an andropause. There are probably many significant factors which results in fracturing, and one of them is reduced bone mass. Also, if you look at fractures in an institutional setting where there is a population which is much more unsteady on its feet, then the incidence of fractures is very much higher. We now have a variety of non-invasive techniques with which to measure bone mass objectively, and this remains our primary indicator of whether someone is at risk of fracture in general. In many studies, bone mass clearly begins to fall in women in almost the same decade as the fracture incidence begins to rise. There is a considerable danger in putting causal effect together with chronic associations – and this I quite understand –, but they do happen coincidentally. As bone mass falls further as a function of age, the fracture frequency increases dramatically in women. The second question concerns a cross-sectional review of two populations. The two groups were matched for age, calcium intake and exercise activity. The only statistically significant difference between these two groups was the use of oral contraception. When I said 6 months, I meant a minimum of 6 months – the majority of users were exposed to moderate doses of 30–50 μg oral contraceptives for about two and a half years. In fact, if you look at menopausal women, you can see the same effect. What the slide didn't show is that, if the women are allowed to go through the menopause without estrogen treatment, then the effect disappears within 5 years. The values revert to the normal slope.

Comment: The many epidemiological studies that have been done on the combined contraceptive pill have shown an association between various cardiovascular events and the therapy. There are now some 12 epidemiological studies of cardiovascular events in women receiving Premarin. I must add that nearly all of them are American studies, and virtually none of them shows any increase in cardiovascular events. In fact, the best of the studies – like the one from Los Angeles and the American nurses study from the Channing Lab. in Boston – showed a decreased risk of coronary events. In view of the great importance of cardiovascular disease, this could well be the most important beneficial effect of estrogen therapy. However, we are now adding progestogens to the estrogens, and this might well alter the situation radically.

Schwartz: What is the role of endogenous progesterone in lipid metabolism?

Tikkanen: I don't think that endogenous progesterone has any effect on lipid metabolism. Studies have been conducted with quite large doses of progestogen, and there has not been much change in the lipids. The studies with progestogens added to estrogen therapy are of two different kinds. There are short-term biochemical-type studies, in which the laboratory tests are almost always performed on the last day of the progestogen treatment period in order to determine the maximum effect. This is all right if you are interested in biochemical matters. From the clinical point of view, however, I would like to mention the studies on the average, effects such as those carried out by Dr. Gambrell in America, who showed in large numbers of women that, on the average, there is no significant difference in HDL-cholesterol even if you combine 19-nortestosterone derived progestogens with estrogen replacement therapy.

Question: There is a trend against claiming depression as a typical climacteric symptom. In data from Danish psychiatric departments, there is no increase of climacteric women with depression compared to the number of younger or older women admitted with depression. Dr. Greenblatt claimed that a correlation exists between the level of serotonin and tryptophane and depression, but is there any proof of this? Dr. Wenderlein stated that depression is a typical climacteric symptom, but what is the definition of depression? Are these women psychotic depressive, are they neurotic depressive – or is it just that their fertile period has ceased, the children have grown up and the marriage is perhaps not as attractive as before? Or are we as doctors influencing these women by asking them whether they are sad now that they have reached the climacteric? In his slide of the cross-over study, Dr. Schneider showed that depression is not one of the symptoms which are relieved by estrogen therapy. Consequently, I believe that depression is not a primary menopausal symptom that should be treated in isolation, but that the depressive signs are an integral part of the whole status of this phase of life.

Wenderlein: I agree, but I still think that the incidence of depression in the perimenopause is a bit higher than in other phases, of life. As regards the other point, you cannot, of course, tell whether the depression is neurotic, psychotic or reactive. However, the incidence of psychotic depression is very rare and assimilates to neurotic depression.

Greenblatt: Depression is, of course, a very common complaint in women from the age of 18 onwards, so we cannot blame all types of depression on states of estrogen deficiency. In the selected group in our study, however, the tryptophane values were definitely lower than in our controls and increased by at least 50% under estrogen therapy. They never reached normal values, but they certainly improved and there was a corresponding improvement of the patient's complaints.

2 Management of the climacteric patient

2.1 General aspects

The influence of nutrition and exercise

M. Notelovitz

Introduction

The climacteric is a natural event that is experienced by all women. Unlike the menopause (the last natural menstrual period) which lasts only a few days, the climacteric spans three decades – between the ages of 35 and 65 years. By making this clear differentiation, attention can be focused on two potential complications of an otherwise physiologic event, which, if undetected, can result in much morbidity and mortality: cardiovascular disease and osteoporosis. In 1980, over 350,000 women died in the United States from some cardiovascular related event, while each year approximately 300,000 women fracture their hips due to osteoporosis. Of this figure, approximately 15% will die within six months due to factors directly attributable to the fracture [1]; only ⅓ of the survivors will regain normal activity [2]. Spinal osteoporosis is even more prevalent and adds its toll of physical and psychologic pain. The net result is a devastating, negative impact on the future well-being of many women in their middle and later years by potentially preventable conditions.

During the period 1963 to 1981 there was an age-specific decrease in coronary mortality that has ranged from 44.8% (at age 35–44) to 38% (at age 55–64 [3]); this has been attributed in large measure to changes in diet and physical activity [3, 4]. Although no definitive studies have as yet been published, the increased prevalence of osteoporosis may be similarly related to inadequate and inappropriate nutrients and other lifestyle habits such as smoking and physical inactivity.

Osteogenesis and bone health

Bone is a living organ. Like tissues elsewhere it is constantly being removed and replaced. Normally these processes are coupled: the amount of old bone removed is replaced with an equal amount of freshly formed bone. Initiation of the cycle is dependant on the recruitment and activation of osteoclasts followed by the formation of osteoblasts. These cells synthesize collagen which is the main component of the newly formed bone matrix or osteoid. The latter matures by mineralizing and forming hydroxyapatite crystals. The elastic and tensile strength of the bone is further determined by the orientation of the collagen fibrils and the three dimensional network of plates and bars commonly found especially in trabecular bone. Interruption of this scaffold-like arrangement, e.g., the loss of the horizontal trabeculae due to aging, impairs the structural integrity of the bone and results in fracture.

Exercise: Mechanical force plays an important role in bone formation and function. There is a physiologic "band" of activity that is site specific: immobilization can lead to severe bone loss at some sites, while repeated loading at high strain magnitudes can result in bone hypertrophy [5]. A number of clinical studies attest to the benefit of exercise: athletes [6], cross-country runners [7], ballet dancers and weight-lifters [8], all have higher than average bone mass. Exercise probably has a systemic and a local effect. Professional tennis players have an overall greater bone mass than age-matched casual tennis players, but in addition have much more cortical bone in their dominant arm – 34.9% and 28.4%, respectively, for men and women [9]. For exercise to be osteogenic it should be vigorous and diverse: relatively few repititions of weight-bearing exercise at load-bearing strains in excess of 1000 micro-strain are optimal [10]. Compressive forces also generate lateral bending of long bones with medial new bone formation and an increase in the cross-sectional diameter of bone; the net result is improved resistance of the bone to bending [11].

The optimum amount and frequency of exercise required is not known; it is, however, possible to exercise too much as illustrated both experimentally and by women marathon runners whose activity has been associated with exercise induced amenorrhea [12, 13]. Amenorrhea may not be the over-riding factor: in a study of women with anorexia nervosa, all of whom were amenorrheic and hypoestrogenic, those who were physically active had significantly greater bone mass than a similar group of inactive anorectics [14].

Nutrition: Nutritionally deprived but exercised rats increase the amount and concentration of collagen in their femora, but not the calcium content [15]. This experiment illustrates a most important point: to benefit from exercise and its osteogenic stimulus, an adequate supply of the substrate (mainly calcium) is needed to mineralize and mature the newly formed bone. This may be the reason why amenorrheic women athletes reported in one study had a lower spinal (but not cortical) bone mineral content. In contrast to the eumenorrheic controls, they fell short of the 1500 mg of elemental calcium required per day [12].

In fully mature bone, the protein matrix accounts for 35% of the intercellular material with minerals occupying the remainder. Although hydroxyapatite crystal has significant amounts of sodium, magnesium, carbonate and citrate ions, calcium and phosphorus are the principle minerals. Factors that regulate their supply, absorption, deposition and withdrawal from the bone are the bases for the importance of nutrition and its role in maintaining bone health. For calcium balance, premenopausal women need 1000 mg of elemental calcium per day; women in the perimenopause require 1200 mg; and post-menopausal women, 1400 mg per day [16]. The average intake of calcium in women between 40–65 years of age in the USA varies between 450–600 mg/day [17]. Thus the average daily intake needs to be increased by 100%!

Whereas 75% of ingested calcium is absorbed during periods of rapid skeletal growth, this rate decreases to 30–50% in adults [18]. Despite contrary opinions, calcium is absorbed as efficiently from calcium supplements as it is from dairy products. The most important point is that the calcium requirement must be fulfilled consistently on a daily basis. As with exercise, individuals need to be given the option of meeting this need by whatever means are convenient, acceptable and affordable. In an on-going study at the Center for Climacteric Studies involving women participating in a two-year exercise program to prevent osteoporosis, only 41% of the women met the RDA of calcium (800 mg) and 12% the desired 1400 mg. With successive interviews and counseling sessions, significant increases were noted: at 12 months 93% met the RDA, and 82% the 1400 mg, requirement. Only 8% of the women met this goal by increasing food sources. Reasons for not increasing calcium-rich food include concern for weight-gain, dislike of certain dairy products, constipation and lactose intolerance. Lactase deficiency is found in 27% of women with post-menopausal osteoporosis versus 3% of normal women [19]. Yogurt is often well tolerated by the lactose-intolerant individual. A group of volunteers with a history of lactase deficiency absorbed 50% of the lactose in milk versus 85% of the lactose in yogurt. Yogurt consumption is thus a convenient and palatable way of overcoming this deficiency [20]. Calcium citrate tablets or meals help with calcium absorption in the elderly and in those prone to achlorhydria – a problem of increasing prevalence in the elderly. Multiple feedings and the taking of calcium supplements at night are other measures recommended as means of maximizing calcium absorption [21].

Bone Robbers: the bioavailability of calcium may be negatively influenced by a number of nutrients and foods [22]: dietary fiber, the phytic acid found in bran and oxalic acid in vegetables such as spinach are such examples. Excess amounts of protein increase the urinary excretion of calcium. Human volunteers given as much as 1600 mg of calcium per day had a negative calcium balance of 140 mg/day on a dietary protein intake of 225 grams. If maintained for one year, this could lead to a loss of 4% of the total skeletal calcium. A 50% increase in protein in premenopausal women is associated with a net calcium loss of 32 mg/day. An excess of dietary sodium – more than 2000 mg/day (1 teaspoonful) – is also associated with an excess excretion of calcium.

Lifestyle also can also have a negative impact: a high caffeine intake (more than 5 cups of coffee per day); smoking and alcohol excess (more than 5 beers per day) are all associated with impaired calcium retention. Inactivity increases calcium excretion and decreases calcium absorption. Finally, there are a host of medications that may also interfere with calcium metabolism: aluminium-containing antacids; glucocorticoids; furosemide; tetracycline and isoniozid.

Vitamin D and Vitamin K, needed for calcium absorption and the synthesis of bone gla-protein respectively, have a clearly defined role and are needed in "normal" amounts to maintain bone homeostasis. Excess amounts of Vitamin D may be harmful and lead to an increase in urinary calcium excretion and a loss of cortical bone. It is currently recommended that Vitamin D intake should not exceed 1000 I.U. per day.

Summary: Osteogensis is a complex multifactorial process. By educating the public about the basic principles of bone physiology, much can be done to ensure against the later development of osteoporosis. Two goals need to be reached: acquisition of as much bone as possible before the menopause; modulation of the rate of bone loss thereafter. This can be achieved in large measure by appropriate and consistent exercise to stimulate new bone, a balanced diet to maximize bone mineralization and moderation of calcium losing lifestyle habits such as smoking, alcohol and caffeine excess.

Cardio-respiratory health

Coronary heart disease causes more than 550,000 deaths per year in the U.S. and a cost $ 60 billion [23]. This is not only a disease of men: the incidence in post-menopausal women is three times greater than in pre-menopausal women [24]. Although we are once again dealing with a multifactorial disease, physically active persons have fewer clinical manifestations of coronary heart disease than their sedentary counterparts. Further, if coronary events do occur in active persons, they are usually less severe and occur at an older age.

Biochemical Benefits of Exercise: Regular exercise – apart from improving physical characteristics such as increasing maximal oxygen uptake – modifies risk factors related to atherogenic heart disease such as hypertension and high blood lipid and lipoprotein levels. In order for physical activity to have a meaningful impact, exercise must be taken regularly and be of sufficient intensity and duration. For example, the blood lipid profile improves (mainly an increase in the cardioprotective HDL-lipoprotein) only after four months of running 10–15 miles per week [25]. With moderate activity such as walking, about 30 miles/week for three months is necessary before a significant increase in HDL cholesterol occurs [26]. Although aerobic endurance activity such as swimming, bicycling and long-distance running have usually been associated with improved lipids and lipoproteins, muscle-strengthening resistance exercises like weightlifting also have a favorable effect on blood lipids and lipoprotein concentrations [27]. Another "hidden advantage" of exercise is an increase in fibrinolytic activity as measured both by plasminogen activity [28] and the synthesis of α_2 antiplasmin inhibitor [29] and by a reduction in platelet aggregation.

Fitness Evaluation: The maximal oxygen uptake ($\dot{V}O_2max$) is the amount of oxygen taken up by the entire body during maximal effort. Physical exercise performed at activity levels less than 50% of $\dot{V}O_2max$ can be maintained for hours; to achieve physical fitness and its associated benefits, training needs to be performed at 70% to 85% of $\dot{V}O_2max$ for at least 20–40 minutes three times a week [30]. Training levels sustained in excess of this range could be harmful to individuals with asymptomatic cardiovascular disease. For sedentary (and middle aged) women who wish to participate in meaningful exercise, the graded exercise test, the treadmill test, is as integral a part of screening a patient as is the medical history. It is also an important key to the determination of a proper exercise program and can serve as a measure of the conditioning effect of training when periodic $\dot{V}O_2max$ testing is included in the program.

There are many protocols for graded exercise testing, all of which accomplish essentially the same thing [30]. A GXT is classified as either maximal or submaximal. A maximal test imposes progressively increasing workloads on the exercising subject until exhaustion is reached. Because this test requires the collection and analysis of expired air samples, it is not suited to everyday clinical practice. Submaximal testing, on the other hand, is better suited to the practicing physician: the patient rides a stationary bicycle against a progressively increasing workload until a given heart rate or workload is achieved. This point is used to estimate the $\dot{V}O_2max$ [31]. Several studies have shown that submaximal testing correlates well with actual maximal testing when corrected for age, but none of these have examined climacteric women. One hundred and sixty three healthy sedentary females between the ages of 35 and 75 years had a maximal $\dot{V}O_2$ test performed at the Center for Climacteric Studies using a modified Balke procedure. The results of these tests were compared with those of the matched group of 121 women tested on an ergometer. The actual and the estimated $\dot{V}O_2$ data and the range of values for subjects in both groups showed no differences [32]. Similarly, a sub-group of 29 climacteric women were tested by both tests, and once again a close correlation was obtained ($r = .789$). Finally, since the onset of the menopause has been linked with an abrupt change in the cardiorespiratory fitness of females, a group of women aged 45–55 years were divided according to whether or not they were still menstruating. Their menopausal status was defined by hormone analysis and a history of amenorrhea. No significant difference in the estimated $\dot{V}O_2max$ was noted, indicating that the menopause per se does not influence cardiorespiratory fitness [32]. Based on the documented decline in both maximal and submaximal testing in our laboratory, we have developed guidelines for evaluating the fitness status of climacteric women using either method. Guidelines such as these are useful for prescribing exercise.

The functional loss in cardiorespiratory function associated with the peri-menopause coincided with age-related changes and can be reversed by a program of regular physical activity. In one recent study, pre-menopausal women (mean age of 41 years) who trained for nine weeks, improved their $\dot{V}O_2max$ by 12.1%, while a similarly trained post-menopausal group (mean age 57 years) improved their $\dot{V}O_2max$ by 19% [33]. We evaluated 38 post-menopausal women (mean age 56 years) before, after six months and after one year of a structured program that involved three weekly 20 minute treadmill, ergometer or Nautilus (muscle strengthening) sessions. Subjects were exercised between 70–85% of the maximal heart rate. Significant improvements in both $\dot{V}O_2max$ and time on the treadmill were recorded and maintained by the bicyclers and treadmill groups.

Summary

In summary, we have determined that submaximal testing can be used as a screen to determine cardiorespiratory fitness in climacteric women. Patients at high risk for cardiovascular disease and those classified as having fair or poor health as measured by ergometry, require more detailed evaluation before embarking on a prescribed exercise program. We have also established that it is possible to train sedentary climacteric women and maintain a state of physical fitness for at least one year. Exercise is probably cardioprotective. Although this effect may not translate into longevity for all who exercise, there is compelling evicence that exercise does enhance the feeling of well-being and, hence, the quality of life.

Conclusion

The ability of dietary manipulation and exercise to prevent osteoporosis and atherosclerosis in women has yet to be proven. We have established that climacteric women can be influenced to alter their lifestyles and be compliant for at least one year. Longer term studies are needed before definitive conclusions can be reached. Widespread consumer education and early lifestyle behaviour modification should, we believe, relegate the image of the shrunken, little old lady to history. This image should be replaced by the image of a woman imbued with vitality and a zest for an active and productive old age.

References

[1] Lewis, A.F., Brit. Med. J. 283:1217 (1981).
[2] Keene, J.S. and Anderson, C.A., JAMA 248:564 (1982).
[3] Walker, W.J., N.Engl. J. Med. 308:649 (1983).
[4] Pfaffenberger, R.S., Hyde, R.T., Wing, A.L. et al. JAMA 252:491 (1984).
[5] Carter, D.R., Calcif. Tissues Int. 36:519 (1984).
[6] Nilsson, B.E. and Westlin, N.E., Clin. Orthop. 77:179 (1971).
[7] Dalen, N. and Olsson, K.E., Acta Orthop. Scan., 45:170 (1974).
[8] Nilsson, B.E., Anderson, S.M., Hardrup T. et al. Amer. J. Roentgenol. 131:539 (1978).
[9] Jones, H.H., Priest, J.D., Hayes, W.C. et al., J. Bone Joint Surg. [AM] 59:204 (1977).
[10] Lanyon, L.E., Calcif. Tissue Int. 36:556 (1984).
[11] Emiola, L., O'Shea, J.P., Nutr. Rep. Int. 17:669 (1978).
[12] Drinkwater, B.L., Nilson, K., Chestnut, C. et al., N. Engl. J. Med. 311:277 (1984).
[13] Cann, C.E., Martin, M.C., Genant, H.K. et al., JAMA 251:626 (1984).
[14] Rigotti, N.A., Nussbaum, S.R., Herzog, D.B. et al., N. Engl. J. Med. 311:1601 (1984).
[15] Chvapil, M., Bartos, D. and Bartos, F., Gerontologia 19:263 (1973).
[16] Heaney, R.P., Gallagher, J.C., Johnston, C.C. et al. AM. J. Clin. Nutr. 36:986 (1982).
[17] Avioli, L.V., Fed. Proc. 40:2418 (1981).
[18] Avioli, L.B., in Cecil Textbook of Medicine. Ed. Beeson, P.B., McDermott, W., and Wyngaarden, J.B., W.B.Saunders, Philadelphia, p.2225 (1979).
[19] Newcomer, A.D., Hodgson, S.F., McDill, D.B. et al., Ann. Int. Med. 89; 218 (1978).
[20] Kolars, J.C., Levitt, M.D., Aouji, M. et al., N. Engl. J. Med. 310:1 (1984).
[21] Recker, R.R., N. Engl. J. Med. 313:70 (1985).
[22] Notelovitz, M., Interrelations of Exercise and Diet on Bone Metabolism and Osteoporosis in Nutrition and Exercise. Ed. Myron Winik. John Wiley and Sons., New York (in Press).
[23] Concensus Conference. JAMA 253:2080 (1985).
[24] Kannel, W.B., Hjortland, M.C., McNamara, P.M. et al., Ann. Int. Med. 85:447 (1976).
[25] Williams, M.H., Nutritional Aspects of Human Physical and Athletic Performance, 2nd ed. Springfield, IL. Charles C.Thomas, (1985).
[26] Sopko, G., Leon, A.S., Jacobs, D.R. et al., Metabolism 34:227 (1985).
[27] Goldberg, L., Elliot, D.L., Schutz, R.W. et al., JAMA 252:504 (1984).
[28] Hedlin, A.M., Mulojevic, J., and Korey, A., Thromb. Haemostas (Stuttgart) 3a:743 (1978).
[29] Huisveld, J.A., Haspen, A.J.H. and Bernink, M.J.E., Appl. Physiol. 53:330 (1982).
[30] Bruce, R.A., Med. Sci. Sports and Exerc. 16:8 (1984).
[31] Åstrand, I., Acta Physiol. (Scand.) 49:45 (1960).
[32] Notelovitz M., Fields C., Caramelli K., Amer. J. Obstet. Gynec. (1986), In Press.
[33] Cowan, M.M., and Gregory, L.W., Med. Sci. Sports and Exerc. 17:138 (1985).

Non-hormonal medication

W. H. Utian

> "Where the patient is delicate and subject to female weakness, night sweats or an habitual purging, with flushing in the face and a hectic fever: For such; ass's milk, jellies and raw eggs, with cooling fruits will be proper. At meals she may be indulged with half a pint of old, clear London porter, or a glass of Rhenish wine."
>
> *John Leake, 1777*
>
> "The bowels must be kept open."
>
> *John Burns, 1814*

Although historical references to non-endocrine treatment of the menopause may sound amusing, it is a sad reflection of the state-of-the-art, that even today we can offer little more in the way of non-hormonal medication to the women suffering severe hot flushes and having a reason not to take hormonal therapy.

The general lack of information on non-hormonal medication of the menopause can best be exemplified by the following analysis. As editor of Maturitas, the International Journal for the Study of the Climacteric, I reviewed the subject of all papers published between 1978 and this meeting. Out of 227 papers published, 96 related directly to hormonal therapy, yet only 7 were on non-hormonal medication (Table I).

Table I Survey of Therapy Papers Published in Maturitas 1978 – 1985

Year	Total Papers Published	Hormonal Medication	Non-Hormonal Medication
1978	16	8	2 Vitamin B-6 Clonidine
1979	19	6	
1980	38	18	
1981	37	16	1 Ethamsylate
1982	39	17	
1983	23	9	1 Opipramol
1984	35	18	1 Naproxen
1985	20 (Half-Year)	4	2 Lofexidine Naloxone
Total	227	96	7

Perhaps the problem really does not lie as much in the realm of therapeutics as it does in the actual definition of "menopausal symptoms".

The climacteric syndrome

The term "menopause" has traditionally been applied in so non-precise a fashion that so-called "menopausal symptoms" have included virtually any complaint a middle aged woman cared to take to her physician. Indeed, until the early 1970's it was almost impossible to differentiate genuine endocrine-generated symptoms truly related to climacteric from those problems that are totally unrelated.

The net result was that clinicians tended to divide symptoms presented by perimenopausal women on an empirical basis into "autonomic" and "metabolic" or, even worse, to simply itemize them grocery-list style without any attempt at explanation. Clinicians were thus truly in the dark as to causation of symptoms and were inevitably forced to treat "effect" on an empirical basis rather than "cause" on a valid scientific basis [1].

The problem was a lack of established scientific data relating to human climacteric. Even much of the published research showed serious deficiencies in patient sampling and methodology [2]. In particular, there was virtually no published information relating to specific symptoms or signs with parameters of estrogen production or secretion. Other notable deficiencies included the differentiation of true drug effects from placebo responses, and the minimal information on the psychologic and sociocultural contributions to symptom formation. The majority of clinical features ascribed to this period in the human life cycle were therefore mere assumptions and could have been no more than coincidental features in a generally aging population.

A virtual flurry of publications from 1970 onward did much to remedy the lack of specific data [3–15]. This is not to decry the attempts of earlier investigators in defining menopausal symptomatology, but rather to state that invariably case selection, controls, or empirical scoring of symptoms were not specific enough to provide the required information [16–19]. Nonetheless, inadequate knowledge of true menopause-related symptoms has virtually excluded the possibility of even estimating the number of women who have sufficient symptoms at the time of menopause to seek medical advice and who would therefore comprise the potential pool for non-hormonal medication.

It is now generally accepted that the symptoms associated with the climacteric can be generated by three etiologic mechanisms:

1. Decreased ovarian activity with subsequent alteration in endocrine profiles and target organ responses.
2. Sociocultural factors determined by the woman's environment.
3. Psychologic factors dependent on the structure of the woman's character.

The broad spectrum of symptoms that manifest at the time of menopause is the result of interaction between these three components [3]. This point needs emphasis. The definitive statement that the varied symptom profile after menopause is caused by an interaction between three components (endocrine, social/environment, psychologic) allows for the fact that the nature and incidence of symptomatology varies in different educational, socioeconomic, racial, and *population* groups. But it lays stress on the actual causal agent of the symptom, thus suggesting that treatment must be selective. For instance, hormone-dependent symptoms will be best treated by appropriate hormonal replacement, which I will mention no more; other symptoms may justify non-hormonal medication, psychotherapy or actual educational programs to alter negative attitudes in specific sociocultural groups.

Some cross-over of therapeutic modalities is inevitable, perhaps even desirable, for example, non-hormonal treatment of the hot flush for the patient adverse to receiving hormones or in whom they are contraindicated. But the above brief discussion does explain the difficulty in evaluating non-hormonal substances for efficacy and therefore, perhaps, the paucity of literature in this area.

Psycho-social-cultural symptoms of climacteric

A host of symptoms such as palpitations, fatigue, vertigo, headaches, dyspnea, irritability, depression, frigidity, and apprehension that are listed as components of the climacteric syndrome are probably manifestations of the psycho-socio-cultural disturbances that may occur at this time of life. There is no evidence that these symptoms are causally related to altered hormone profiles [20, 21]. There is also no evidence that libido is affected by menopause, although it is possible that hysterectomy may deleteriously affect this function [22].

The actual verification and classification of these symtpoms within the sphere of climacteric has proven exceptionally difficult. Not only do social and ethnic differences exist [23], but outside influences such as work and play also modify responses to climacteric [24]. Above all, it has been almost impossible to define the problem and to undertake inter-study or cross-cultural comparisons because of the lack of adquate tools to measure changes in behavior. For example, the gynecologist refers to postmenopausal depression but really understands this as an altered mood up to the point where normal behavior ends and clinical depression begins. The psychiatrist, on the other hand, has a different perception of the problem.

It is generally accepted that climacteric does not precipitate any major psychiatric illness. The following psychologic symptoms have been reported to accompany the climacteric [25, 26]:

Fatigue or diminished drive	Loss of ability to concentrate or apathy
Vertigo (dizziness)	Headache

Irritability	Depression
Apprehension	Tension or anxiety
Insomnia	Dyspnea
Altered libido	General fluctuations in mood
Feeling of inadequacy or non-fulfillment	

Unfortunately, a list such as this contains many vague and ill-defined terms, most of which are not exclusive to psychiatric problems, but could occur in organic illnesses where no psychiatric disorder is suspected.

Table II Perimenopausal Symptoms

1. *Specific: True hormonal-related symptoms*
   Early: Hot flushes; perspiration (night sweats)
   Later: Relate to the metabolic change in the target organ affected, e. g. osteoporosis causing backache, vaginal atrophy causing dyspareunia, etc.
2. *Nonspecific: Psycho-socio-cultural symptoms*
   Determined by the woman's environment and the structure of her character; e. g., depression, irritability, insomnia, frigidity, headache, apprehension, etc.

From Utian, WH: Menopause in Modern Perspective, 1980. Courtesy of Appleton-Century-Crofts, New York

The overall symptom production at the climacteric is summarized in **Table II.** It can be concluded that the climacteric, whether artificial or spontaneous, is associated with certain specific symptoms. Contrary to popular opinion, however, the number and variety of direct, true homone-related effects are fewer than generally assumed. The following classification of perimenopausal symptoms summarizes current thought and, being practical, is easily related to the clinical situation:

1. Specific: true hormone-related symptoms
   Early: hot flushes; perspiration (night sweats)
   Later: relate to the metabolic change in the target organ affected; e.g., osteoporosis causing backache, vaginal atrophy causing dyspareunia, etc.
2. Nonspecific: Psycho-socio-cultural symptoms
   Determined by the woman's environment and the structure of her character; e.g., depression, irritability, insomnia, frigidity, headache, apprehension, etc.

It therefore follows that a case can be made for hormonal treatment of specific symptoms but not for the nonspecific ones.

It is in this context that non-hormonal medication can be considered in greater detail.

Non-hormonal medication for climacteric

Correctly, non-hormonal drugs have a secondary role in the management of the climacteric syndrome. That is, specific hormone-dependent symptoms or metabolic factors respond best to selected hormones and should be treated primarily with these substances provided no contraindication to their use exists. Symptoms that develop as a result of psycho-socio-cultural factors necessitate an educational and psychotherapeutic approach, with the use of drugs as an adjunct only. It is, of course, obvious that unexplained symptoms should always be investigated for a specific cause and be treated according to accepted principles of practice dependent upon that cause.

There are specific instances when non-hormonal drugs may be indicated in the management of the climacteric syndrome and these include:

1. The patient in whom sex-steroid therapy is contraindicated.
2. The patient who does not respond to sex-steroid therapy.
3. The patient who does not want hormone therapy but does request symptom relief.
4. The patient who cannot tolerate sex steroids because of side effects such as nausea or fluid retention.

The selection of a non-hormonal drug for treatment of the climacteric syndrome is based more on empirical observation than on satisfactory documentation for therapeutic effect. The literature is striking for its paucity of well-controlled, randomized, double-blind, prospective studies of the therapeutic efficacy of non-hormonal agents. A brief discussion of some of the more frequently prescribed drugs or groups of drugs follows.

Sedatives

Sedatives may help in reducing the number of hot flushes. They are less useful for the symptoms associated with irritability and emotional upset. Clinical experience appears to have been greater with the barbiturate sedatives than with the nonbarbiturates. In particular, phenobarbital USP, alone or in combination with other drugs, seems to be effective. For example, based on the concept that functional disorders may involve hyperactivity of the sympathetic and parasympathetic nervous systems, phenobarbital USP 20 to 40 mg is combined with ergotamine tartrate, a sympathetic inhibitor, and levoratatory alkaloids of belladonna, a parasympathetic inhibitor. In the author's personal experience, this combination is less effective than estrogen in relief of hot flushes, but is a satisfactory alternate when estrogens cannot be used. It is commercially available as Bellergal tablets.

Tranquilizers

The tranquilizers now comprise a large group of drugs, the description of which is outside the scope of this presentation. It can be stated that these drugs have often been abused in relation to the postmenopausal patient. It has been used excessively and all too often in the absence of a well-defined indication. Nonetheless, in appropriately selected patients tranquilizers are of value as adjuncts to educational and psychotherapeutic programs, particularly in the presence of excessive anxiety, irritability, insomnia, and related agitational states.

The most frequently prescribed drugs include diazepam (Valium), chlordiazepoxide (Librium), benzodiazepine (Ativan), hydroxyzine (Atarax), meprobamate, and some of the phenothiazines.

Antidepressants

Remarks similar to those on the tranquilizers discussed above also apply to the antidepressants. Antidepressants are indicated for true psychiatric depression. They are less likely to be of value in situations with marginal mood changes not severe enough to be classified as depression. Among the most commonly used antidepressants are amitriptyline (Elavil), some of the phenothiazines, monamine oxidase inhibitors (e.g., phenelzine sulfate – Nardil; tranylcypromine sulfate – Parnate), the dibenzoxepin tricyclic compounds (doxepin HCL – Sinequan), and the imipramines (imipramine pamoate – Tofranil).

Non-hormonal treatment for hot flushes

Vasomotor symptoms (VMS) are the most visible and disabling of the early problems facing the perimenopausal woman. Parallel research has been directed at exploring the mechanism of the hot flush and at evaluation nonhormonal medications, but so far with limited success.

1. Clonidine

Clonidine, an imidazoline derivative, is worthy of discussion because of the attention it has received as an alternate to estrogen in the treatment of hot flushes. Introduced in a low dose as an antimigraine drug [27], and in a higher dose as an antihypertensive [28, 29] clonidine was reported by Clayden to be effective in reducing perimenopausal flushing [30, 31]. Clonidine appears to inhibit sympathetic nervous system function at least in part by interacting with a central alpha adrenergic receptor [32].

Personal experience has been less promising and most recent reports in the literature conflicting [33, 34].

2. Propranolol

Propranolol, a drug which causes both central and peripheral betablockade, has also been studied for its effect on menopausal hot flushes, but has generally been shown to be no more effective than a placebo [35].

3. Lofexidine

Lofexidine, an orally administered alpha-adrenergic agonist, has been shown to be of limited value in treating vasomotor flushes. Unfortunately, the side effects may become intolerable at doses which completely eliminate fluhes [36].

4. Opipramol

Opipramol is a relatively potent inhibitor of catecholamine uptake in the rat. However, in a double-blind placebo-controlled study the drug did not induce a significantly different response than a placebo [37].

5. Ethamsylate

Ethamsylate, a non-hormonal agent acting to promote capillary integrity, has also not been demonstrated to have any markedly superior effect over placebo in controlling hot flushes [38].

6. Naloxone

The endogenous opiates have been incriminated as causing hot flushes, the essential evidence being that naloxone, an opiate antagonist, significantly reduces the incidence of hot flushes [39, 40].

Further research into the exogenous opiate mechanism is likely to be most fruitful with regard to development of satisfactory non-hormonal antiflushing medications.

7. Naproxen

Prostaglandin inhibitors have also been tested for relief of hot flushes but responses do not differ dramatically from those induced by placebo [41].

8. Vitamin B-6 (Pyridoxine)

As in the oral contraceptive, there is some evidence to show that ethinyl-estradiol and possibly progestogens lead to a disturbance of tryptophan metabolism and a deficiency of vitamin B-6 (pyridoxine) [42, 43, 44]. Adams et al have reported that the clinical consequences include depression, emotional instability, fatigue, disturbances in concentration, and loss of libido [43]. The same problem has been reported by Haspels et al to occur in postmenopausal women on estrogen therapy [45]. These symptoms apparently respond to vitamin B-6, 250 mg per day [43, 45]. Altered tryptophan metabolism with sex-steroid therapy appears to warrant further investigation.

Conclusion

The selection of pharmacologic agents, hormonal and non-hormonal, for use after menopause needs to be specific. Misuse or abuse of drugs can no longer be justfied. This does not imply that physicians and patients should shun their use, an opposite extreme that also cannot be supported. When a definitive indication exists, and the basic principles of drug therapy and follow-up are observed, then the use of such agents will often generate extremely gratifying results and should not be unduly withheld. There is an urgent need for further research in this area.

References

[1] Utian, W. H.: Menopause in Modern Perspective. Appleton-Century-Crofts, New York 1980.

[2] McKinlay, S. M., McKinlay, J. B.: Selected studies of the menopause. J. Biosoc. Sci. 5:533, 1973.

[3] Utian, W. H., Serr, D.: The climacteric syndrome. In: van Keep, Greenblatt, Albeaux-Fernet (eds): Consenus on Menopause Research, Lancaster, MTP Press 1976, p. 1.

[4] Utian, W. H.: The true clinical features of postmenopause and oophorectomy, and their response to oestrogen therapy. S. Afr. Med. J. 46:732, 1972.

[5] Utian, W. H.: The mental tonic effect of oestrogens administered to oophorectomized females. S. Afr. Med. J. 46:1079, 1972.

[6] Utian, W. H.: Definitive symptoms of postmenopause – incorporating use of vaginal parabasal cell index. Front. Horm. Res. 3:74, 1975.

[7] Utian, W. H.: Effect of hysterectomy, oophorectomy and estrogen therapy on libido. Int. J. Gynaecol. Obset. 13:97, 1975.

[8] Utian, W. H.: The scientific basis for postmenopausal estrogen therapy. The management of specific symptoms and rationale for long-term replacement. In: Beard, R. (ed.): The Menopause. Lancaster, MTP Press, 1976, p. 175.

[9] Stone, S. C., Mickal, A., Rye, P. H.: Postmenopausal symptomatology, maturation index and plasma estrogen levels. Obstet. Gynecol. 45:625, 1975.

[10] Jaszmann, L.: Epidemiology of climacteric and postclimacteric complaints. Front. Horm. Res 2:22, 1973.

[11] Van Keep, P. A., Prill, H. J.: Psycho-sociology of menopause and postmenopause. Front. Horm. Res. 3:32, 1975.

[12] Kruskemper, G.: Results of psychological testing (MMPI) in climacteric women. Front. Horm. Res. 3:105, 1975.

[13] Thompson, B., Hart, H. A., Durno, S.: Menopausal age and symptomatology in a general practice. J. Biosoc. Sci. 5:71, 1973.

[14] Abe, T., Furuhashi, N., Yamaya, Y., et al.: Correlation between climacteric symptoms and serum levels of estradiol, progesterone, follicle-stimulating hormone, and luteinizing hormone. A. J. Obstet. Gynecol. 129:65, 1977.

[15] Hutton, J. D., Jacobs, H. S., Murray, M. A. F., James, V. H. T.: Relation between plasma oestrone and oestradiol and climacteric symptoms. Lancet 1:678, 1978.

[16] Heller, C. G., Farney, J. P., Myers, G. P.: Development and correlation of menopausal symptoms, vaginal smear and urinary gonadotropin changes following castration in 27 women. J. Clin. Endocrinol. 4:101, 1941.

[17] Kupperman, H. S., Blatt, M. H. G., Weisbader, H., Filler, W.: Comparative clinical evaluation of estrogenic preparations by menopausal and amenorrhoeal indices. J. Clin. Endocrinol. Metab. 13:688, 1953.

[18] Newton, M., Odom, P. L.: The menopause and its symptoms. South. Med. J. 57:1309, 1964.

[19] Serr, D. M., Rabau, E., Mannor, S.: Correlation of menopausal symptoms with oestrogen deficiency. Clin. Trials J. 5:91, 1968.
[20] Van Keep, P. A., Kellerhals, J.: The aging woman. Front Horm. Res. 2:160, 1973.
[21] Utian, W. H.: Current status of menopause and postmenopausal estrogen therapy. Obstet. Gynecol. Survey 32:193, 1977.
[22] Utian, W. H.: Effect of hysterectomy, oophorectomy and estrogen on libido. Int. J. Gynecol. Obstet. 13:97, 1975.
[23] Maoz, B., Antonovsky, A., Apter, A., Wijsenbeek, H., Datan, N.: The perception of menopause in five ethnic groups in Israel. Acta Obstet. Gynecol. Scand. Suppl. 65:69, 1977.
[24] Maoz, B., Antonovsky, A., Apter, A., et al.: The effect of outside work on the menopausal woman. Maturitas 1:43, 1978.
[25] Dennerstein, L., Burrows, G. D.: A review of studies of the psychological symptoms found at the menopause. Maturitas 1:55, 1978.
[26] Brown, J. R. W. C., Brown, M. E. C.: Psychiatric disorders associated with the menopause. In Beard, R. (ed.): The Menopause. Lancaster, MTP Press, 1976, p. 57.
[27] Shafar, J., Tallett, E. R., Knowlson, P. A.: Evaluation of clonidine in prophylaxis of migraine. Double-blind trial and follow-up. Lancet 1:403, 1972.
[28] Haeusler, G.: Cardiovascular regulation by central adrenergic mechanisms and its alteration by hypotensive drugs. Circ. Res. Suppl. 36–37:223, 1975.
[29] Van Zwieten, P. A.: The central action of antihypertensive drugs mediated by central α-receptors. J. Pharm. Pharmacol. 25:89, 1973.
[30] Clayden, J. R.: Effect of clonidine on menopausal flushing. Lancet 2:1361, 1972.
[31] Clayden, J. R., Bell, J. W., Pollard, P.: Menopausal flushing – double-blind trial of a non-hormonal medication. Br. Med. J. 1:409, 1974.
[32] Metz, S. A., Halter, J. B., Porte, D., Robertson, R. P.: Suppression of plasma catecholamines and flushing by clonidine in man. J. Clin. Endocrinol. Metab. 46:83, 1978.
[33] Lindsay, R., Hart, D. M.: Failure or response of menopausal vasomotor symptoms to clonidine, Maturitas 1:21, 1978.
[34] Lauter, L. R., Erlik, Y. et al.: Effect of clonidine on hot flashes in postmenopausal women. Obstet. Gynecol. 60:583, 1982.
[35] Coope, J., Williams, S., Patterson, J. S.: A study of the effectiveness of propranolol in menopausal hot flushes. Br. J. Obstet. Gynaecol. 85:472, 1978.
[36] Jones, K. P., Ravnikar, V., Schiff, I.: A preliminary evaluation of the effect of lofexidine on vasomotor flushes in postmenopausal women. Maturitas 7:135, 1985.
[37] VanLith, N. D. and Motke, J. C. T.: Opipramol in the climacteric syndrome. Maturitas 5:17, 1983.
[38] Harrison, R. F.: Ethamsylate in the treatment of climacteric flushing. Maturitas 3:31, 1981.
[39] Lightman, S. L., Jacobs, H. S. et al.: Climacteric flushing: clinical and endocrine response to infusion of naloxone. Brit. J. Obstet. Gynaecol. 88:919, 1981.
[40] Hendy, M. S., Cockrill, B., Sherwood, B. P.: The effects of naloxone infusion and stellate ganglion blockade on hot flushes in the human male. Maturitas 7:169, 1985.
[41] Haataja, M., Paul, R. et al.: Effect of prostaglandin inhibitor and oestrogen on climacteric symptoms and serum free fatty acids. Maturitas 5:263, 1984.
[42] Rose, D. P.: Excretion of xanthurenic acid in the urine of women taking progestogen-oestrogen preparations. Nature 210:196, 1966.
[43] Adams, P. W., Rose, D. P., Folkard, J., et al.: Effect of vitamin B6 upon depression associated with oral contraception. Lancet 1:897, 1973.
[44] Coelingh Bennink, H. J. T., Schreurs, W. H. P.: Disturbance of tryptophan metabolism and its correction during hormonal contraception. Contraception 9:347, 1974.
[45] Haspels, A. A., Coelingk Bennink, H. J. T., Schreurs, W. H. P.: Disturbance of tryptophan metabolism and its correction during oestrogen treatment in postmenopausal women. Maturitas 1:15, 1978.

Discussion

Hammerstein: Dr. Notelovitz, you have shown how exercise influences bone mass in postmenopausal women. Is anything similar known for men?

Notelovitz: Yes, in fact that is one of the main reasons why we believe that exercise works. There are a number of reasons why men don't get osteoporosis, and one of them is related to muscle mass. Men have greater muscle mass than women and are normally more active physically. I think this is one of the more important reasons why men do not suffer from osteoporosis.

Upton, USA: I should like to make a comment on Dr. Utian's paper. I think that the area of non-hormonal medication for the relief of hot flushes in particular is not only interesting, but also in need of research. There are so many women who may have contraindications or who prefer not to take hormones.

Utian: If you look at the literature on non-hormonal drugs, none of the evidence for the use of any of the substances is based on a prospective randomised double-blind study. All the evidence is narrative and unsubstantiated. I should like to stress that there is an urgent need for research in this area.

Hammerstein: I am convinced that everybody here in the hall who practices as a gynaecologist had experience with sedatives and some sort of drugs in climacteric women who are unable to tolerate sex hormones. The experience is there, probably throughout the world. The point is, however, that nobody has checked this; there are no prospecitve studies. Thus, I think it is time for somebody to grasp the initiative.

Question: I come from a country where estrogen replacement therapy is farily infrequent, being employed in about 10% of the women of this age group. My question relates to osteoporosis. Is there any indication that women with severe climacteric symptoms are at higher risk of developing osteoporosis and, if so, would the dosage that we usually give, 1 or 2 mg estradiol, be sufficient to protect their skeletons?

Notelovitz: Unfortunately, there is no correlation between the presence and severity of symptoms and the incidence of osteoporosis. If there were, it would be an ideal means of discrimination. As far as the dosage that you mention is concerned, I think both would be adequate for prevention in the management of osteoporosis.

Hammerstein: I should like to return to these runners, the women who run themselves into amenorrhoea. I thought that the loss of bone mass was just the result of becoming amenorrhoeic and of ceasing to produce estrogens. Is this right or is there also some other explanation?

Notelovitz: I think the generally accepted explanation is that it is the amenorrhoea associated with a loss of body weight which causes the decrease in estrogen levels to the point where the protective effect of estrogens is lost. However, as I mentioned in the one paper, when you look at other aspects such as the presence of an adequate intake of calcium, you certainly find that these women happen to be deficient in calcium as well. I am not too sure what the answer to the problem really is, because when you have women who have become amenorrhoeic for other reasons, e.g. the anorectics, and you exercise them – and I think it is the degree of exercise which is important –, you find that you can improve the bone mass. However, I think the real answer to the question is that, if a woman is exercising excessively to the extent that she causes amenorrhoea, then she is putting herself at greater risk. The problem with these individuals is getting them to cut back on exercising. It is a very difficult thing to do and, consequently, can be an indication for the use of estrogen therapy.

Question: My question concerns something I haven't heard mentioned today. Is there a minimum effective dose for estradiol valerate in respect of calcium metabolism or its effectiveness in the prevention of osteoporosis?

Lindsay: That is a very difficult question to answer, but my understanding of the literature is that 2 mg of estradiol valerate clearly lowers urinary calcium, while 1 mg is less, but probably still, effective.

Question: Dr. Lindsay, what is the present status of fluoride in the possible prevention of osteoporosis?

Lindsay: I believe that fluoride has a clear but undefined role place in the therapy of oesteoporosis, and this will probably be borne out by the two prospective studies being conducted in the United States in the Mayo Clinic and the Henry Ford Hospital.

Question: This question also concerns the preventive treatment of osteoporosis. If it is decided to give preventive treatment, then what is the optimum duration of treatment? I think this is important because there is some disagreement as to what happens when the treatment is discontinued. How fast will the bone mass then be lost?

Notelovitz: It depends on what modality of prevention is being used. I think I mentioned in my presentation that, if you are using lifestyle and exercise as a means of prevention, then this has to be continued ad infinitum. The question of hormonal therapy is very interesting, as Dr. Lindsay pointed out earlier this morning. The use of oral contraceptives in the younger woman also seems to have a bone-conserving effect. If this hidden benefit means that osteoporosis can be prevented later in life, then I think this is another reason for the use of oral contraceptives in women of reproductive age. As regards the use of estrogen therapy in postmenopausal women – in those who have not yet developed osteoporosis –, I would agree with John Studd that you really need to keep the treatment going until the age of 60 or 65. Dr. Lindsay will be able to answer the question in terms of long-term usage at the end of 10 years, but I think he is beginning to see a slight decrease in the bone mineral content. Nevertheless, if it were up to me, I think I would still advocate continuation of the therapy up to the age of 65. I choose this age because it is the time when the natural decrease in bone mineral content ceases.

Lindsay: I have just one comment to make, and that is that the retrospective case control data suggest that a minimum of 5 years of therapy commenced as close as possible to the menopause is effective at least in the prevention of hip fractures. I think that these data are a little looser than some of the prospective data that will come out, and I suspect that we'll end up with a minimum time of about 10 years of treatment if we want to see a significant impact on the incidence of facture in the over-65 age groups.

Hammerstein: We should leave the subject of osteoporosis and its related problems now and turn to a point that is true not only for this symposium but also for the FIGO congress as a whole, and that is that psychology is totally underrepresented. Even here we have only one lecture on psychological aspects – despite the fact that many of the troubles of climacteric patients lie in this direction. I should therefore like to ask my co-chairman what the psychologist can do to help the patients and to save estrogens?

Frick-Bruder: A few remarks first on the question of climacteric depression and its medical management. I believe that most depressive reactions in the climacteric are quite normal and not a sign of sickness or illness. Most if not all of us here in this room have experienced these depressive reactions at some time of our lives when we have been faced with limits and loss. It helps a lot to get this across to the patients – that they must accept their depressive reactions and that they are transient. We have a special term for this coping behaviour in Germany – Trauerarbeit, or affliction work. It is essential in the process of growing older that the patients accept that this contributes to limits and losses. I think it is something quite different from so-called endogenous depression, which has nothing to do with the climacteric. So, although the use of hormones can be helpful, getting the patient to understand this is, in my experience, also very helpful.

2.2 Hormonal treatment

Selection of patients – kind and duration of treatment

J. W. W. Studd, H. M. Andersen, J. C. Montgomery

The long-term metabolic benefits of estrogen therapy related to bones (Christiansen), the bladder (Versi) and the skin (Brincat) are covered in this symposium. This chapter will deal principally with selection of patients and selection and duration of the appropriate estrogen therapy.

It is clear that before any therapy can be considered, the correct diagnosis must be made. This essential principle of medicine is especially important when considering the climacteric because of the large overlap between true symptoms of estrogen deficiency and those of psychological or behavioural disorders occurring in the fourth and fifth decades of life.

There is no doubt that a significant increase in psychiatric morbidity occurs at this time. It is a time of many life stresses related to children leaving home, marital problems, aging and disenchantment with life and career. However, the peak incidence of psychiatric morbidity occurs in women aged 45 to 50 years and is directly related to the menopause, a time of profound hormonal changes [1]. Women are often prescribed psychiatric drugs at this time. Forty to fifty percent of new patients attending the Dulwich Hospital Menopause Clinic are receiving psychotropic drugs [2]. This sort of treatment with tranquillizers and anti-depressants must be quite inappropriate. On the other hand estrogen therapy for the climacteric, in spite of its clear benefits and few disadvantages, should not be used in a wayward fashion or become a prop for the psychoneurotic who would abuse and discredit such therapy [3].

Symptoms

The most characteristic symptoms of estrogen deficiency are the vasomotor symptoms which consist of hot flushes, night sweats, palpitations and headaches. These invariably respond to estrogen therapy within three weeks of commencement.

Another characteristic group of symptoms is due to pelvic atrophy. Vaginal dryness and dyspareunia are the most common. Urinary symptoms of frequency, urgency and incontinence (due to urethral and trigonal atrophy) are also common in climacteric women. These symptoms should be treated with estrogens and not antispasmodics or antibiotics which rarely work.

Although hot flushes are the most common symptoms, the most disturbing complaints are the psychological manifestations. These consist of loss of sleep, tiredness to the point of exhaustion, irritability, loss of energy, loss of libido and sometimes profound depression. These occur in an insidious way in women who have been in control of their lives, their families and their career. The occurrence of these disabling emotional problems is to them an incomprehensible nadir of their lives.

The fourth group of menopausal symptoms are the musculo-skeletal ones, which consist of aches and pains that may result from osteoporosis or the loss of collagen from the ligaments and other soft tissues. It is frequent for women to complain of thin, dry skin, brittle nails and loss of hair and it is easy to attribute these complaints to introspection and anxiety about body image. However, these symptoms are real and are the result of the profound loss of collagen from the body, particularly the skin, that occurs following decrease in estrogen levels [4].

Attitudes

Unfortunately, the attitude persists that the menopause is natural and all things natural must be good. The corollary to this which seems to be more a spiritual comment than a medical one is that these women do not need any estrogen therapy as the problems for some patients with enough fortitude will simply go away. Although this is bad enough, it is probably even worse when, although a problem is recognized, antidepressants or tranquillizers are prescribed. These powerful psychoactive drugs have no place whatsoever in the treatment of the menopause as they only confuse the patient. Their use should be specifically reserved for depression and anxiety neurosis, and should be withhold in patients with suspected climacteric problems until estrogen has been implemented for an adequate period.

Choice of patients

Women can experience wretched, disabling symptoms. The menopause, although easily diagnosed, can only be recognised if it is considered. In women who no longer have periods or who have had a hysterectomy and bilateral oophorectomy, the diagnosis is usually straightforward. Although the symptoms of the climateric syndrome are varied, the finding of hot flushes and sweats are virtually diagnostic. The complaint of vaginal dryness is also a strong indicator. If these characteristic symptoms occur in combination with loss of libido, loss of energy, headaches or depression, the diagnosis is almost sure to be the climacteric, and estrogen therapy can be started. Estrogen therapy can also serve as a diagnostic test when the diagnosis has not been made with confidence.

Frequently symptoms occur in women having periods [5]; often these are more severe than those seen in women whose periods have ceased. These women who do not have the diagnostic feature of amenorrhoea are frequently not considered for treatment because the diagnosis, for obvious reasons, is often missed. However, it should be apparent from a careful history and, once again, the presence of flushes within the symptom complex that the patient is perimenopausal and will respond to estrogen therapy. If confirmation is required, a single determination of blood FSH level solves the problem if FSH is higher than 15 U/l, then they are perimenopausal [6]. Conversely, if women have FSH levels below 15 U/l, they are not truly perimenopausal and do not have hot flushes. These women do not usually have estrogen responsive symptoms.

Levels of LH, on the other hand, are not helpful for diagnosis since the postmenopausal levels of LH never reach the high levels found in the pre-ovulatory surge in younger women. Treatment of patients with no symptoms is perhaps more controversial. Enthusiasts see no problem here and would certainly treat women after hysterectomy and bilateral oophorectomy either by oral administration of estrogen or by insertion of pellets of estradiol, and perhaps testosterone, in the wound at the time of closure [7]. Similarly a woman in good health with no symptoms who is merely anxious about future osteoporosis may request estrogen therapy. In practice, this occurs quite infrequently, because the informed patient conjures up a few symptoms, real or imaginary, to avoid any conflict. Nevertheless if the attending physician believes in the overall benefits, including the prophlactic effect upon the skeleton it is very difficult for him to justify the denial of estrogen replacement to such a healthy asymptomatic woman.

Contraindictions

As with all therapies, estrogen therapy requires consideration of the severity of the illness to be treated and the possible side-effects. Most workers would accept that breast carcinoma and recent endometrial carcinoma are contraindications, but scientific support of both these objections is hard to find. It is not unusual to find a woman with such an estrogen-dependent tumour who claims that her life is made so wretched by the menopausal symptoms that she would be prepared to take the risk of estrogen therapy. Frequently she would commence medication with oral estrogens and attend the clinic with this a fait accompli. There is in fact little evidence that estrogen therapy produces a recurrence of breast or endometrial carcinoma (Creasman W. T., personal communication) but if a recurrence does occur it is likely that estrogens will be blamed.

Hypertension, varicose veins, a previous thrombotic episode, diabetes, endometriosis and fibroids are classically regarded as contra-indications, but this is almost certainly result of over cautiousness. There is no evidence that natural estrogens, i.e., estrone, estradiol or estriol, cause any elevation of blood pressure in a normotensive or hypertensive woman [8]. The apparent objections to this treatment in the presence of varicose veins are based on the assumption that estrogens have a thrombogenic potential. However, there is no evidence that natural estrogens either affect coagulation, fibrolysis or platelet behaviour or cause deep vein thrombosis [9, 10]. If estrogen therapy avoids the first-pass liver effect by employing a percutaneous estradiol implant or estradiol cream, there is no reason why synthesis of coagulation factors from the liver should be stimulated. A great deal of work comparing the effect of various hormones on glucose tolerance makes it possible to state confidently that although synthetic ethinylestradiol and mestranol are diabetogenic, "natural estrogens" such as estrone, estradiol and estriol are not [11].

Endometriosis and fibroids are certainly responsive to endogenous and exogenous estrogens and it is possible that such therapy will stimulate activity of these benign gynaecological conditions. This does not, in practice, represent any clinical problem because treatment can easily be discontinued. Patients who have undergone a hysterectomy with or without oophorectomy for these conditions do not have any contra-indication for estrogen therapy. This is particularly true for endometriosis when the woman is quite young, and may have suffered a surgical castration. The surgeon has a compelling but illogical reluctance to prescribe replacement estrogens in case the pain of this condition recurs.

Preliminary investigations

After the establishment of the diagnosis, the examination should be no more than the routine annual check-up that women should undergo. This should include a check of blood pressure and weight, urine analysis, pelvic examination, cervical cytology and palpation of the breasts. It is possible that in the future pelvic ultrasound and mammography may be added to these routine annual checks, but this is really a statement about the need for routine screening rather than a comment on any putative risks of estrogen therapy.

Because the staff at the Dulwich Hospital Menopause Clinic is energetically involved in research, we need to draw a clear distinction between investigations required for scientific study and examinations required for supervision of therapy. Fundamentally the climacteric is easily diagnosed and its treatment is safe and straightforward. It must not be made difficult, exclusive or expensive [12].

These comments are particularly relevant to the investigations of plasma hormone profiles and the endometrial status in women before beginning therapy. Such investigations are expensive, time consuming and create an obstacle between patient and the fulfillment of her simple therapeutic needs. It is rarely necessary to perform assays of FSH or estradiol and never necessary to assay the other half a dozen hormones which are frequently offered as a package deal. Occasionally the difficult diagnosis in a woman with menstruation and atypical symptoms may need to be clarified by a single FSH assay. The younger woman with a premature menopause will also need this investigation to clarify the cause of her amenorrhoea.

A preliminary endometrial biopsy, whether done under general anaesthesia or as an outpatient Vabra curettage, is not necessary unless there is a history of irregular or post-menopausal bleeding. Nobody would recommend routine endometrial biopsy in postmenopausal women in order to diagnose early endometrial pathology. The plan to prescribe estrogens to such a woman does not create this need.

Choice of treatment

The consultation is clearly an important event; it provides not only the opportunity to make the diagnosis but also to reassure the woman that these many distressing and incomprehensible symptoms are indeed due to the menopause and that they are easily treatable. This support is of especially great value when the woman and her family think that she is psychiatrically disturbed and doctors who resist estrogen therapy have done nothing to dissuade them from that conclusion. Estrogen therapy is not one of just reassurance, is not one of placebo therapy and is certainly not one of tranquillizers or anti-depressants. Estrogens are not only the most effective therapy – they are the only therapy which to our current knowledge effectively treats the symptomatic and the metabolic sequelae of the menopause.

Some women with minimal symptoms may be happy with reassurance and not wish to receive hormone therapy. The vasomotor symptoms of the climacteric syndrome may be mild and may last for less than a year. In these cases, a conservative attitude may be adopted by both physician and patient, although the prevention of the long-term skeletal problems should be considered. Most patients need and request some form of symptomatic relief by estrogen therapy.

At its simplest this treatment involves the application of estrogen tablets for 3 weeks out of 4, using natural estrone, estradiol or estriol, a weak estrogen. Most oral preparations contain various esters of estrone or estradiol (Harmogan, Premarin and Progynova). Synthetic estrogens such as ethinylestradiol or mestranol should not be prescribed as they produce long-term metabolic side effects. The non-steroidal oral preparations of stilboestrol or dienoestrol should also not be used. If estrogens are given in this cyclical manner without added progestogen, bleeding may or may not occur in the week off, hyperplasia occurs in 7 to 14.8% (Table 1) and irregular bleeding is a not-infrequent occurrence [13]. Therefore it is justifiable to

Table 1 Total number of biopsy specimens, type of specimen and number showing abnormal histology in 745 women receiving hormone replacement.

Regimen	No	Biopsy specimens Unsatis.	Satis.	No (%) of abn. specimens
Low Estrogen	76	33	43	3 (7.0)
High Estrogen	232	56	176	26 (14.8)
Estrogen and Progestogen	366	41	325	4 (1.1)
Estrogen implant and Progestogen	328	45	286	42 (14.8)
Total	1002	175	827	75 (9.1)

use unopposed estrogens for short-term therapy for up to one year. For longer therapy progestogens should be added [14].

Estrogen skin creams, although used extensively in France, have not yet assumed much popularity elsewhere in spite of high patient acceptability and lack of side effects. Current developments in research on estrogen patches will encourage further studies of this interesting route of administration.

Another means of administration which avoids the first-pass liver effect is the percutaneous implantation of estradiol as pioneered by Greenblatt 1949 [15]. Implants have been used extensively by our team and have become our first-choice means of therapy. Ten years ago 7% of patients had estrogen implants; this has risen to 85%. The technique is quick, simple, and performed in the surgery [16]. After the skin of the abdomen or buttock is infiltrated with local anaesthetic, a small 4 mm incision is made to facilitate entry of the trocar and cannula, which are then pushed into the subcutaneous fat, avoiding the rectus sheath, muscle and any old scar tissue. The hormone pellets are then introduced into the cannula and pushed by the obturator into the fat. The instrument is gently withddrawn with pressure exerted over the track for a short time to prevent any oozing of blood and haematoma formation. The usual dose is 25 mgs, 50 mgs or 100 mgs of estradiol with or without 100 mgs of testosterone.

Pellet implantation is particularly appropriate for those patients with no uterus and ovaries who have no risk of any irregular bleeding. In these cases there is a need to add testosterone because of the lack of ovarian androgens. Other indications for implantation are unsatisfactory oral therapy due to inadequate response or gastro-intestinal side effects. Implantations are also particularly useful for women complaining of loss of libido, loss of energy and depression who respond to testosterone. Our double-blind randomised trial of patients on placebo, estradiol and estradiol and testosterone implants showed that testosterone offers additional benefits in treating the above symptoms. [17].

The symptomatic relief following implantation begins in approximately 3 weeks and last for 5 to 6 months, when a repeat implant is usually needed. The pharmacokinetics of this treatment are outlined by Cardozo [2] in this symposium.

Whether the form of administration is tablets, skin cream or percutaneous implants, there is a considerable risk of irregular bleeding if progestogen is not added. There is no doubt that unopposed continuous and prolonged estrogen stimulation from a source as powerful and effective as an estradiol pellet will invariably result in cystic hyperplasia. A study of more than *700* patients on various regimens of hormone replacement therapy demonstrated that failure to take progestogens with an implant led to hyperplasia in 55.8% of cases (Table 2).

Although patients with oral therapy can be allowed cyclical unopposed estrogen therapy for a short period of time, patients receiving continuous estrogens by implant must take a course of progestogens every month to ensure regular bleeding and to prevent hyperplasia. Thirteen days of progestogen ensures virtually a zero percent incidence of hyperplasia whether estrogen administration is oral or percutaneous. Seven days of progestogen is associated with a 5.9% incidence of hyperplasia when used in conjunction with oral therapy (Tables 2 and 3). This protective

Table 2 Abnormal histology in satisfactory endometrial biopsy samples in women with estradiol implants receiving treatment with progestogen.

Duration of Progestogen (days)	Satisfactory biopsy	Abnormal histology total (%)
0	43	24 (55.8)
5	144	12 (8.3)
7	40	5 (12.5)
10	33	1 (3.0)
>10	23	0 (0)
Total	283	42 (14.8)

Table 3 Abnormal histology in satisfactory endometrial biopsy samples in women receiving oral estrogen and progestogen

Regimen	Days of Progestogen	Satisfactory Biopsy	Abnormal Histology Total (%)
Prempak	7	17	1 (5.9)
Cyclo-Progynova	10	54	1 (1.9)
Syntex Menophase	13	139	0 (0)

effect of progestogen has been recognised and various combination preparations are available commercially. These include: Cyclo-Progynova 1 mg or 2 mg. (Estradiol-valerate and levonorgestrel for 10 days.)

Prempak and Prempak C 0.625 mg or 1.25 mg. (Conjugated equine estrogens and norgestrel for 7 or 12 days.)

Trisequens (estradiol and estriol and norethisterone for 10 days.)

Problems with progestogens

Although there is no doubt that progestogens protect the endometrium, there is a fear that, as in the combined oral contraceptive, progestogens may have a deleterious effect upon the cardiovascular system [18, 19]. The effect upon lipids varies, but in general it seems to involve the lowering of the lipoproteins and in particular HDL [20, 21]. Moreover, progestogen causes many unpleasant symptomatic problems which are both dose and duration dependent. These include depression, irritability, bloated feelings, headaches and protean cyclical symptoms consistent with the premenstrual syndrome [22]. Women taking cyclical progestogens do not usually object to the necessary monthly period, but if this period is associated with

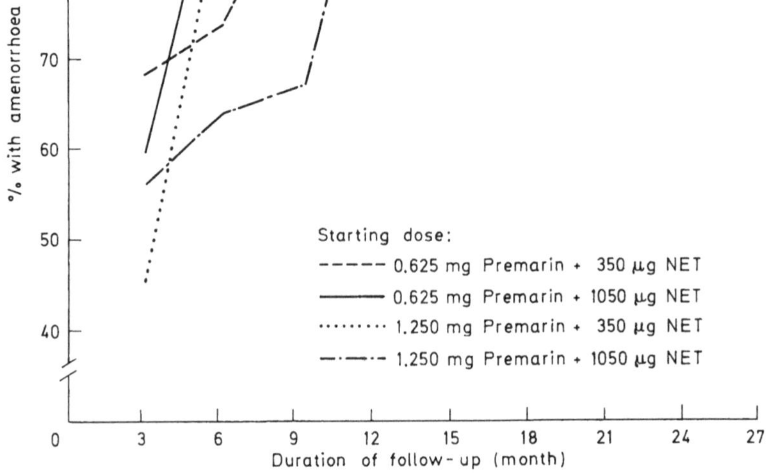

Figure 1 Bleeding Patterns after Continuous Oral Estrogens and Low Dose Progestogen

premenstrual symptoms, uterine cramps and dysmenorrhoea, the benefits of this therapy may be more difficult to appreciate.

We have attempted to reduce the dose of progestogen and the bleeding periods by prescribing oral estrogens in combination with very low but continuous doses of progestogens, in the belief that endometrial atrophy should be produced. Low and medium doses of oral estrogens were used in connection with 0.35 mg tablets of norethisterone (as in the progestogen-only contraceptive) using 1 to 3 per day. Figure 1 indicates that amenorrhoea is achieved in all patients by 9 months, and that the lower the dose of estrogen, the easier it is to achieve amenorrhoea [23]. Before amenorrhoea is established, the patient may experience occasional spotting which is not heavy and is usually acceptable as long as an end can be seen. Most patients prefer this continuous therapy with amenorrhoea, rather than therapies which result in cyclical bleeds. The progestogenic side effects were also avoided by using this continuous low dose of norethisterone.

This continuous estrogen/progestogen medication requires further evaluation as it would appear to be a logical regimen of oral therapy for the future. The patients no longer have to bleed, no longer have the behavioural disadvantages of oral progestogen, and have an atrophic endometrium.

The various options of estrogen therapy with or without progestogen are shown graphically in Figure 2.

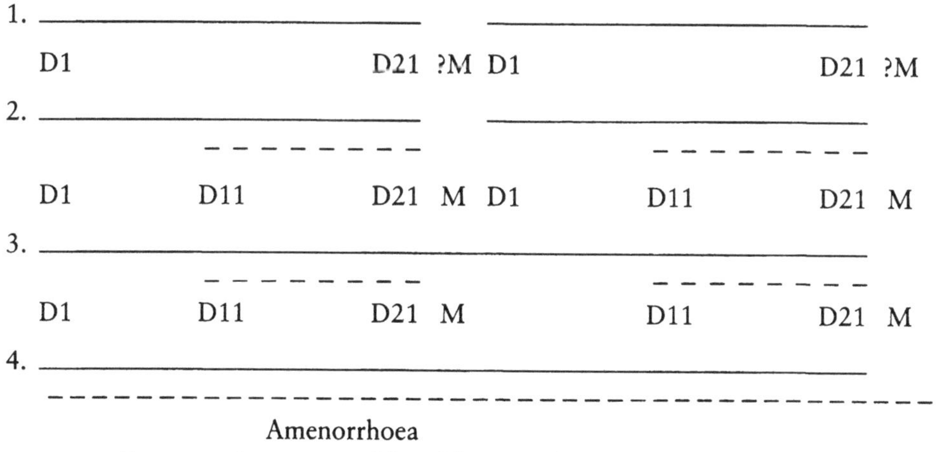

——— Estrogen therapy M = Menstruation

– – – – Progestogen therapy D = Days of Cycle

1. Cyclical unopposed estrogens, e.g., Premarin, Progynova
2. Cyclical opposed estrogens, e.g., Prempak, Cyclo-Progynova
3. Continuous estrogen & cyclical progestogens, e.g., implant
4. Continuous estrogen and continuous progestogens

Figure 2 Estrogen Therapy with or without Progestogens.

Although our team supplied much of the data showing the protective effect of progestogen [13, 14], we believe that because there are so many clinical and theoretical problems with progestogen, we prefer to use it sparly. For example we do not insist on full thirteen day courses and would accept 7 days of norethisterone 5 mgs, or even half that daily dose, if unacceptable symptoms still occurred.

The same philosophy is applied to the more controversial issue of the protective effect of progestogen on the breasts in women who have had a hysterectomy. Although Gambrell [24] has recently suggested that progestogen does have a protective effect, his evidence should be considered in conjunction with Pike's less convincing evidence that progestogen in the oral contraceptive pill increases the risk of the development of breast cancer [25]. More information is required before any clear statement on this can be given. Until then we would suggest that patients who have no uterus do not need progestogens.

Duration of therapy

The duration of estrogen replacement therapy is either an easy or a difficult problem according to one's philosophical point of view. Our belief is that if the long-term protective effect of estrogen therapy is accepted, then there seems to be no reason to limit the length of therapy. In practice, the patient decides this issue herself. If she is getting relief from climacteric symptoms with no side effects and is not distressed by any cyclical bleeding, it is certain that she will continue. She may well omit therapy for an occasional month, but the return of symptoms will firm up her view on this matter. On the other hand, if she feels no better on therapy, does not feel she needs estrogens, or has unpleasant side effects, that she will probably abandon this treatment. The confident physician should be willing to supervise this therapy for at least a decade of the patient's post-menopausal life.

During the time of long-term therapy it is necessary to sample the endometrium and this inconvenience might be unacceptable to both patient and doctor. The necessary frequency of endometrial sampling, most conveniently performed by outpatient curettage, is open to debate. Current opinion favors endometrial biopsy in the event of irregular bleeding. For patients taking cyclical unopposed estrogens biopsy may be necessary every year. The protective effect of progestogen for 7 to 12 days, can reduce the necessity of sampling to once every five years. Because it is likely that 13 days of progestogen removes all excess risk of serious endometrial pathology, the use of this regimen can eliminate the necessity of endometrial sampling altogether.

References

[1] Ballinger, C.B. (1975): Psychiatric Morbidity and the Menopause. Screening of General Population Sample. BMJ 1975:3; 344–346.

[2] Cardozo, L.D., Gibb, D.M.F., Tuck, S.M., Thom, M.H., Studd, J.W.W. and Cooper, D.J. (1984): The effects of subcutaneous hormone implants during the climacteric. Maturitas 1984:5; 177–184.

[3] Studd, J.W.W., Chakravati, S. and Oram, D. (1977): The Climacteric in the Menopause. In: Clinics in Obstetrics and Gynaecology 4, 1, 3–29. Ed.: Greenblatt, R.B. and Studd, J.W.W. W.B. Saunders & Co.

[4] Brincat, M., Moniz, C.J., Studd, J.W.W., Darby, A., Magos, A.L., Emburey, G. and Versi, E. (1985): Long term effects of the Menopause and Sex Hormones on Skin Thickness. Brit. J. O. & G. 1985:92; 256–259.

[5] Jazzman, L. (1973): Epidemiology of Climacteric and Post-Climacteric Complaints. Frontiers Hormone Research 1973:2; 22–34 (Karger, Basel).

[6] Chakravati, S., Collins, W.P., Thom, M.H. and Studd, J.W.W. (1979): Relationship between plasma hormone profiles, symptomatology and response to estrogen in women approaching the menopause. Brit. Med. J. 1979:1; 983–985.

[7] Studd, J.W.W., Chakravati, S. and Collins, W.P. (1978): Plasma Hormone Profiles after the Menopause and Bilateral Oophorectomy. Postgraduate Mecial Journal 54 (2), 25–30.

[8] Hammond, C.B., Jelovsek, F.R., Lee, K.L., Creasman, W.T. and Parker, R.J. (1979): Effects of long term estrogen replacement therapy. 1 Metabolic effects: Am. J. Obstet. Gynecol. 1970:133; 5, 525–535.

[9] Thom, M., Dubiel, M., Kakkar, V.V. and Studd, J.W.W. (1978): The effects of different regimens of estrogen on the Clotting and Fibronolytic system of the postmenopausal woman. Frontier Hormone Research 1978:5; 192–202 (Karger, Basel).

[10] A report from the Boston Collaborative Drug Surveillance Program (1974): Surgically confirmed gall bladder disease venous thromobembolism and breast tumours in relation to post-menopausal estrogen therapy. New Engl. J. Med. 1974:290! 15–19.

[11] Thom, M., Chakravarti, S., Oram, D.H. and Studd, J.W.W. (1977): Effect of Hormone Replacement Therapy on Glucose Tolerance in Postmenopausal Women. Brit. J. Obstet. Gynaecol. 1977:84; 776–784.

[12] Studd, J.W.W. and Thom, M. (1981): Ovarian Failure and Ageing. Clinics in Endocrinology and Metabolism **10**, 1, 89–113. W.B. Saunders & Co.

[13] Paterson, M.E.L., Wade-Evans, T., Sturdee, D.W., Thom, M.H. and Studd, J.W.W. (1980): Endometrial disease after treatment with estrogens and progestogens in the climacteric. B.M.J. 1980:280; 822–827.

[14] Studd, J.W.W. and Thom, M. (1981): Estrogen and Endometrial Cancer. Progress in Obstetrics and Gynaecology. Vol. 1, 182–198. Ed.: Studd, J.W.W. Churchill Livingstone, London.

[15] Greenblatt, R.B. and Duran, R.R. (1949): Indications for hormone pellets in the therapy of endocrine and gynaecological disorders. J. Obst. Gynecol. Brit. Emp. 1949: 51; 294–301.

[16] Thom, M.H. and Studd, J.W.W. (1980): Hormone Implantation B.M.J. 1980:280; 848–850.

[17] Montgomery, J.C., Appleby, L., Versi, E., Brincat, M., Tapp, A. and Studd, J.W.W. (in press): Prospective randomised study of Estradiol and Estradiol and Testosterone implants in the treatment of pschiatric and psychosexual problems at the menopause.

[18] Royal College of General Practitioners' Oral Contraceptive Study (1977): Effect on hypertension and benign breast disease of progestagen component in combined oral contraceptives. Lancet 1977:1:624.

[19] Meade, T.W., Greenberg, G. and Thompson, S.G. (1980): Progestogens and cardiovascular reactions associated with oral contraceptives and a comparison of the safety of 50 and 30 μg estrogen preparations. B.M.J. 1980:280; 1157–1161.

[20] Hirvonen, E., Malkonen, M. and Manni-

nen, V. (1981): Effect of different progestogens on lipoproteins during post menopausal replacement therapy. New Eng. J. Med. 1981:304; 560–563.

[21] Silfverstolpe, G., Gustafson, A., Samsioe, G. and Svanborg, A. (1979): Lipid metabolic studies in oophorectomized women; effects of three different progestogens. Acta Obstetrica et Gynaecologica Scand. 1979: Suppl. 88; 89–95.

[22] Magos, A. L., Brincat, M. and Studd, J. W. W. (1985): Treatment of the Premenstrual Syndrome by Subcutaneous Estradiol Implants and Cyclical Oral Norethisterone. (Submitted).

[23] Magos, A. L., Brincat, M., Studd, J. W. W., Wardle, P., Schlesinger P. and O'Dowd, T. (1985): Amenorrhea and Endometrial Atrophy with continuous oral estrogen and progestogen therapy in postmenopausal women. Obstet. Gynecol 1985:65; 496–499.

[24] Gambrell, D. (1985): The Protective Effect of Progestogen on the Breasts in Women who have had a hysterectomy. Personal Communication.

[25] Pike, M. C., Henderson, B. E., Krailo, M. D., Duke, A. and Roy, S. (1983): Breast cancer in young women and use of oral contraceptives: possible modifying effect of formulation and age at use. Lancet 1983:II; 926–929.

Routes of estrogen administration

L. Cardozo

Now that it is widely accepted that estrogen replacement therapy is the appropriate treatment for the climacteric syndrome our aim must be to provide the most effective treatment with the fewest side-effects. Estrogens may be given orally as tablets; parenterally as a cream – percutaneously or directly to the vagina; as a subcutaneous implant, vaginal ring or transdermally. Although the pharmacodynamic properties have been studied for all routes of administration there is, as yet, little comparative data regarding the efficacy of the different types of treatment in terms of symptom relief and patient acceptability. In the majority of cases estrogens in any form will give adequate symptom control because of the high plasma levels achieved.

Oral estrogen therapy is the most popular form of treatment although this is not necessarily always the best route of administration. Parenteral estrogens differ from oral estrogens because they by-pass the gastrointestinal tract. This fundamental difference is important as the passage of estrogens through the liver causes certain changes. Oral estrogens are absorbed through the gut wall and enter the liver via the portal system before continuing on into the general circulation. In the liver about a third of the dose of oral estrogen is converted to estrone-3-glucuronide which is excreted in the urine and bile without producing the desired effect; thus the dose of orally administered estrogen needs to be significantly higher than the dose of parenterally administered estrogen required to provide the same symptom relief.

A study by Campbell and Whitehead (1982) has shown that during a 24 hour period the plasma levels of estrone-3-glucuronide were not elevated above the baseline following the administration of parenteral estrogens. After an oral dose of estradiol valerate the mean levels of estrone-3-glucuronide at least doubled throughout the 24 hours, with a peak following ingestion of the preparation. This correspondend almost exactly with an increase in the plasma estrone level following oral administration. This fluctuation in plasma level may be a problem if one dose of estrogen is to be given to control symptoms for 24 hours. The rate of absorption and release of the active estrogen from creams and implants occurs without peaks and troughs so that the dose can be kept at a minimum for maximum effect.

In pre-menopausal women the physiological ratio of plasma estradiol to estrone is greater than one. This is maintained by the natural production of estrogens by the ovary. When estradiol is administered orally a large proportion is converted, by dehydrogenation, to estrone. Thus the ratio of estradiol to estrone in women treated with oral estrogens is reversed. This is not so for women treated with parenteral estradiol, which is absorbed as such and only later partially converted to estrone as part of the normal metabolism of estradiol. Since both estrone and estradiol relieve symptoms of the climacteric, the higher level of estrone achieved with oral therapy may be unimportant.

Because of their passage through the liver, oral estrogens cause certain hepatocellular effects which do not occur when estrogens are prescribed parenterally. Oral estrogens produce an increase in sex-hormone binding globulin, cortisol binding globulin and renin substrate. Mashchak and colleagues (1982) have shown that this increase is much greater following oral administration of synthetic estrogens such as diethylstilbestrol and ethinylestradiol than with natural estrogens.

Synthetic estrogens are also associated with an increased incidence of thrombo-embolic disease due to increased platelet aggregation and reduced anti-thrombin III, so their use should be avoided in post-menopausal women requiring hormone replacement therapy. Even natural estrogens, given orally, cause a reduction in the level of anti-thrombin III activity (Elkik et al., 1982). With parenteral estrogen there is no change in anti-thrombin III activity.

Estrogens are thought to protect against ischaemic heart disease by increasing the high density/low density lipoprotein ratio. Although both oral and parenteral estrogens have been shown to decrease low density lipoprotein, only oral estrogens have been shown to increase high density lipoprotein (Fahraeus et al., 1981). Thus oral estrogen therapy may have more beneficial effect on lipid metabolism than parenteral therapy. As yet, however, no studies have shown a difference in the incidence of ischaemic heart disease.

The incidence of endometrial hyperplasia and the probability of causing a well-differentiated adenocarcinoma of the endometrium is increased whatever route of administration is used. Assessment of estrogen concentration within the nuclei of endometrial cells has shown a higher level of estradiol than estrone (Whitehead, et al., 1981), so it is likely that estradiol has a greater effect on cell proliferation. In this respect, therefore, oral estrogens, when unopposed, may be preferable as they are probably associated with a lower incidence of endometrial hyperplasia than are parentally administered estrogens. However, the addition of cyclical progestogen therapy for 13 days each month has been shown to virtually abolish endometrial hyperplasia (Studd et al., 1980).

The use of oral estrogens for replacement therapy is well established and in North America it is still the preferred route (Judd et al., 1981). In a large double-blind crossover study in 1977, Campbell and Whitehead showed that significant relief of climacteric symptoms was achieved using 1.25 mg conjugated estrogens daily.

From the patient's point of view, oral therapy requires daily patient compliance and if given cyclically there may be a return of symptoms in the treatment-free week. Some patients develop nausea and even vomiting with oral estrogens. However, it is possible to vary the dose of oral therapy to suit the individual patient and, if necessary, therapy can be stopped abruptly with very little carryover effect. Very occasionally oral estrogens are not effective because of de-activation in the liver. This has been shown in patients taking hydantoin for epilepsy (Englund and Johansson, 1978). Such patients will benefit from parenteral therapy if their symptoms are purely due to hypoestrogenism.

Vaginal estrogen creams have long been used in the treatment of atrophic vaginitis. They were originally thought to produce a local effect only, but more recent studies have shown that the plasma levels of estrone and estradiol achieved using a standard daily dose of 1.25 mg of conjugated estrogen cream are the same or higher than those produced by the same dose of oral conjugated estrogen (Whitehead et al., 1978). The only difference is the time at which the peak plasma levels occur, since the vaginal epithelium allows a much faster absorption than the gastrointestinal tract. Very low doses of vaginal estrogens (0.1 mg daily) are capable of producing significant changes in vaginal cytology and do not cause a rise in plasma estrogen levels (Dyer et al., 1982). However, there is no long-term study to show that such low doses vaginal estrogens are completely safe in patients for whom estrogens are contra-indicated. Despite the low plasma levels it is still not certain that there is no associated systemic effect. Certainly if vaginal estrogens are prescribed in the normal manufacturer's recommended dose, cyclical progestogens should also be prescribed to women with a uterus to protect the endometrium.

The rate of absorption of estrogens from the vagina is affected by the state of the vaginal epithelium. In women with atrophic vaginitis, absorption is poor during the first week of treatment but improves during the second and third weeks because of the improved cytological status of the vagina and the increased vascularity (Whitehead et al., 1978). Thus after estrogenisation has taken place, a very small maintenance dose of estrogen cream should be sufficient to maintain the improved status.

Another factor affecting the rate of absorption of locally applied estrogens is the medium in which it is suspended. Estradiol in saline has been shown to give much higher plasma levels than the same dose in ointment (Schiff et al., 1977); the usual vaginal creams, such as conjugated estrogen cream, slow down the rate of absorption so that one application gives increased plasma levels throughout 24 hours without peaks and troughs. However, some women find the slowly absorbed cream messy and it has been known to produce gynaecomastia in their male sexual partners (Di Raimondo et al., 1980).

Percutaneous estrogen cream is relatively new and is not yet marketed worldwide. Estradiol is suspended in a hydroalcoholic gel which is rubbed into the skin of the lower anterior abdominal wall from which it is easily absorbed. The standard manufacturer's recommended dose is 5 g of cream containing 3 mg of estradiol daily. As previously explained, this method of administration gives a physiological serum estradiol to estrone ratio by by-passing the entero-hepatic circulation. Various studies have shown that it produces good symptomatic relief and is a safe form of hormone replacement therapy in postmenopausal women which appears to mimick the physiological state (Strecker et al., 1980).

Lyrenas et al. (1981) showed that compared to oral estrogens the percutaneous cream produced a quite slow increase in serum estrogens which was maintained longer (48 hours). Furthermore, as anticipated, with percutaneous cream there was a much higher rise in serum estradiol and a less marked increase in serum estrone. The estradiol to estrone ratio after three days treatment with percutaneous estradiol cream was 1.51. However, the daily application of cream does require some patients compliance and some patients find the cream rather sticky, although it dries quite quickly.

Percutaneous estrogen can also be administered as a transdermal estradiol patch. This consists of two membranes about 3 cm in diameter enclosing a reservoir of estradiol. The lower membrane is covered by adhesive tape and is permeable to estradiol. Various strengths of patch are available which deliver 25, 50 or 100 µg of estradiol daily. They are designed to stay in place for three days. Evaluations of transdermal estradiol patches have shown that they produce all the usual changes associated with parenteral estrogen therapy. They are well tolerated by patients and have not been shown to produce any systemic side effects (Padwick et al., 1985). However, long-term use may reveal local skin reactions and the patches may become detached prematurely.

Continuous parenteral delivery of estradiol has the theoretical advantage of mimikking physiological conditions. This can be achieved using vaginal rings or subcutaneous implants. Cylindrical silicone vaginal rings impregnated with estradiol have proved effective in the treatment of the climacteric syndrome. Although they produce an initially high level of plasma estradiol, thereafter a relatively constant level is maintained for several weeks. The estimated daily delivery of estradiol is 0.2 mg (Englund et al., 1981). The rings are easy to insert and remove and do not interfere with coitus. They have not, however, gained widespread popularity.

The use of subcutaneous estrogen implants which release their active component over several months is not new (Bishop, 1938). For over 30 years implants have been used to treat the climacteric syndrome (Greenblatt and Buran, 1949). However, this form of therapy has never gained the same popularity as oral estrogens. The technique of implantation is simple and can be done in the office or out-patients' clinic under local anaesthetic. Thom et al. (1981) studied the effect of 50 mg and 100 mg estradiol on the hormone profiles of postmenopausal women undergoing implant therapy. They showed that in response to 100 mg of estradiol the plasma follicle stimulating hormone and luteinising hormone fell dramatically within two weeks of implantation and that the levels were lowest two to three months after implantation. After this they gradually rose but did not yet return to their pre-treatment level at six months. The rise in serum estrogens corresponded to the fall in gonadotrophins, which was maximal at two to three months after implantation. Although there was a good rise in serum estrogens, the level did not exceed the physiological pre-menopausal range and the serum estradiol to estrone ratio was physiological. Estradiol implants have also been shown to improve vaginal cytology within 14 days of treatment (Nagamani et al., 1977).

The use of subcutaneous hormone implants avoids the need for daily patient compliance. A methyl testosterone pellet which is useful for the treatment of psychosexual symptoms but hepatotoxic when administered orally, can be inserted at the same time.

Hormone implant therapy gives good symptomatic relief and is acceptable to climacteric women. Side-effects and complications of therapy are rare (Cardozo et al., 1983).

In a prospective study of 55 post-menopausal women Brincat et al. (1983) compared the symptom relief from estradiol 50 mg and testosterone 100 mg with that obtained by a placebo implant. They assessed a selection of symptoms at two, four and six months after implantation. All symptoms apart from "aches and pains" were initially improved by a hormone implant. At four months improvement in the urethral syndrome was no longer significant and at six months only six symptoms (flushes, headaches, irritability, insomnia, depression and lethargy) were significantly improved. By contrast there was no improvement in symptoms at any time with placebo implants and many of the patients in that group demanded further treatment before the end of the study. From the results of this study it would seem that 50 mg estradiol implants require replacement at about four months if the return of troublesome symptoms is to be avoided.

With such a wide range of good estrogen preparations available it is difficult to know how to choose the right one for each patient. Estradiol implants are useful for those women who have a predominance of psychosexual symptoms since it allows testosterone to be given concurrently, and for those women who have undergone a hysterectomy since, as then no tablets are required, treatment can be forgotten for months at a time.

Oral therapy or percutaneous cream may be more suitable for first-time estrogen users as the dose can be adjusted and therapy stopped if problems arise, whereas an implant, once in situ may be difficult to remove. Patients who have a predisposition for arterial disease or a family history of myocardial infarction or cerebrovascular accidents may be better treated oral estrogens because of their beneficial effect on lipid metabolism. Similarly women who have developed cystic glandular hyperplasia might benefit from the reversed serum estrone to estradiol ratio produced by oral therapy.

For those patients who develop nausea or vomiting with oral estrogens or in whom symptomatic relief is inadequate parenteral therapy with implants or percutaneous cream may be more helpful. Parenteral therapy is also more appropriate for patients with previous histories of thromboembolic disease if estrogen therapy is required.

It is usually advisable to treat localised atrophic changes of the lower genital tract with vaginal creams. Providing the dose is small enough, it is probably safe to withhold progestogens which makes treatment more acceptable to the older woman who has long since stopped menstruating and would find the return of vaginal bleeding difficult to cope with.

Whichever route of administration is used for estrogen replacement therapy, it is important to remember that treatment should be given for an adequate time span, usually at least two years, for the relief of symptoms and that when therapy is stopped it should be withdrawn gradually to prevent a recurrence of distressing climacteric symptoms.

References

[1] Bishop, P. M. F. (1938): A clinical experiment in estrogen therapy. Brit. Med. J. 1:939–941.

[2] Brincat, M., Magos, A., Studd, J. W. W., Cardozo, L. D., O'Dowd, T., Wardle, P., Cooper, D. J. (1984): Subcutaneous hormone implants – A prospective study. The Lancet. 8367, 16–18.

[3] Campbell, S., Whitehead, M. I. (1977): Estrogen therapy and the menopausal syndrome. Ed. Greenblatt, R. B., Studd, J. W. W. Clinics in Obstetrics and Gynaecology 4 (1) (The Menopause). W. B. Saunders 31–47.

[4] Campbell, S., Whitehead, M. I. (1982): Potency and hepato-cellular effects of estrogens after oral, percutaneous and subcutaneous administration. Ed. van Keep, P. A., Utian, W. H., Vermeulen, A. The Controversial Climacteric. M.T.P. Press 103–125.

[5] Cardozo, L. D., Gibb, D. M. F., Studd, J. W. W., Tuck, S. M., Thom, M. H., Cooper, D. J. (1984): The effects of subcutaneous hormone implants during the climacteric. Maturitas. 5:177–184.

[6] Di Raimondo, C. V., Roach, A. C., Meador, C. K. (1980): Gynaecomastia from exposure to vaginal estrogen cream. New Engl. J. Med. 302:1089–1095.

[7] Dyer, G., Townsend, P. T., Jelowitz, J., Young, O., Whitehead, M. I. (1982): Dose related changes in vaginal cytology after topical conjugated equine estrogens. Br. Med. J. 284:789–790.

[8] Elkik, F., Gompel, A., Mercier Bodard, C., Kutten, F., Guverne, P. N., Corvol, P., Marvais Jarvis, P. (1982): Comparative effects of percutaneous and conjugated estrogens on the level of plasma proteins and triglycerides in the post-menopausal woman. Am. J. Obstet. Gynecol. 143:888–892.

[9] Englund, D. E., Johansson, E. D. B. (1978): Plasma levels of estrone, estradiol and gonadotrophins in post-menopausal women after oral and vaginal administration of conjugated equine estrogens. Brit. J. Obstet. Gynaecol. 85:957–954.

[10] Englund, D. E., Victor, A., Johansson, E. D. B. (1981): Pharmacokinetics and pharmaco-dynamic effects of vaginal estradiol administration from silastic rings in postmenopausal women. Maturitas. 3:125–129.

[11] Fahraeus, L., Wallentin, L., Larsson

Cohn, U. in Campbell, S. and Whitehead, M.I. (1982): Potency and hepatocellular effects of estrogens after oral, percutaneous and subcutaneous administration. Ed. van Keep, P.A., Utian, W.H., Vermeulen, Al. The controversial climacteric. M.T.P. Press 103–125.

[12] Greenblatt, R.B., Buran, R.R. (1949): Indications for hormone pellets in the therapy of endocrine and gynecological disorders. Am. J. Obstet. Gynecol. 57:294–301.

[13] Judd, H.L., Cleary, R.E., Creasman, W.T., Figge, D., Kase, N., Rosenwaks, Z., Tagatz, G. (1981): Estrogen replacement therapy. Obstet. Gynecol. 58:267–275.

[14] Lyrenas, S., Carlström, K., Backström, T., von Schoultz, B. (1981): A comparison of serum estrogen levels after percutaneous and oral administration of estradiol 17B, Brit. J. Obstet. Gynaecol. 83:181–187.

[15] Mashchak, C.A., Lobo, R.A., Dozono-Takano, R., Eggena, P., Nakamura, R.M., Brenner, P.F., Mishell, D.R. (1982): Comparison of pharmacodynamic properties of various estrogen formulations. Am. J. Obstet. Gynecol. 144:511–518.

[15] Nagamani, M., Lin, T.J., McDonough, P.G., Watatani, H., McPherson, J.C., Mahesh, V.B. (1977): Clinical and endocrine studies in menopausal women after estradiol pellet implantation. Obstet. Gynecol. 5:541–547.

[17] Padwick, M.L., Endacott, J., Whitehead, M.I. (1985): Efficacy, acceptability and metabolic effects of transdermal estradiol in the management of postmenopausal women. Am. J. Obstet. Gynecol. 152:1085–1091.

[18] Schiff, I., Tulchinsky, D., Ryan, K.J. (1977): Vaginal absorption of estrone and 17B estradiol. Fertility and Sterility. 28:1063–1065.

[19] Strecker, J.R., Lauritzen, C.H., Nebelung, T., Musch, K. (1980): Climacteric symptoms, estrogens and gonadotrophins in plasma and urine after application of estradiol ointment on the abdominal skin of oophorectomized women. Ed. Mauvais-Jarvis, P., Vickers, C.F.H., Wepierre, J. Percutaneous absorption of steroids. 267–272.

[20] Studd, J.W.W., Thom, M.H., Paterson, M.E.L., Wade-Evans, T. (1980): The prevention and treatment of endometrial pathology in postmenopausal women receiving exogenous estrogens. Ed. Pasetto, N., Paoletti, R., Ambrus, J.L. The menopause and postmenopause. M.T.P. Press 127–139.

[21] Thom, M.H., Collins, W.P., Studd, M.W.W. (1981): Hormone profiles in postmenopausal women after therapy with subcutaneous implants. Brit. J. Obstet. Gynaecol. 88:426–433.

[22] Whitehead, M.I., Minardi, J., Kitchin, Y., Sharples, M.J. (1978): Systemic absorption of estrogen from Premarin vaginal cream. Ed. Cooke, I.D. The Role of Estrogen/Progestogen in the management of the menopause. M.T.P. Press, 63–71.

[23] Whitehead, M.I., Lane, G., Dyer, G., Townsend, P.T., Collins, W.P., King, R.J.B. (1981): Estradiol: the predominant intranuclear estrogen in the endometrium of estrogen-treated postmenopausal women. Br. J. Obstet. Gynaecol. 88, 914–918.

Sex steroids and lipoproteins

U. Larsson-Cohn, L. Wallentin

Effects of exogenous sex steroids on the lipoprotein pattern

Table 1 summarizes the main effects of sex steroids on lipoproteins. Table 2 lists additional factors that are of importance for the effects of sex steroid treatment on the plasma lipoproteins. These will be discussed in detail below. The present discussion will be based mainly on the investigations of our own group [1–7].

Tab. 1 Effects of sex steroids on lipoproteins.

	HDL	LDL	VLDL
Estrogen	↑	↓	↑
Progestogen	↓	↑	↓
Androgen	↓	↑	↓

Tab. 2 Additional factors of importance for effects of sex steroids on lipoproteins.

Quantity – dose and potency of the drug
Quality – chemical structure of the drug
Route of administration
Basic hormonal and metabolic state of the recipient

Dose and potency of the estrogen

In the mid-seventies we showed that 50 μg of ethinylestradiol had a more pronounced influence on the lipoprotein pattern than 2 mg of estradiol valerate [1]. The former drug raised the HDL 20–40% and reduced the atherogenic cholesterol, e.g., the cholesterol within the two lighter lipoprotein fractions, by 25%. Estradiol valerate produced only a 10% increase of the HDL-cholesterol and had no influence on the other lipoproteins. Since 50 μg of ethinylestradiol has a much higher estrogen potency than 2 mg of estradiolvalerate, the varying influences on the lipoproteins seemed quantitative rather than qualitative. A more recent study [2] employing increasing levels of estradiol-17 β has given further support to the opinion that plasma lipids respond to estrogen treatment in a does-related way.

Route of administration

Oral estradiol-17 β is rapidly absorbed and thus generates high initial estrogen concentrations in the liver. Part of the estradiol is immediately metabolized to estrone, so that plasma levels of estrone are considerably higher than of those of estradiol.

Percutaneously administered estradiol-17 β is absorbed more slowly and less of it is converted into estrone. Thus percutaneous treatment gives lower but more stable and lasting levels of estrone and estradiol. The plasma concentrations of the two estrogens are about equal.

In order to investigate whether the two routes of administration had different metabolic consequences, we treated postmenopausal women with estradiol-17 β either orally (daily dose 2–4 mg) or percutaneously (daily dose 3 mg) [2]. Both regimens had beneficial effects on postmenopausal symptoms and gave comparable reductions of the plasma gonadotrophin levels. The women on oral medication showed a 15% increase of HDL-cholesterol and a similar reduction of LDL-cholesterol; however, the percutanous treatment had no significant influence on the plasma lipoproteins.

We conclude that percutaneous estrogens have less effect on the lipoprotein metabolism than oral treatment. The difference is probably related to lower estradiol levels and to the fact that the first pass effect of the liver is avoided during percutaneous treatment.

Quality of the progestogen

Metabolic effects of progestogens may vary due to the chemical structure of the hormones. Hirvonen et al. [8] reported that the testosterone-derived progestogens norethisterone and levonorgestrel reduced the plasma HDL-levels of postmenopausal women. The progesterone-derived medroxyprogesterone acetate had no such effect. We [3] have obtained similar results in estrogen-treated postmenopausal women: 120 μg of levonorgestrel reduced the HDL-2-levels by about 30%, where as 300 mg of oral progesterone had no influence on this lipoprotein. Levonorgestrel, but not progesterone, also reduced the VLDL-triglycerides.

The effects of progestogens on the lipoprotein metabolism are dose-dependent. In women receiving danazol in the very high, but common, anti-endometriosis dose of

600 mg daily, the HDL-cholesterol levels were reduced by 60% and the HDL-2-cholesterol by as much as 80–90% [4].

It can be concluded that testosterone-derived progestogens reduce the HDL and VLDL levels while progestogens of the progesterone-type have less influence on the lipoprotein metabolism. The alterations are dose-dependent.

Basal hormonal and metabolic situation

Estrogens given to women with hereditary lipid-metabolic disturbances can dramatically influence the lipoprotein metabolism. Subjects with hypertriglyceridaemia, Type IV, can respond with a severe rise of the triglyceride levels. Similar reactions have been reported in pregnant women with hereditary hypertriglyceridemia, Types IV or V. On the other hand, females with hyperlipidemia, Type III, and postmenopausal women with hypercholesterolemia, Type II, may show an amelioration of the hyperlipoproteinemia following estrogen administration [9]. There are also data that suggest that sex steroids may influence the lipoprotein pattern differently in pre- and postmenopausal subjects [10].

Combined oral contraceptive treatment

The influence on the lipid metabolism of combined oral contraceptives depends on the absolute and relative doses of the two components. In a randomized prospective study [5] the effects of four different combinations of levonorgestrel and ethinylestradiol were compared. Combinations with a high dose of levonorgestrel and a high weight-per-weight ratio between the progestogen and the estrogen reduced the HDL-cholesterol significantly. However, it was shown that it was possible to balance the doses of the progestogen and the estrogen in such a way that the combination had no effect on the HDL-cholesterol level.

Effects of the endogenous sex steroid production

Both male puberty and exogenously given steroids with androgenic properties reduce the HDL levels. It could, therefore, be expected that endogenous testosterone production should diminish HDL. However, this has not, so far, been proven. On the contrary, several investigators have found a positive correlation between the plasma levels of HDL and testosterone [11]. In one study concerning males with carcinoma of the prostate, orchidectomy strongly reduced the plasma testosterone but had no significant effect on the plasma lipoprotein levels [6].

The physiological reduction of estrogen production in the postmenopause could be expected to increase the LDL and reduce the HDL levels. In fact, in the postmenopause the LDL levels are increased while the HDL concentration remains unchanged. It might be asked if the simultaneous loss of progesterone production would explain the unaltered HDL level in the postmenopause.

Pregnancy offers an opportunity to study the effects of changes in production of endogenous hormones. In a truly prospective investigation, in which all participants were enrolled in the study before they conceived, 20 women were followed throughout their pregnancy and during lactation [7]. From early in pregnancy until term, triglyceride levels were raised in all the lipoprotein fractions. There was also increased cholesterol in the HDL fraction. During the latter part of the gestational period there was a marked elevation of the LDL level. The rises of triglycerides and HDL are probably consequences of raised estrogen production. The cause of the high LDL level in pregnancy is at present less clear.

It can be concluded that there are physiological situations during which alterations of the endogenous sex steroid production do not effect the lipoprotein metabolism as expected.

References

[1] Wallentin, L. and Larsson-Cohn, U. (1977): Metabolic and hormonal effects of postmenopausal estrogen replacement treatment. II. Plasma lipids. Acta Endocrinol. 86, 597

[2] Fåhraeus, L., Larsson-Cohn, U. and Wallentin, L. (1982): Lipoproteins during oral and cutaneous administration of oestradiol-17 β to menopausal women. Acta Endocrinol. 101, 597

[3] Fåhraeus, L., Larsson-Cohn, U. and Wallentin, L. (1983): L-Norgestrel and progesterone have different influences on plasma lipoproteins. Eur. J. Clin. Invest. 13, 447

[4] Fåhraeus, L., Larsson-Cohn, U. and Wallentin, L. (1984). Profound alterations of the lipoprotein metabolism during Danazol treatment in premenopausal women. Fertil. Steril. 42, 52

[5] Larsson-Cohn, U., Fåhraeus, L., Wallentin, L. and Zador, G. (1981): Lipoprotein changes may be minimized by proper composition of a combined oral contraceptive. Fertil. Steril 35, 172

[6] Wallentin, L. and Varenhorst, E. (1981): Plasma lipoproteins during antiandrogen treatment by estrogens or orchidectomy in men with prostatic carcinoma. Horm. Metab. Res. 13, 293

[7] Fåhraeus, L., Larsson-Cohn, U. and Wallentin, L. (1985): Plasma lipoproteins including HDL subfractions during normal pregnancy. Obstetrics & Gynaecology. 66, 468

[8] Hirvonen, E., Mälkönen, M. and Manninen, V. (1981): Effects of different progestogens on lipoproteins during postmenopausal replacement therapy. N. Engl. J. Med. 304, 560

[9] Tikkanen, M. J., Nikkilä, E. A. and Vartiainen, E. (1978): Natural oestrogen as an effective treatment for type-II hyperlipoproteinaemia in postmenopausal women. Lancet 2, 490

[10] Heiss, G., Tamir, I., Davis, C. E., Tyroler, H. A., Rifkind, B. M., Schonfeld, C., Jacobs, D. and Frantz, I. D., (1980): Lipoprotein-cholesterol distributions in selected North-American populations: The lipid research clinics programm prevalence study. Circulation 61, 302

[11] Mendoza, S. G., Osuna, A., Zerpa, A., Gartside, P. S. and Glueck, C. J. (1981): Hypertriglyceridemia and hypoalphalipoproteinemia in azoospermic and oligospermic young men: Relationships of endogenous testosterone to triglyceride and high density lipoprotein cholesterol metabolism. Metabolism 30, 481

Discussion

Question: Mr. Studd, in view of Dr. Gambrell's statement about breast cancer and the protective effect of progestogen addition, do you still maintain your position for the woman – no uterus, no progestogen, no problem?

Studd: Yes, I think that is right, but one needs more confirmation on that work and a very careful controlled long-term study. Until then, however, I don't think it makes any sense to use progestogens – knowing their side effects – to protect the breast. As you know, there was a paper from Los Angeles in the Lancet which stated that progestogens can cause breast cancer. Of course, you and I think it is nonsense, but that is the balance. So, until we have better information, I would stick to my belief that we should avoid progestogens if we can.

Diczfalusy: What makes you believe that the risk of endometrial cancer in menopausal estrogen therapy has been overstated?

Studd: The alleged risk stems from an epidemic that occurred only in North America – and only in one part of North America. There was no such epidemic in other countries which were deeply involved in menopausal therapy for a long time. I am also convinced that many of the stage I cancers were, in fact, severe hyperplasia. The evidence for this is in the two papers by Stanley Roboy and Lightwood. In their long follow-up of patients with estrogen-dependent tumours, there was a 5-year survival rate of 100% and a 10-year survival rate of 100%. It therefore strikes me that the whole risk has been overestimated and, of course, the disease overdiagnosed.

Hammerstein: What about the type of progestogen – you only mentioned medroxyprogesterone acetate? Are there any other progestogens you would administer?

Studd: I would say that norethisterone is a reasonable progestogen as well, but women often display an idiosyncratic response in that they cannot tolerate one of them. In these cases, we switch them to another progestogen.

Question: No use of androgens at all? After the patients pass the age of 60 and you balance a litte light androgen against the estrogen for, say, 5 days of the week, there is certainly no cancer and the patients feel very well. I don't believe there is any hepatic toxicity. Have you had any experience with it?

Studd: The internist's view of methyltestosterone is so alarming that I don't think we could use it.

Question: I wonder that you recommended cytology but did not recommend mammography before commencing estrogen therapy.

Studd: I did, in fact. I mentioned breast palpations and, sometimes, mammography. I am rather more convinced of the safety benefits of cytology than the safety benefits of mammography. That, I think, is the answer. I understand the problems of the breast, but you may well be right – although I say palpation, mammography might be the better routine.

Question: Would you recommend repeated mammography after a year?

Studd: I am really not sure about that. I am not convinced that it is a totally safe procedure. Useful, no doubt, but I am just not sure whether repeated mammography is safe. And that will be the view of most breast surgeons in my country.

Haspels: I reduce the dose of progestogens by giving 2 months unopposed and the third month opposed.

Studd: Yes, that is a reasonable compromise.

Lachnit: The problem with prolonging the additional progestogen treatment from 10 to 13 days is that some women complain of spotting before the withdrawal bleeding – one of the unpleasant progestogen symptoms. Because of this I was glad to hear that you are not as strict on the 13-day regimen as some of your colleagues in the U.K., but suggest a progestogen intake of 10–13 days.

Studd: I am pleased you mentioned that because, as you know, the 13-day protection was my data of 5 or 6 years ago, and I am not strict about it. It is merely a guideline, and I recognise the dangers of progestogens as much as their safety. As Dr. Vessey said, we are in danger of protecting the endometrium with 13 days of progestogen but, perhaps, of causing a lot of cardiovascular symptoms and certainly a lot of general psychiatric problems.

Comment: I should like to point out that the progestogenic side effect applied to higher doses than are used by Whitehead. As far as endometrial suppression is concerned, he will show tomorrow that 75 μg of levonorgestrel is sufficient for that purpose. Now, I don't think we should assume that a 14-day course or longer of 75 μg daily will have the same subjective effects as 250 μg.

Lachnit: Strangely enough, even very low doses of progestogen given for longer than 10/12 days have unfavourable side effects, and they cause spotting.

Question: I have a question for Dr. Cardozo. Why not use a simple alcoholic solution? I had one made up 8 years ago, and I still use it as a first choice in climacteric therapy. Just 20 drops daily on the skin is sufficient. It is the cheapest way, forceful, and the solution remains stable for 2 years.

Cardozo: I believe that, if you use only alcohol, the rate of absorption and the amount absorbed are variable in different women. This is why it has been incorporated into a sticky cream rather than a pure alcoholic solution – because of the unpredictability of absorption.

Question: Could you comment on why you did not mention the parenteral use of intramuscular estrogen as one of the alternatives particularly in patients who cannot take oral estrogens and don't really want a pellet implanted?

Cardozo: That is a fair question, but I can't really comment on it because I haven't used it. However, patients are loath to accept frequent injections even for diabetes, never mind anything else. At least, when you give a hormonal implant, it is only once every six months.

Crosignani: Have you observed any local reactions to the implantation of the pellets?

Cardozo: Patient do sometimes have local reactions. The site has become infected on one or two occasions, and one patient returned to the casualty department because the pellet had come out. In most cases, however, there is no reaction at all and bleeding is rare. We just make a small skin incision and put the pellet in. We don't suture it afterwards – we just press on it and it all settles down. If you put it in below the hair line, it doesn't show and, if you tell them not to get it wet for 24 hours, it heals completely very quickly.

Lachnit: After you had done your estradiol/testosterone implantation, you gave relatively high doses of norethisterone cyclically. Did you do any lipid profiled in these patients? I ask because I suspect that some pronounced decreases in HDL could show up with this combination.

Cardozo: Yes, we did do lipid profiles in these patients, and no, there were no pronounced changes in the lipid profile or in blood pressure or weight. In fact, we looked at a lot of parameters.

Greenblatt: Dr. Lachnit, we have studied dozens and dozens of patients who have had pellet implants. We studied high und low density and very low density lipoproteins, and there were no changes as long as the estrogen levels were high enough – regardless of what progestogen was used.

Schwartz: I wanted to comment on Dr. Larsson-Cohn's presentation. Just recently Dr. Shargil of Israel published the results of a 3-year prospective study* on the use of a triphasic contraceptive in women aged 41 to 49. He found an increase of HDL cholesterol and a decrease of LDL cholesterol administering the same preparation as in women of reproductive age.

Hammerstein: Something has been bothering me for quite some time. Why are we so afraid of oral contraceptives in women and approaching the forties – and especially in those in their forties – as regards the induction of cardiovascular disease, and not all afraid of this once the menopause has occurred? I think there are at least three possible explanations and I would be very interested to hear which one you would give prevalence. The first is that we use different types of estrogen before and after menopause. The second is that, in the postmenopausal women, we use sequential formulations and not combined therapy. The third explanation is that lipids increase in the forties and that women at, let's say, 50 benefit from the depression of lipids. Are there still others?

Larsson-Cohn: Yes, I think we have to realise that what we are measuring in the

* Shargil, A.A., Int. J. Fertil. 30:15, 1985.

blood are just biochemical changes, the relevance of which is based on long-term epidemiological studies showing that subjects who have a certain disease – cardiovascular or whatever – have taken this, that or the other. As regards OC's, it is the thrombogenic side effect, which is quite another matter. And I think that, with the lipids, it has nothing to do with a risk of cardiovascular disease, a risk of developing arteriosclerosis. Women who have had myocardial infarction in young ages on the pill do not usually have any changes in their arteries.

Vessey: Something that must be realised from the start is that the types of epidemiological study that have been done in premenopausal women taking the pill are just the same as the types of study that have been done in postmenopausal women under replacement therapy. Indeed, for the most part the studies have been done by the same groups, i.e. the groups that have shown cardiovascular disease/pill associations in young women are the same groups that have shown no association (or a protective association) with replacement therapy in postmenopausal women. I believe this is an important methodological point. A very important factor must be the combination of estrogen and progestogen. In the combined pill, women are taking estrogen and progestogen, and this combination is important in relation to myocardial infarction and cerebrovascular disease. In relation to venousthrombosis and embolism, estrogen is more important. If you look for studies of venousthrombosis in women taking Premarin, you will find that there are very few of them. Most of the studies actually deal with myocardial infarction and stroke. I think it might be quite useful to do some more studies of venousthrombosis in postmenopausal women – and not only in those under Premarin. We really do need some studies dealing with some of these other preparations.

Hammerstein: If my memory is right, your paper in 1970 together with the Danish and Swedish people stated that the cardiovascular risk of sequential preparations was the same as that for the combined pill. Is that right?

Vessey: That study was principally concerned with venousthrombosis and embolism and, of course, the numbers too were quite small there. I think the way many people now think is that the venous events are probably estrogen-related, while the arterial events are estrogen plus progestogen-related.

2.3 Risk-benefit evaluation of hormonal therapy

Prospective study on long term risk of hormone replacement therapy

K. Hunt, M. Vessey

Introduction

The level of use of hormone replacement therapy (HRT) has fluctuated considerably over the past fifteen years in response to both favourable and adverse publicity. In the mid-1970's a considerable increase in the number of prescriptions for HRT was seen in Britain which continued up to the peak year of prescribing in 1977 (Figure 1). Thereafter use declined in response to the publication of papers indicating an increased risk of endometrial cancer amongst post-menopausal women taking unopposed HRT (i.e. estrogen replacement therapy without added progestogens).

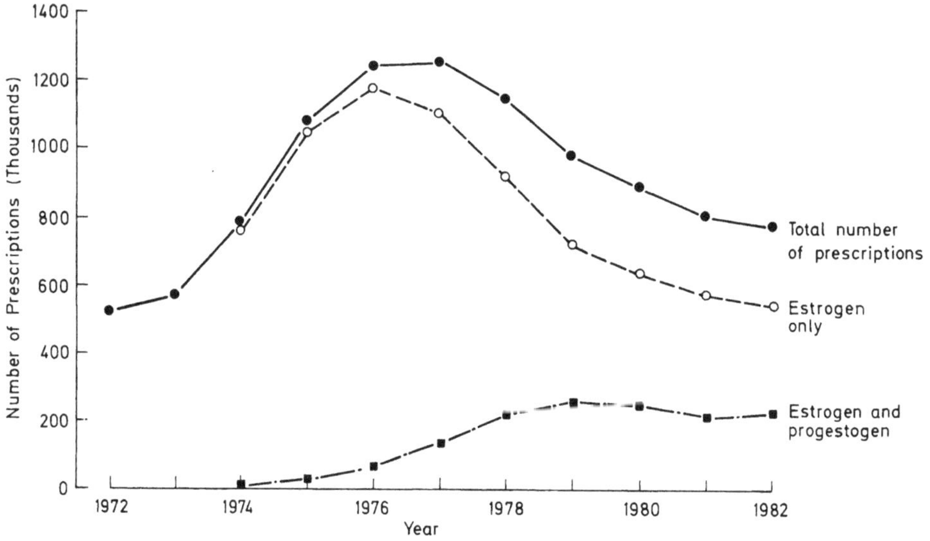

Fig. 1 Hormonal Preparations Issued for Treatment of Menopausal Symptoms (United Kingdom) (1972–1982)

Similar fluctuations in prescribing of HRT have been seen in the USA [1] and in Sweden [2] and reflect the continuing discussion about the appropriate use of treatment.

Randomised controlled trials of short-term use of HRT have shown that it is effective in alleviating the vasomotor symptoms of the menopause [3] and many studies have been reported which indicate that prolonged therapy is important in the prevention of post-menopausal osteoporosis [4, 5, 6, 7].

As HRT has been much more extensively used in the USA than in other countries where epidemiology flourishes, most studies of long-term risks and benefits have been conducted there. The finding that use of unopposed estrogens increases the risk of endometrial cancer has been independently and consistently reported in at least 17 case-control studies [see, for example, 8, 9, 10, 11, 12], although many of these have also shown that the lesions found in estrogen users tend to be low grade, early stage tumours with a good prognosis [see, for example, 13, 14, 15]. Furthermore, even this risk seems to be avoidable by the use of adequately opposed treatment regimens. The evidence on breast cancer is more controversial; while some studies have reported no relationship with HRT use [see, for example, 16, 17, 18], others have indicated that there may be an excess risk of the order of 20–50% [19, 20]. More encouraging is the developing consensus that unopposed estrogens used as HRT may provide some protection against coronary heart disease [21].

In 1977, the British Medical Research Council (MRC) decided to establish a survey of mortality and cancer incidence in a cohort of over 5000 long-term users of HRT. Brief details of the study are presented here.

Methods

The MRC survey is collaborative and multi-center and began in 1978. With the co-operation of the gynaecologists concerned, 4544 women using HRT were recruited from 24 leading specialist menopause clinics around the UK by the end of 1982. Essential details of obstetrical, gynaecological and medical histories, together with data about social and physical characteristics, were recorded for each woman at recruitment. In addition, histories of past and present use of HRT were obtained. To be included in the survey a woman had to have used HRT continuously for at least one year.

All participants in the study are 'flagged' in the British National Health Service Central Registries (NHSCRs). Notifications of deaths and cancers occuring among the cohort members are automatically forwarded from the NHSCRs to the study co-ordinating center at Oxford University. In addition, use of treatment during the follow-up period and women's views about the role of HRT have been investigated via a postal questionnaire.

Subjects

The majority of women in the study were aged 45–54 years at recruitment (60.0%) and at their first use of HRT (63.3%) (Table 1). About 6% of women had never been married and about 20% were nulliparous.

Table 1 Age at First Use of Hormone Replacement Therapy and at Entry to the Survey (%)

Age (Years)	At first HRT	at Entry
–39	9.0	5.5
40–44	14.6	9.3
45–49	32.8	24.6
50–54	30.5	35.5
55+	13.1	25.1
Total	100.0	100.0

Age at menopause and type of menopause (natural or surgical) are thought to play an important role in the etiology of many of the diseases of interest in this study. Menopausal status at first use of HRT is given in Table 2. Almost 36% of women in the cohort had already undergone hysterectomy at that time, about 2 to 2½ times the proportion in the general British population [22]. This is not surprising since hysterectomy (particularly with concurrent bilateral oophorectomy) is seen as an indication for replacement therapy by some physicians. Of the women with intact uteri, roughly equal numbers were either naturally post-menopausal or were pre- or peri-menopausal at their first use of HRT.

Table 2 Menopausal Status at First Use of HRT

Menopausal Status	no. of Women	%
Hysterectomy:		
with bilateral oophorectomy	859	18.9
at Least One Ovary Intact	765	16.8
Natural Menopause	1318	29.0
Radiation Menopause	9	0.2
Irregular Menses	1085	23.9
Regular Menses	356	7.8
Status Uncertain	152	3.4
	4544	100.0

Women in the cohort tended to be of higher social class than the general population (Table 3); this may be related to the fact that the results of the postal questionnaire showed that many women had had to pressurise their doctors in order to receive HRT. With respect to parity and smoking patterns, the women in the cohort appeared to be similar to the general population.

Table 3 Social Class Distribution

Social Class (Registrar-General's Classification)	Social Class of Husband for Married Women in Study	Social Class Distribution for Men in Great Britain (1971 Census)
I	12.5	5
II	33.9	18
III N	13.4	12
III M	25.5	38
IV	8.1	18
V	1.2	9
Other	1.4	
Not Known	4.0	
Total	100.0	100

Table 4 Use of 5 Major HRT Preparations in the Cohort

Major Preparation (taken alone or in combination with another preparation)	Per Cent of Overall Accumulated Use
Premarin (Conjugated Equine Estrogens)	39.4
Estradiol Implants	12.9
Harmogen (Piperazine Estrone Sulphate)	8.6
Ethinyl Estradiol	8.5
Progynova (Estradiol Valerate)	5.7
Other	24.9
	100.0

One striking feature of the MRC study is the great variety of HRT preparations (and combinations of preparations) which were used by the participants. Table 4 shows that Premarin (conjugated equine estrogens) accounts for only 40% of the overall accumulated use. Furthermore, Table 4 gives a greatly simplified impression of the diversity of treatment regimens and combinations used; indeed, over 175 different treatments are included in the survey coding schedule! Many women have taken opposed HRT and many different progestational agents have been used. This provides a marked contrast with North America, where Premain has been predominantly used, and where, until recently, the addition of a progestogen to estrogen replacement therapy has been uncommon [1]. Treatment histories of individuals in our cohort of users are also characterised by many changes of preparation or regimen.

Results

Although some detailed results were presented at the symposium, they are not reproduced here as they are to be published elsewhere. It may be noted, however, that the mortality observed in the cohort so far is only about half that expected at the national rates. The extent to which this reflects an effect of therapy, on the one hand, and the selected nature of the population under study, on the other, was discussed. The incidence of endometrial cancer was significantly higher than expected (relative risk about 3.0), as was the incidence of breast cancer (relative risk about 1.5).

Conclusion

The mortality results are generally reassuring. The incidence figures for endometrial cancer are not surprising although some patients had taken (inadequately) opposed therapy. The slight excess of breast cancer incidence is more worrying and we are continuing our analysis of the relevant data in more detail.

Acknowledgements

We would like to thank those working in the specialist menopause clinics who have made it possible for us to undertake this study. We are also grateful to the Medical Research Council for financial support.

References

[1] Kennedy, D. L., Baum, C., Forbes, M. B.: Non contraceptive estrogens and progestins: use patterns over time. Obstet. Gynecol. 1985; 65:441–446.

[2] Persson, I., Adami, H.-O., Lindberg, B. S., Johansson, E. D. B., Manell, P.: Practice and patterns of estrogen treatment in climacteric women in a Swedish population. A descriptive epidemiological study. Part 1. Acta Obstet Gynecol Scand 1983; 62:289–296.

[3] Campbell, S., Whitehead, M.: Oestrogen therapy and the menopausal syndrome. Clinics in Obstetrics & Gynaec 1977; 4:31–47.

[4] Lindsay, R., Hart, D. M., Aitken, J. M.,

MacDonald, E. B., Anderson, J. B., Clarke, A. C.: Long-term prevention of postmenopausal osteoporosis by oestrogen. Evidence for an increased bone mass after dealyed onset of oestrogen treatment. Lancet 1976; i:1038–1041.

[5] Horsman, A., Gallagher, J. C., Simpson, M., Nordin, B. E. C.: Prospective trial of oestrogen and calcium in postmenopausal women. British Medical Journal 1977; ii:789–792.

[6] Recker, R. R., Saville, P. D., Heaney, R. P.: Effects of oestrogens and calcium carbonate on bone loss in postmenopausal women. Annals of Internal Medicine 1977; 87:649–655.

[7] Horsman, A., Jones, M., Francis, R., Nordin, C.: The effect of estrogen dose on postmenopausal women. New England Journal of Medicine 1983; 309:1405–1407.

[8] Smith, D. G., Prentice, R., Thompson, D. J., Hermann, W. L.: Association of exogenous estrogen and endometrial carcinoma. New England Journal of Medicine 1975; 293:1164–1167.

[9] Ziel, H. K., Finkle, W. D.: Increased risk of endometrial carcinoma among users of conjugated estrogens. New England Journal of Medicine 1975; 293:1167–1170.

[10] Mack, T. M., Pike, M. C., Henderson, B. E., Pfeffer, R. I., Gerkins, V. R., Arthur, M.: Estrogens and endometrial cancer in a retirement community. New England Journal of Medicine 1976; 294:1262–1267.

[11] McDonald, T. W., Annegers, J. F., O'Fallon, W. M., Dockerty, M. B., Malkasian, G. D., Kursland, L. T.: Exogenous estrogen use and endometrial carcinoma. Case-control and incidence study. American Journal of Obstetrics & Gynecology 1977; 127:572–580.

[12] Gray, L. A., Christopherson, W. M., Hoover, R. N.: Estrogens and endometrial cancer. Obstetrics & Gynecology 1977; 49:385–389.

[13] Antunes, C. M. F., Stolley, P. D., Rosenshein, N. B., Davies, J. L., Tonascia, J. A., Brown, C., Burnett, L., Rutledge, A. Pokempner, M., Garcia, R.: Endometrial cancer and estrogen use. Report of a large case-control study. New England Journal of Medicine 1979; 300:9–13.

[14] Jick, H., Watkins, R. N., Hunter, J. R. Dinan, B. J., Madsen, S., Rothman, K. J. Walker, A. M.: Replacement estrogens and endometrial cancer. New England Journal of Medicine 1979; 300:218–222.

[15] Hulka, B. S., Kaufman, D., Fowler, W. C., Grimson, R. C., Greenberg, B. G.: Predominance of early endometrial cancers after long-term estrogen use. JAMA 1980; 244:2419–2422.

[16] Kelsey, J. L., Fischer, D. B., Holford, T. R., Livolsi, V. A., Mostow, E. D., Goldenberg, I. S., White, C.: Exogenous estrogens and other factors in the epidemiology of breast cancer. Journal of National Cancer Institute 1981; 67:327–333.

[17] Gambrell, R. D., Maier, R. C., Sanders, B. I.: Decreased incidence of breast cancer in post-menopausal estrogen-progestogen users. Obstetrics & Gynecology 1983; 62:435–443.

[18] Kaufman, D., Miller, D. R., Rosenberg, L., Helmrich, S. P., Stolley, P., Schottenfeld, D., Shapiro, S.: Non contraceptive estrogen use; the risk of breast cancer. JAMA 1984; 252:63–67.

[19] Hoover, R., Gray, L. A., Cole, P., MacMahon, B.: Menopausal estrogens and breast cancer. New England Journal of Medicine 1976; 295:401–405.

[20] Brinton, L. A., Hoover, R. N., Szklo, M., Fraumeni, J. F.: Menopausal estrogen use and risk of breast cancer. Cancer 1981; 47:2517–2522.

[21] Vessey, M., Hunt, K.: The menopause, hormone replacement therapy and cardiovascular disease; epidemiological aspects. In 'The Menopause' (eds. J. Studd & M. Whitehead). Blackwell. In the press.

[22] Alderson, M., Donnan, S.: Hysterectomy rates and their influence upon mortality from carcinoma of the cervix. Journal of Epidemiology & Community Health 1978; 32:175–177.

Long-term metabolic effects of estrogen therapy

F. Husmann

Several metabolic processes are influenced or controlled by estrogens, either directly or in cooperation with other hormones such as growth hormone and cortisol. Thus, after the menopause, the lack of estrogens causes important alterations in estrogen-mediated metabolic pathways which include carbohydrate, lipid, lipoprotein, and protein metabolism.

One of the major mechanisms responsible for the development of metabolic abnormalities is the disturbed balance between cortisol, on the one hand, and estrogens on the other. The secretion of estrogens decreases rapidly after the menopause, whereas the formation of cortisol by the adrenal glands remains almost unchanged. From that point on metabolic pathways which are stimulated by cortisol predominate so that liponeogenesis and gluconeogenesis is increased while the synthesis of protein is diminished. In the postmenopausal period more and more catabolic pathways gain predominance. Estrogens have no anabolic activity, but they do act as anti-catabolic substances. This mechanism can be explained by cortisol antagonism (Husmann, 1984).

There are also other factors which are of importance in the development of metabolic alterations. The synthesis of various proteins, such as transcortin, sex hormone-binding globulin, and ceruloplasmin, is directly induced by estrogens. In the case of other proteins it is the growth hormone which is responsible for the induction of their synthesis. The release of growth hormone decreases after the menopause and increases under estrogen replacement therapy (von Schoultz and Damber, 1984).

Carbohydrate metabolism

The effects of estrogen deficiency on carbohydrate metabolism are explained by the gluconeogenetic activity of cortisol. After the menopause this effect of cortisol is no longer antagonized by estrogens. Thus, the age of manifestation of diabetes mellitus reaches its maximum a few years after the menopause (Fig. 1).

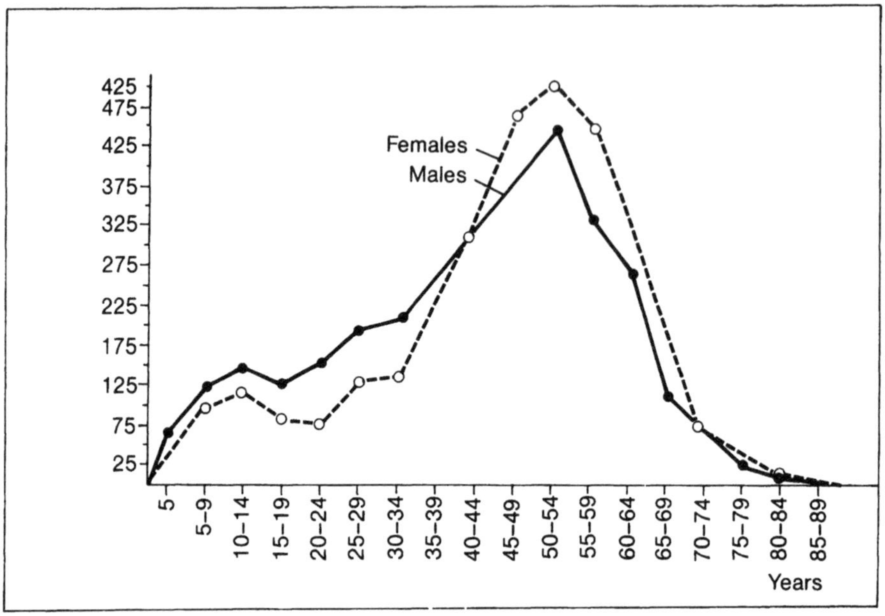

Fig. 1 Age dependent manifestation of diabetes mellitus.

Lipid and lipoprotein metabolism

Atherosclerotic vascular disease (AVD) morbidity and mortality rates are higher in males than in females during the reproductive years. However, AVD morbidity and mortality rates tend to increase substantially after the menopause in a manner unrelated to age (World Health Organization, 1981). These findings suggest that during the reproductive years women are partly protected against AVD, which raises the question whether the risk of AVD is related to estrogen deficiency. During the past years most of the mechanisms involved in the development of AVD have been identified and the influence of estrogens on some of them is now well known. Thromboxane – derived from arachidomic acid via the cyclo-oxigenase pathway (Fig. 2) – causes thrombocyte adhesion to the blood vessel wall with subsequent transformation into fibrin and liberation of smooth muscle proliferating factor (SMPF). SMPF enters the vessel wall and stimulates the formation of numerous myofibrils. VLDL and LDL then enter the vessel wall from the blood stream and are bound by the corresponding receptors present in the membranes of the myofibrils. Finally, the lipoproteins are incorporated into macrophages and, after rupture of the membranes due to overloading of the macrophages, free lipids appear in the vessel wall (Fig. 3).

The first step in AVD genesis, the formation of thromboxane, is inhibited by estrogens, as was demonstrated by Silfverstolpe and co-workers (1984a).

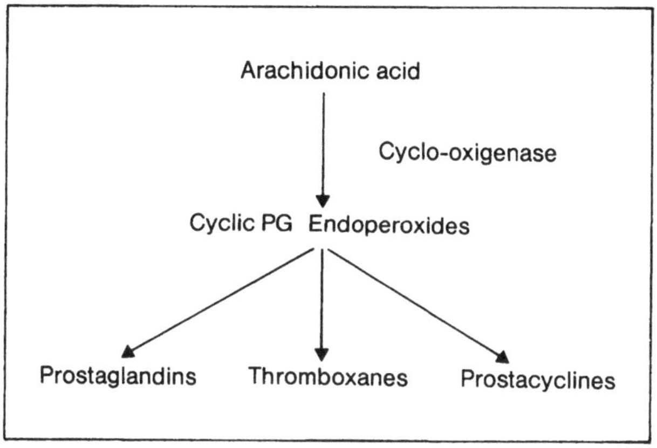

Fig. 2 Cyclo-oxigenase pathway of arachidonic acid.

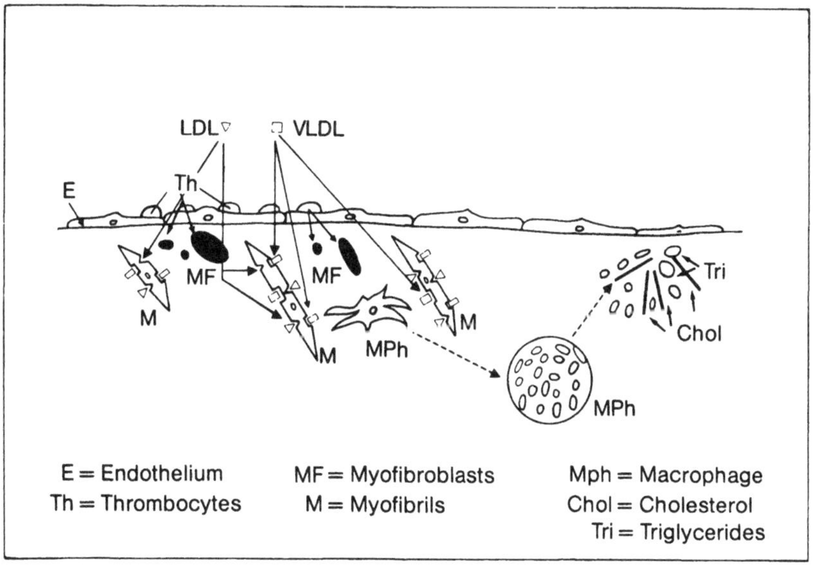

Fig. 3 Development of atherosclerotic blood vessel wall alterations. Adhesion of thrombocytes, proliferation of myofibrils, and interaction of lipoproteins with the corresponding receptors in myofibrils.

HDL counteracts the immigration of VLDL and LDL into the vessel wall. Thus, HDL is able to inhibit one of the last steps in AVD genesis. This explains the findings of the Framingham Study which imply that high HDL blood levels are indicative of minimal arteriosclerotic alterations. Thus, HDL seems to have vasoprotective properties: However, when this parameter is examined, the levels of total cholesterol, triglycerides, VLDL und LDL have to be considered as well since the counteractive potency of HDL is not unlimited.

Table 1 Alteration of Triglycerides, Cholesterol and Lipoproteins during Estrogen Replacement (mg/dl).

Alteration of Triglycerides, Cholesterol and Lipoproteins during Estrogen Replacement (mg/dl).

	Tri	Chol	HDL	LDL	VLDL
Group of Age 20–44 Years					
Untreated	93 ± 83.2	189 ± 58.1	52 ± 11.9	123 ± 56.1	13 ± 10.9
conj. Estrogens	141 ± 59.9	227 ± 52.7	65 ± 18.9	142 ± 51.6	20 ± 9.3
Group of Age 45–65 Years					
Untreated	114 ± 66.9	230 ± 44.3	61 ± 15.6	154 ± 43.8	16 ± 13.8
conj. Estrogens	141 ± 71.5	219 ± 33.9	69 ± 17.7	133 ± 33.9	18 ± 12.5
Ethinyl-estradiol	168 ± 56.7	229 ± 29.7	86 ± 19.3	121 ± 23.7	22 ± 9.0

Wahl. P. et al.: New Engl. J. Med **308** (1983) 862–867

In estrogen-deficient women the blood levels of lipids and lipoproteins are elevated. They can, at least in part, be normalised by estrogen replacement therapy (Tab. 1).

Table 1 shows that the response of lipids and lipoproteins to estrogen treatment is clearly age-dependent. Furthermore, the data reveal that the degree of HDL increase depends on the estrogenic activity of the hormone preparation administered. The ratio of total cholesterol to HDL is of particular importance. If we use the above data to calculate the percentage of total cholesterol present as HDL before, and during, treatment with conjugated estrogens, we obtain 27.5% and 28.6%, respectively, for the group of younger women; and 26.5% and 31.5% for the group of older women. Ethinylestradiol raised this percentage to 37.6%.

These findings, together with Silfverstolpe's observation, support the assumption that estrogens are able to protect from AVD. The first investigations in this field were published by Ross and co-workers (1981) who found out that the administration of conjugated estrogens to postmenopausal women over a period of 5 years reduced the relative mortality rate from ischaemic heart disease to 0.43.

However, the administration of estrogens and progestogens in combination, as is now recommended in order to prevent the development of endometrial cancer, the vasoprotective effects of estrogens may be abolished. Several progestogens, espec-

Table 2 Alteration of Lipoproteins by Different Estrogens and Progestagens

Alteration of Lipoproteins by Different Estrogens and Progestagens

	VLDL	LDL	HDL
Non-alkylated Estrogens	–	(↓)	↑
Alkylated Estrogens	(↑)	(↓)	↑
17-OH-Progesterone	–	–	–
Norethisterone	–	↑	↓↓
Levonorgestrel	–	–	↓
OD 14	↓	–	↓

ially 19-nor testosterone derivatives with inherent androgenic activity, produce the opposite effect and are able to reverse the influence exerted by estrogens on lipid and lipoprotein metabolism. Table 2 summarises the findings obtained by several authors (Crona and co-workers 1984; Davely and co-workers, 1984; Silfverstolpe and co-workers 1984b).

Natural progesterone has no influence on lipid and lipoprotein metabolism (Fig. 4). In the female organism this substance is partly converted into deoxycorticosterone (Ottoson and co-workers, 1984). This substance is a steroid with distinct mineralocorticoid activity. It increases the retention of sodium at the distal renal tubulus which leads to a rise in blood pressur. Concomitantly, water retention increases. Progesterone itself has a distinct anti-mineralocorticoid activity which completely antagonises the effect of deoxycorticosterone. Thus, Brincat and co-workers (1984b) found that many patients became hypotensive under treatment with progesterone. Due to these properties progesterone may be a real alternative to synthetic progestogens in the treatment of postmenopausal women. Judged by the fall in HDL seen under treatment with OD 14, this newly developed steroid has a considerable androgenic activity.

Obviously, the androgenic activity of a progestogen is responsible for the unfavorable effects on lipids and lipoproteins. One should, therefore, expect that cyproterone-acetate, with its strong anti-androgenic activity, could be very useful in the treatment of postmenopausal women when estrogens and progestogens are administered in combination. Investigations of this hypothesis are in progress.

Estrogens exert an influence on lipoprotein composition, especially on LDL, as measured by the alterations in the cholesterol/triglyceride ratio (Knopp and co-workers, 1981, Tab. 3).

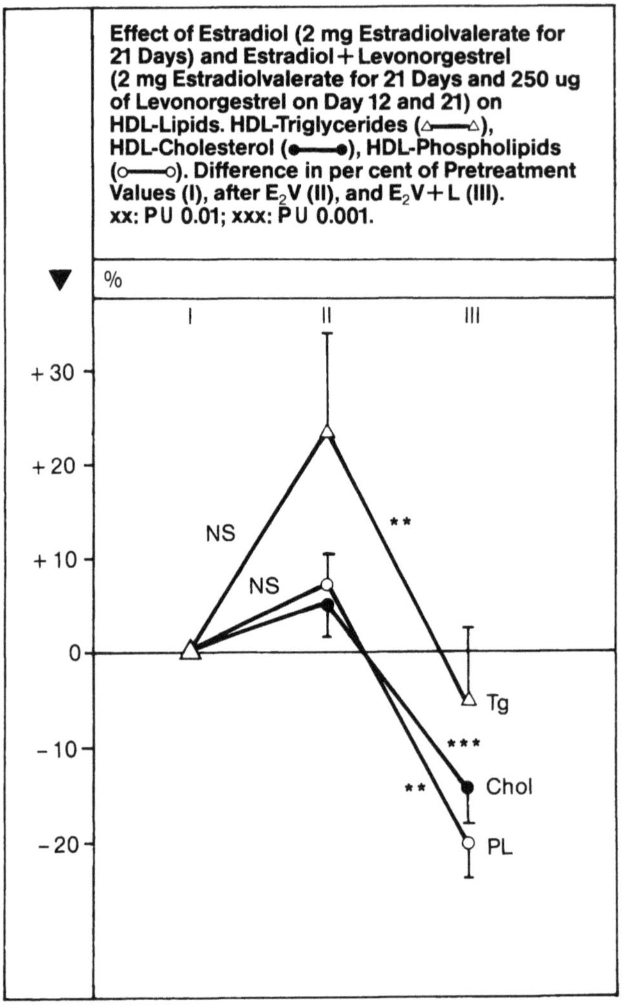

Tikkanen, M. J. et al.: J. Clin. Endocrinol. Metab. **54** (1982) 1113–1117

Fig. 4

Under estrogen replacement therapy an increase occurs in triglycerides in the LDL fraction. This is a desirable effect. In the case of elevated cholesterol concentration, cholesterol-rich LDL would be formed. LDL of this type are preferentially incorporated into blood vessel walls as is seen in Type III hyperlipoproteinemia.

The mechanism of the estrogen-induced increase of HDL has been investigated in several studies. The HDL_2 subfraction increases during estrogen replacement therapy while HDL_3 is not influenced to a significant degree (Tikkanen and co-workers, 1982). HDL_2 degradation is mainly controlled by a lipase present in the endothelial

Table 3 Effect of Estrogens on Lipoprotein Composition Measured by Cholesterol-Triglyceride-Ratio

Effect of Estrogens on Lipoprotein Composition Measured by Cholesterol-Triglyceride-Ratio

	VLDL	LDL	HDL
Unreated	0.30 ± 20.24	8.35 ± 6.50	3.73 ± 1.24
conjug. Estrogens	0.29 ± 0.22	5.95 ± 2.36	3.41 ± 1.34

Knopp, R. H. et al.: J. clin. Endocr. Metab. **53** (1981) 1123–1132

cells of liver sinusoids. The administration of estradiol-valerate results in a reduction of lipase activity of 25%. Thus, the increase in HDL by estrogens is mainly caused by an inhibition of their degradation. This effect is reversed by levonorgestrel, even when it is given in combination with estrogens. Increased lipase activity is accompanied by a decrease in HDL.

Furthermore, estrogens have a considerable influence on lipoprotein structure and composition (Schaefer and co-workers, 1983, Tab. 4).

Table 4 Alteration of Lipoprotein Composition by 0.1 mg Ethinylestradiol per Day

Alteration of Lipoprotein Composition by 0.1 mg Ethinylestradiol per Day

	Proteins	Cholesterol	Phospholipids	Triglycerides
VLDL				
Untreated	8.8 ± 4.1	13 ± 6	13 ± 7	28 ± 15
0.1 mg EE_2	17.8 ± 9.8*	28 ± 12*	27 ± 9	68 ± 38*
LDL (1.006–1.019 g/ml)				
Untreated	2.1 ± 1.9	3 ± 2	3 ± 1	7 ± 5
0.1 mg EE_2	3.0 ± 2.9	6 ± 4*	6 ± 3*	16 ± 9*
LDL (1.019–1.063 g/ml)				
Untreated	60 ± 17	96 ± 11	55 ± 19	15 ± 6
0.1 mg EE_2	57 ± 8	93 ± 15	65 + 16	21 ± 4
HDL (1.063–1.21 g/ml)				
Untreated	144 ± 17	47 ± 5	48 ± 8	11 ± 2
0.1 mg EE_2	168 ± 9*	65 ± 5*	86 ± 23*	30 ± 3*

* < 0.05

Schaefer, E. J. et al.: clin. Endocrinol. Metab. **57** (1983) 262–267

Estrogens stimulate the elimination of cholesterol via the liver and bile. The disadvantage of this positive effect is the accumulation of cholesterol in the bile and thus increased risk of gallstone formation. For the formation of cholesterol gallstones, the mobility of the gall bladder and its ability to take up bile are of importance. During the normal menstrual cycle about 79% of hepatic bile are taken up by the gall bladder. In the second half of the cycle, under the influence of progesterone, this percentage decreases to 65%. Under 10 mg medroxyprogesterone acetate per day only 47% of hepatic bile is taken up by the gall bladder. This steroid diminishes the tonus of the gall bladder and the sphincter of Oddi, thereby prolonging the depletion time of this organ. These mechanisms should make it possible that medroxyprogesterone acetate could induce stone formation. However, the dosages used in these experiments exceedes by far the therapeutic dose (Shaffer and co-workers, 1984).

Magnesium

Only few studies have investigated the metabolism of magnesium after the menopause and the alterations produced by estrogens. In 1984 it was shown that in postmenopausal women the excretion of magnesium in the urine increases, while the plasma levels remain almost unchanged. Under estrogen replacement therapy, a significant decrease in renal magnesium excretion occurs without alteration of the plasma levels. It is assumed that estrogen deficiency leads to increased mobilisation of magnesium from the sceletal system. On the other hand, the loss of magnesium via the kidney is at least partly compensated for by an increase in absorption of magnesium from the intestine. It is still not known whether estrogen deficiency is, by itself, responsible for the increase in intestinal magnesium absorption. The alterations in magnesium metabolism found in postmenopausal women completely disappear under estrogen replacement therapy (McNair et al., 1984).

Neurotransmitter substances

The formation of neurotransmitters, for example serotonin, is estrogen- and vitamin B_6-dependent. Estrogens stimulate the activity of essential decarboxylases such as 5-hydroxytryptophane decarboxylase. Vitamine B_6 is a cofactor of decarboxylases and transaminases such as kynurenine transaminase which catalyses intermediary steps in the formation of serotonin from tryptophane.

Contraceptive steroids sometimes cause an abnormally high urinary excretion of xanthurenic acid which can be normalised by administering pyridoxine-hydrochloride. These observations are in agreement with reports on the possibility of inhibiting kynurenine transaminase by application of estradiol, via a competitive displacement of pyridoxyl-phosphate from its apo-enzyme binding position. The conversion of tryptophane to serotonin is thereby inhibited and thus results in a lack of serotonin which brings about psychic depression. Some estrogens inhibit the absorption of vitamine B_6 and are, therefore, most prone to cause depressions.

The administration of vitamine B_6 in high doses leads to increased vitamine B_6 plasma levels and, according to the law of mass and effect, to a displacement of estrogens from the apo-enzyme binding site of kynurenine transaminase. As a consequence, the formation of serotonin normalises, and the depression fades away. For this, doses of 600 to 900 mg vitamine B_6 administered daily for 10 to 12 days are necessary (Haspels et al., 1975).

On the other hand, estrogen deficiency can, by itself, elict severe depressive states either by inhibiting the activity of 5-hydroxytryptophane decarboxylase or by lowering the plasma level of free tryptophane (Teran et al., 1984). Estrogen replacement therapy normalizes the activity of the enzyme and raises the levels of free tryptophane from 3.76 ± 0.09 to 4.41 ± 0.19.

Thus, in the treatment of depressions in postmenopausal women, estrogens occasionally have to be combined with high doses of vitamine B_6.

Protein metabolism

The synthesis of some proteins in the liver is directly stimulated by estrogens. Obviously, hepatocytes are equipped with estrogen receptors (Laurell and Rannevik, 1979). Table 5 shows how the synthesis of some important proteins is stimulated or impaired by estrogens.

Estrogen replacement therapy produces a rise in growth hormone levels. That this is an estrogen-specific effect is shown by the fact that the increase in growth hormone can be prevented by simultaneous administration of tamoxifen, an anti-estrogenic substance. Further evidence for an estrogen-mediated increase in growth hormone is

Table 5 Alterations in plasma concentrations of various proteins under 0.05 mg ethinylestradiol or mestranol + 1.0 mg norethisterone in percent (Baseline level = 100 percent).

Ceruloplasmin	203.0 ± 28
Sex hormone-binding globulin	202.0 ± 28
Transcortin	202.0 ± 21
Thyroxine-binding globulin	167.0 ± 27
Transferrin	163.0 ± 31
Alpha-lipoprotein	130.0 ± 15
Plasminogen	127.0 ± 12
Albumin	80.4 ± 13

given by the fact that 1-DOPA stimulates the secretion of this hormone in estrogen-treated women much more than in untreated women.

Preliminary results obtained by von Schoultz and Damber (1984) suggest that growth hormone mediates the effects of estrogens on hepatocytes. Growth hormone, by itself, raises the levels of sex hormone-binding globulin, ceruloplasmin and somatomedin C. In animal experiments, it was demonstrated that growth hormone induces the formation of estrogen receptors and estrogen-binding protein in hepatocytes.

The elevated level of hydroxyproline found in the urine of postmenopausal women is caused either by increased collagen degradation or by inhibition of collagen synthesis with diminished hydroxyproline incorporation. Estrogen replacement therapy raises the collagen content of the skin statistically significantly, from 156.21 μg/mm² to 230.89 μg/mm², which is an increase of 48% (Brincat et al., 1983). The question whether testosterone could be responsible for this increase has

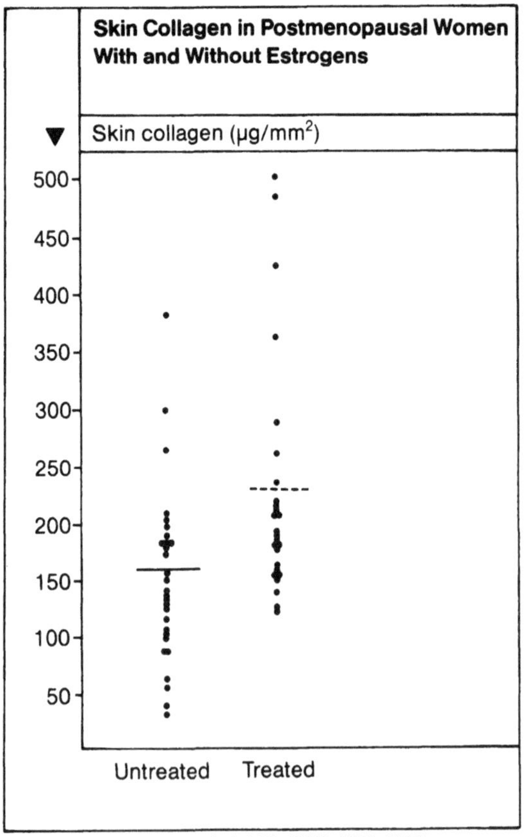

Brincat, M. et al.: Brit. med. J. 287 (1983) 1337–1338

Fig. 5

been discussed. However, testosterone levels are not substantially lower in postmenopausal women and do not rise under estrogen treatment.
The influence of estrogens on fibroblasts and on the epidermis can be impressively demonstrated in skin biopsies. In untreated postmenopausal women, very few fibroblasts are present in the corium (Fig. 5). These show hardly any signs of activity, and almost no fiber formation is to be detected. The chromatin of the cell nucleus is very dense and clotted. Estrogen replacement therapy stimulates the formation of fibroblasts. The chromatin of the cell nucleus becomes loose and vacuolated. These cells produce fibers and are able to incorporate thymidine and hydroxyproline into proteins.

Similar alterations can be seen in epidermal cells. The cell nucleus looses its vacuoles. The chromatin becomes more and more clotted and the synthesis of protein declines gradually. The epidermis is then thin and consists of few cell layers with decreased turgor. The stratum germinativum is fibrous and blurred. Estrogen therapy normalises the histological findings with loose und vacuolated chromatin and normally shaped cell nucleus. Again epidermis thickens, it shows numerous cell layers with restored intra- und extracellular water and fluid balance (Aertgeerts, 1974).

These skin alterations develop over months or years following the menopause. It is obvious that estrogen replacement therapy must be continued for several months to normalise the far-reaching alterations caused by estrogen deficiency.

These fundamental alterations which take place in the skin of postmenopausal women should not be regarded as merely a cosmetic problem. The findings obtained so far clearly indicate that repair mechanisms also decline. Furthermore, fibroblasts and related cell structures are present not only in the skin but also in all other tissues of mesenchymal origin, including cartilage and bone.

It is assumed that the activity of fibroblasts in all these tissues is stimulated by estrogens. This assumption is supported by the findings of Brincat and co-workers (1984a) from which the authors concluded that postmenopausal osteoporosis was not a disorder of metabolism. The results they obtained indicate that the decline in bone density observed in normal, untreated, post-menopausal women is rather due to a decline in bone collagen matrix. This graduated loss of bone collagen with postmenopausal age is paralleled by a similar loss of skin collagen.

Summary

Several metabolic processes are influenced by estrogens, either directly or in connection with other hormones such as, for example, growth hormone. Thus, after the menopause the lack of estrogens will cause significant alterations in estrogen-mediated metabolic pathways such as carbohydrate, lipid, lipoprotein, and protein metabolism. The age of manifestation of diabetes mellitus reaches its maximum a few years after the menopause. The HDL fraction decreases significantly leading to accelerated progression of atherosclerotic vascular disease. Estrogens exert a vasoprotective effect by inhibiting HDL degradation. In estrogen deficiency, the vasoprotective effect can be maintained by replacement therapy. However, the protective effect is at least partly counteracted by the addition of progestogens with inherent androgenic activity, such as 19-nor testosterone derivatives. Progesterone derivatives do not have this unfavourable effect. Protein metabolism is mediated by estrogens either directly or in connection with growth hormone. Estrogens induce the synthesis of various proteins, for instance sex hormone-binding globulin, transcortin and ceruloplasmin. In the skin and other tissues of mesenchymal origin, estrogens stimulate the activity of fibroblasts and the synthesis of collagen. Normally thymidine incorporation, as well as protein synthesis in general, are increased in these tissues, resulting in normal repair mechanisms, normal cell turgor, normal elasticity, and normal intra- and extracellular water and fluid balance. In estrogen deficiency, the impaired mechanisms can be restored by estrogen replacement therapy. The loss of calcium and magnesium and the resulting loss of bone mass can be prevented by estrogen replacement. Estrogens are involved in the formation of neurotransmitters, such as serotonin by activating the enzymes necessary for their formation. The normalisation of enzyme activity by replacement therapy explains the benificial effect of estrogens observed in depressive postmenopausal women.

References

Aertgeerts, J.: Wirkung oraler Oestrogene auf die Haut der Frau in der Postmenopause und nach Kastration. Ther. d. Gegenw. 113 (1974) 1739–1748.

Brincat, M., C. F. Moniz, J. W. W. Studd, A. J-. Darby, A. Magos and D. Cooper: Sex hormones and skin collagen content in postmenopausal women. Brit. med. J. 287 (1983) 1337–1338.

Brincat, M., C. Moniz, A. L. Magos, E. Versi and J. W. Studd: Correlation between skin collagen content, skin thickness and a index of bone density: effect of years since menopause on these indices. 4th Int. Congr. Menopause. Abstr. 20, Maturitas 6 (1984a) 93–94.

Brincat, M., P. Rylance, V. P. Parsons and J. W. Studd: Progesterone as an antihypertensive. 4th Int. Congr. Menopause. Abstr. 21, Maturitas 6 (1984b) 94.

Crona, N., G. Samsioe and G. Silfverstolpe: Lipoprotein lipids and apolipoprotein A 1 – effects of ORG OD 14. 4th Int. Congr. Menopause. Abstr. 29, Maturitas 6 (1984) 100–101.

Davey, D. A., G. M. Berger, D. Yon and F. E. Hardie: Continuous combined oral oestradiol and norethistosterone acetate in postmenopausal women: effect on vasomotor symptoms, plasma lipids and lipoproteins. 4th Int. Congr. Menopause. Abstr. 32, Maturitas 6 (1984) 103.

Haspels, A. A., H. J. T. Coelingh-Bennink, P. A. van Keep und W. H. P. Schreus: Oestrogene und Vitamin B 6. In: Östrogene in der Postmenopause. Hrsg.: P. A. van Keep and Ch. Lauritzen. Karger: Basel, München, Paris, London, New York. 1975. S. 214–220.

Husmann, F.: Climacterium feminale. Gyne 5 (1984) Heft 4, S. 8–12.

Knopp, R. H., C. E. Walden, P. W. Wahl, J. Hoover, G. R. Warnick, J. J. Albers, J. T. Ogilvie and W. R. Hazzard: Oral contraceptive and postmenopausal estrogen effects on lipoprotein triglyceride and cholesterol in an adult female population: relationships to estrogen and progestin potency. J. clin. Endocr. Metab. 53 (1981) 1123–1132.

Laurell, C.-B., Laurell and Rannevik, G.: A comparison of plasma protein changes induced by danazol, pregnancy, and estrogens. J. Clin. Endocrinol. 49 (1979) 719–725.

McNair, P., C. Christiansen and I. Transbøl: Effect of menopause and estrogen substitutional therapy on magnesium metabolism. Mineral Electrolyte Metab. 10 (1984) 84–87.

Ottoson, U.-B., K. Carlström, J. E. Damber, B. Nilsson and B. von Schoultz: Absorption of oral progesterone and its conversion into deoxycorticosterone during oestrogen replacement therapy. 4th Int. Congr. Menopause. Abstr. 100. Maturitas 6 (1984) 159.

Ross, R. K., A. Pagnani-Hill, T. M. Mack, M. Arthur and B. E. Henderson: Menopausal oestrogen therapy and protection from death from ischaemic heart disease. Lancet I (1981) 858–860.

Schaefer, E. J., D. M. Foster, L. A. Zech, F. T. Lindgren, H. B. Brewer and R. I. Levy: The effects of estrogen administration on plasma lipoprotein metabolism in premenopausal females. J. Clin. Endocr. Metab. 57 (1983) 262–267.

Schoultz, B. von and M.-G. Damber: Growth hormone, oestrogens and liverprotein synthesis. 4th Int. Congr. Menopause. Abstr. 120, Maturitas 6 (1984) 177.

Shaffer, E. A., P. J. Taylor, K. Logan, S. Gadomski and B. Corenblum: The effect of a progestin on gallbladder function in young women. Am. J. Obstet. Gynecol. 148 (1984) 504–507.

Silfverstolpe, G., L. Enk, B. Källfelt, G. Samsioe and N. Crona: Effects of exogenous oestrogens on the prostacyclin/thromboxane balance in oophorectomized women. 4th Int. Congr. Menopause, Abstr. 129. Maturitas 6 (1984a) 184–185.

Silfverstolpe, G., L. Enk, U.-B. Lindberg, G. Samsioe and N. Crona: Effects on serum lipoproteins of 2 mg and 4 mg doses of oestradiol valerate. 4th Int. Congr. Menopause, Abstr. 130. Maturitas 6 (1984b) 185–186.

Teran, A.-Z., J. S. Chadda, R. A. Roesel and R. B. Greenblatt: Tryptophane studies in depressed post-menopausal women. 4th Int. Congr. Menopause, Abstr. 144. Maturitas 6 (1984) 197.

Tikkanen, M. J., E. A. Nikkilä, T. Kuusi and S. Sipinen: High density lipoprotein-2 and hepatic lipase: reciprocal changes produced by estrogen and norgestrel. J. Clin. Endocr. Metab. 54 (1982) 1113–1117.

Wahl, P., C. Walden, R. Knopp, J. Hoover, R. Wallace, G. Heiss and B. Rifkind: Effect of estrogen/progestin potency on lipid/lipoprotein cholesterol. New Engl. J. Med. 308 (1983) 862–867.

Hormonal replacement therapy and breast cancer

R. D. Gambrell, Jr.

Abstract

Breast cancer is the most frequent malignancy in females, accounting for 26% of all cancers in women in the U.S.A. It is also the leading cause of cancer death, causing 18% of all female cancer deaths in the U.S.A. The mortality rate from carcinoma of the breast varies from a high of 37.7:100,000 women per year in Great Britain to a low of 0.2:100,000 in Honduras; it is 22.1:100,000 women in the U.S.A., which ranks 13th in the world. The incidence of mammary malignancy increases throughout the female life span and will strike one in 11 women in the U.S.A. Numerous long-term studies of large numbers of postmenopausal women have failed to incriminate estrogen replacement therapy for any significantly increased risk of breast cancer except in small subgroups of hormone users. There is increasing evidence that adding progestogen to estrogen therapy significantly decreases the risk of carcinoma of the breast. In the Wilford Hall USAF Medical Center studies, the lowest incidence of breast cancer was observed in the estrogen-progestogen users (66.8:100,000) which was significantly lower than that of the non-users (343.5:100,000), and that expected from both the Third National Cancer Survey (188.3:100,000) and the National Cancer Institute SEER data (229.2:100,000) with $P \leq 0.01$. The incidence of breast carcinoma in the estrogen-progestogen users was not significantly lower than that of the unopposed estrogen users (142.3:100,000) but did indicate a trend in that direction with $P \leq 0.08$. There is also some evidence that progesterone deficiency may increase the risk for mammary malignancy.

Introduction

Women in the United States fear getting breast cancer as much, if not more, than any other malignancy. Rightfully so, since carcinoma of the breast will strike one in 11 women in the United States. Breast cancer is the most frequent malignancy in females, accounting for 26% of all cancers in women [1]. It is also the leading cause of death from malignancy in women, causing 18% of all female cancer deaths in the

United States. The American Cancer Society estimated that 119,000 new cases of breast carcinoma would be diagnosed in the United States in 1985 and that 38,400 women would die from this tumor that year. This is 13 times the number of deaths each year from endometrial cancer. The mortality rate from carcinoma of the breast around the world varies from a high of 37.7:100,000 women per year in Great Britain to a low of 0.2:100,000 in Honduras. The death rate from breast cancer in the United States, which ranks thirteenth in the world, is 22.1:100,000. Unfortunately, this mortality has not changed during the past 45 years, even though death from uterine cancer has declined from 31.5:100,000 in 1930 to 8.4:100,000 in 1979. The incidence rates of breast malignancy have increased only slightly during the past 25 years, with an incidence of 70:100,000 female population in 1947 and 75:100,000 in 1975. This may be related to increased longevity, since the risk of mammary malignancy increases progressively with age.

The incidence of breast cancer increases throughout the female life span (Figure 1).

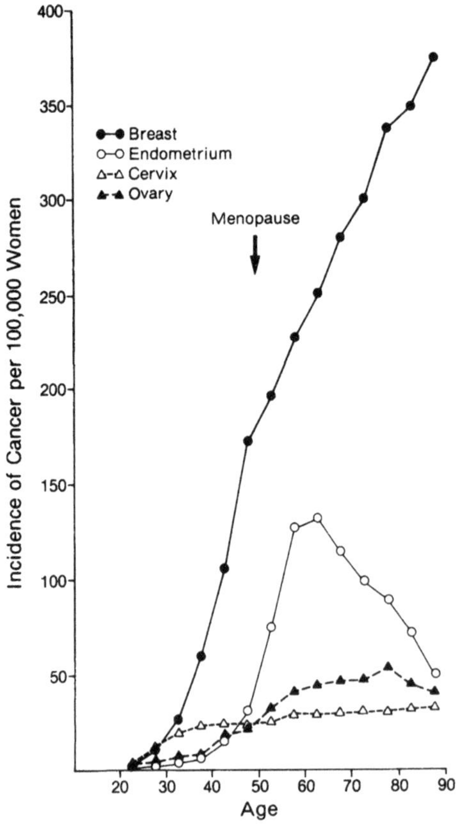

Fig. 1 Incidence of breast endometrial, cervical, and ovarian cancer in women by age. (Reproduced by permission from the published [7]).

In this respect, the incidence of this malignancy differs from cervical, endometrial, and ovarian cancer, which peak in the 40's, 50's, and 60's, respectively, and then either decline or plateau [2]. The sharpest increase in the frequency of breast cancer occurs between the mid-30's and age 50, or about the time of menopause. Then the incidence continues to rise steeply throughout the postmenopausal years, when estrogen levels are lower. Some studies have found a plateau in this progressive increase between the ages of 45 and 55 years [3]; however, no such pause was observed in either the Third National Cancer Survey or the National Cancer Institute SEER data, [2,4]. On the other hand, the incidence of endometrial cancer begins to rise in the late 40's and peaks during the 60's, at about 130:100,000 women. Carcinoma of the cervix increases during the reproductive years and the incidence remains relatively constant at about 38:100,000 throughout the menopause. Ovarian malignancy progressively increases from age 40 to the 70's, to a maximum incidence of 50:100,000 women.

Epidemiologic studies of breast cancer

That estrogen replacement therapy may be causally related to breast cancer has been debated for many years. However, recent reports have failed to incriminate exogenous estrogen use as a cause of mammary malignancy in postmenopausal women. The most recent study concluded that estrogen use did not increase the risk of breast cancer [5]. The relative risk (RR) for estrogen use more than 18 months prior to diagnosis of breast carcinoma was 0.8, when compared with 'never-use' of any estrogens. The results were similar when known risk factors for mammary malignancy were taken into account: Estrogen use by postmenopausal women did not appear to increase the risk of breast cancer, even when taken for many years or in the distant past.

Of the seven groups that have looked at both endometrial and breast cancer in estrogen users, five found a moderate association between unopposed estrogen therapy and adenocarcinoma of the endometrium (Table 1). However, in all studies the association found between estrogens and carcinoma of the breast was considerably less convincing. The study from Ulm, Germany, did not observe an increase in either endometrial or breast carcinoma in unopposed estrogen users and the study from New York found only in placebo users [16, 22]. Only two studies have observed any significantly increased risk of breast carcinoma from estrogen therapy, and in both of these the only increased risk occurred in subgroups of estrogen users. In the first, there was a slightly increased risk in a small subgroup of estrogen users with intact ovaries and a total milligram dose (TMD) of estrogens of greater than 1,500 mg (RR = 2.5; P = 0.02) [6]. A TMD greater than 1,500 mg is equivalent to 0.625 mg of estrogens daily for 25 days each month for eight or more years. As in

Table 1 Relative Risk of Cancer in Estrogen Users

Authors	Endometrial Cancer	Breast Cancer
Mack, Ross et al.[6,20]	8.0	0.7–2.5
Gray, Hoover et al.[11,21]	3.1	1.3
Jick et al.[9,10]	20.0	1.1–3.4
Hammond et al.[12]	9.3	1.1
Nachtigall et al.[22]	0/1*	0/4*
Gambrell[19]	1.8	0.4
Lauritzen and Meier[16]	0.78	0.92

* Estrogen-progestogen therapy: No endometrial or breast cancers were detected in hormone users but one endometrial and four breast cancers were detected in the placebo group.

our study [7] and others [8] a lower RR of mammary malignancy was observed in four other subgroups of estrogen users: prior oophorectomy, ever-estrogen use, RR = 0.8; prior oophorectomy with TMD less than 1,500 mg, RR = 0.9; prior oophorectomy with TMD greater than 1,500 mg, RR = 0.7; and intact ovaries with TMD less than 1,500 mg, RR = 0.9.

In the second study, there was no association between current estrogen use and breast cancer in women with previous hysterectomy (RR = 1.1) [9]. Only slightly more than 50% of the hysterectomized women had also undergone oophorectomy, and the risk of breast cancer in those who had had oophorectomy and those who had not had oophorectomy was similar. In women with an intact uterus undergoing a natural menopause, there was a positive association between current estrogen use and carcinoma of the breast (RR = 3.4). This association varied by age, with an RR of 10.2 in naturally perimenopausal women aged 45–54 years and an RR of 1.9 in those aged 55–64 years. It should be emphasized that this was the study that found the highest risk of endometrial cancer in estrogen users (RR = 20) [10]. It should also be remembered that these case-control studies can never show a true cause and effect but only a possible association. Although oophorectomy may lower the risk for breast carcinoma, it is difficult to understand why hysterectomy with conservation of the ovaries would also lower the risk. Both of the above studies can be criticized because they limited their study population to women up to age 65 and 75 years, respectively [6, 9]. However, the incidence of breast cancer continues to increase with each 5-year increment as long as women live (Figure 1). Since more women are treated with estrogens in the early menopausal years and fewer are so treated after age 60, this alleged increased risk of mammary malignancy probably reflects greater estrogen use in younger postmenopausal women rather than a true association.

In a private practice in Kentucky, an insignificantly increased risk (RR = 1.3) of breast carcinoma was observed in postmenopausal estrogen users [11]. In a follow-up study of these patients with additional patients added from the University of

Louisville, a decreased risk of breast cancer from estrogen replacement therapy was found [8]. These investigators followed 405 postmenopausal women (mean age, 59.7 years) from three to more than 28 years with serial mammography, utilizing xeromammography in the later years of study. The 206 estrogen users received therapy for a minimum of 18 months (mean, 6.5 years) and had fewer carcinoma of the breast than the non-users. It was concluded that long-term estrogen replacement does not significantly alter mammographic parenchymal patterns and that estrogen use does not increase the risk of breast cancer. In a study from Duke University, four cases of breast cancer were found among 301 estrogen users followed five to 25 years; an equal number was found in the 309 non-users, not a statistically significant difference [12]. There were 11 cases of endometrial cancer in the 301 unopposed estrogen users. In the 10-year double-blind study from New York, four breast cancers were detected in the 84 placebo users but none in the 84 estrogen-progestogen users, a statistically significant difference ($P \leq 0.05$).

Another prospective study, from Vanderbilt University, observed that mortality decreased by 25% in estrogen-treated women who did develop breast cancer [13]. In this long-term study of 1,000 estrogen users followed for 15 years, 33 patients developed carcinoma of the breast during, 14,318 patient-years of observation, for an incidence of 300.3:100,000, slightly more, but statistically not significant, from what would be expected. Although 9 to 11 women from this group would be expected to die of mammary malignancy, only 6 succumbed to their disease. The authors concluded that fewer deaths than anticipated suggested either greater host resistance or less virulence. Two earlier reports from Southern California indicate that exogenous estrogens do not increase the risk of breast cancer [14, 15]. In the first, estrogen use was "clearly associated with a reduced risk of breast cancer" [14]. In the second, it was concluded that women with a natural menopause have no increased risk of mammary malignancy from estrogen use after the onset of menopausal symptoms [15]. Two studies from Germany have observed lower incidence of breast cancer in long-term estrogen users [16, 17]. In one, the incidence of mammary cancer in the estrogen users was 123:100,000 compared to 154:100,000 in the non-users; however, this difference was not significantly [16]. In the other, a significantly decreased risk of breast carcinoma ($RR = 0.89$) was observed with estrogen use ($P \leq 0.05$) [17].

Vessey, in his recent review of the case-control studies, wrote that there was some evidence that estrogen therapy carries an increase in breast cancer risk but the effects were generally small [18]. He points out the difficulties in this type of study with many variables. Women with early oophorectomy are at low risk for breast cancer, but are particularly likely to receive estrogen therapy. It has been reasoned that any adverse effect of estrogens on the breast might be apparent in oophorectomized women. He concludes that the adverse effect of estrogen therapy on breast cancer risk is clearly not demonstrated in those with oophorectomy.

Decreased incidence of breast cancer in estrogen-progestogen users

During the five years of prospective study and four years of follow-up at Wilford Hall USAF Medical Center, 69 postmenopausal women were diagnosed with breast cancer (Table 2) [19]. There were a total of 5,563 patients registered in the hormone use survey for a total of 48,669 patient-years of observation, so the overall incidence of breast carcinoma was 141.8:100,000 women per year. The lowest incidence of breast malignancy was observed in the estrogen-progestogen users, including two past users, with 11 patients diagnosed with cancer during 16,466 patient-years of observation, for an annual incidence of 66.8:100,000 women. During 19,676 patient-years of observation, there were 28 breast cancers in the unopposed estrogen users, including four in past users, for an incidence of 142.3:100,000. With 22 breast cancers during 6,404 patient-years of observation, the incidence in the non-users was 343.5:100,000. There were also five breast cancers in the estrogen vaginal cream users, including two past users, during 4,298 patient-years of observation for an incidence of 116.3:100,000. With three cancers during 1,825 patient-years of observation, including one past user, the incidence was 164.4:100,000 in the progestogen users.

Table 2 Incidence of Breast Cancer at Wilford Hall Usaf Medical Center: 1975–1983

Therapy Group	Patient-Years of Observation	Patients with Cancer	Incidence (per 100,000)
Estrogen-Progestogen Users	16,466	11*	66.8
Unopposed Estrogen Users	19,676	28*	142.3
Estrogen Vaginal Cream Users	4,298	5*	116.3
Progestogen Users	1,825	3*	164.4
Non-Users	6,404	22	343.5
Total Patients	48,669	69	141.8

* Includes past users

The expected incidence of breast cancer in this age group, according to the Third National Cancer Survey [4], is 188.3:100,000, and for ages 55 to 59 according to the National Cancer Institute SEER data [2], it is 229.2:100,000. The incidence of breast cancer in the estrogen-progestogen users (66.8:100,000) was statistically significantly lower than that of the non-users (343.5:100,000) and from that expected from both the National surveys in the U.S. with $P \leqslant 0.01$. It was not significantly lower than that of the unopposed estrogen users (142.3:100,000) but does indicate a trend in that direction ($P \leqslant 0.08$). The incidence of mammary malignancy in the unopposed estrogen users (142.3:100,000) was significantly lower than that of the non-users with $P \leqslant 0.01$; however, it was not significantly lower than that expected from the Third National Cancer Survey and only barely so when compared to the National Cancer Institute SEER data expected incidence ($P \leqslant 0.05$). The incidence of breast carcinoma in the estrogen vaginal cream users (116.3:100,000) was significantly lower ($P \leqslant 0.05$) when compared to non-users. None of the other differences were statistically significant except that the non-users (343.5:100,000) had a significantly higher incidence than that expected, both according to the Third National Cancer Survey ($P \leqslant 0.01$) and the NCI SEER data ($P \leqslant 0.05$).

These same data are shown graphically year by year in Figure 2. Of the 11 breast cancers occuring in the estrogen-progestogen users, including two past users, seven occurred during the first four years of study. Only two patients continuing estrogen-progestogen therapy developed carcinoma of the breast during the last year of

INCIDENCE OF BREAST CANCER

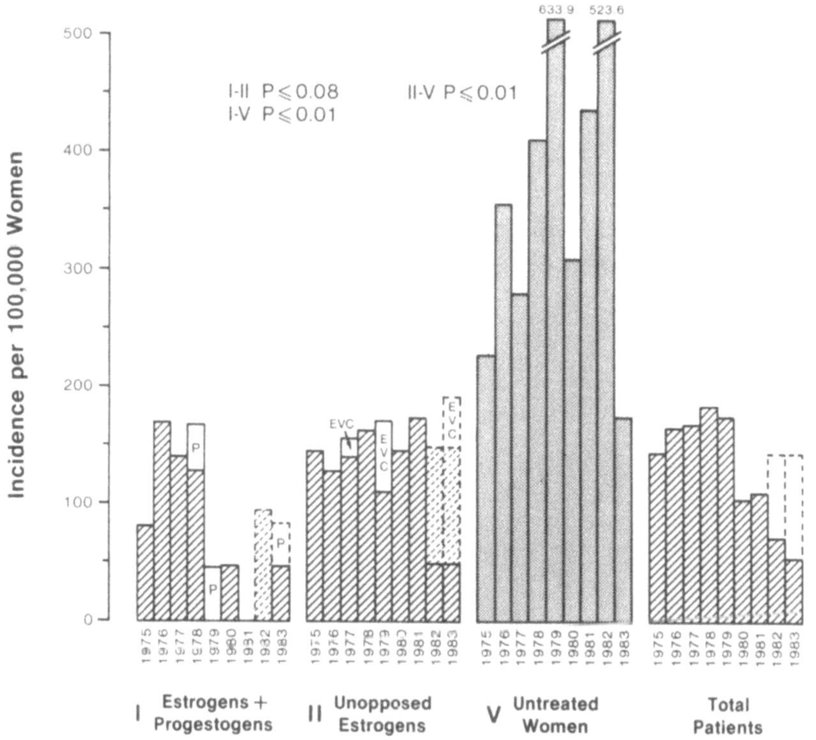

Fig. 2 Incidence of breast cancer by year, 1975–1983, in hormone users compared with the untreated women. Solid lines indicate current users while broken lines indicate past users. EVC = estrogen vaginal cream users; P = progestogen users. (Reproduced by permission from the publisher [19]).

prospective study and the four years of follow-up. The incidence of this malignancy in the unopposed estrogen users was remarkably consistent throughout the entire nine years. During the last two years of follow-up, 6 patients had discontinued either the oral estrogen or estrogen vaginal cream four to six years before detection of cancer. The incidence of breast cancer was highest in the non-users (untreated women), varying from a low of 174.5:100,000 in 1983 to a high of 633.9:100,000 during 1979. Overall, the incidence of breast carcinoma increased slightly from 143.9:100,000 in 1975 to a high of 183.3:100,000 in 1978, followed by significant decreases to 104.2:100,000 in 1980 and 110.4:100,000 in 1981. During the last two years, if the 9 patients who had discontinued their hormones for three to six years are excluded, this incidence further decreases to 52.9:100,000 in 1983. If all 9 past hormone users are included, the incidence of mammary malignancy rises to 143.8:100,000.

The concept of adding progestogens to estrogen replacement therapy was introduced at Wilford Hall USAF Medical Center in 1971. Figure 3 compares the number of estrogen and estrogen-progestogen treated women with the incidence of breast cancer for the 12 years from 1972 through 1983, including three years of retrospective data from 1972–1974. With increasing estrogen usage from approximately 1,320 patients in 1972 to 3,940 estrogen-tested women during 1975, there was a decline in the incidence of breast carcinoma from 189.4:100,000 in 1972 to 143.4:100,000 in 1975, however, this was not statistically significant. With increasing usage of added progestogen from approximately 9.1% of the estrogen users in

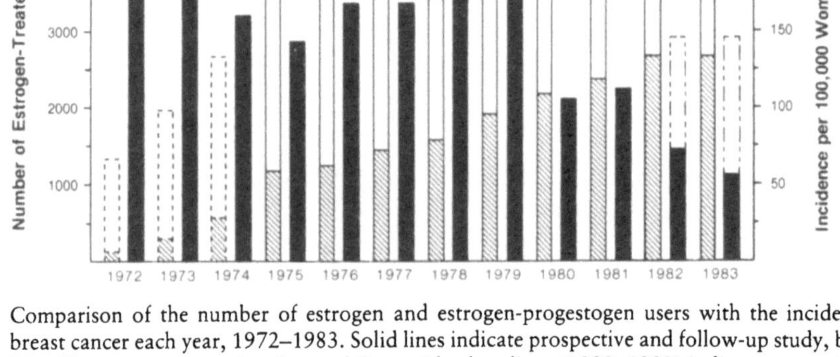

Fig. 3 Comparison of the number of estrogen and estrogen-progestogen users with the incidence of breast cancer each year, 1972–1983. Solid lines indicate prospective and follow-up study, broken lines illustrate retrospective data, while semi-broken lines (1982–1983) indicate cancer in past hormone users. (Reproduced by permission from the publisher [19]).

1972 to 61.1% of the estrogen users by 1983, a significant decrease in the incidence of breast cancer occurred in the ninth and tenth year of follow-up. Carcinoma of the breast declined from 183.8:100,000 in 1978 to 104.2:100,000 in 1980 and 110.4:100,000 in 1981. Excluding the 9 patients who had discontinued hormone use for three to six years prior to 1982 and 1983, the incidence of breast cancer further declined to 71.9:100,000 in 1982 and 52.9:100,000 during 1983. If these 9 past hormone users are included, the incidence for these two years was 143.8:100,000. These women hat not used any hormones for three to six years; the mean interval of discontinuance was 4.5 ± 0.87 years.

It took 12 years of increasing progestogen usage to confirm the protective effect of added progestogen on the breast. Apparently, it takes long-term estrogen-progestogen usage to reduce the risk of breast cancer in postmenopausal women. The reduction in risk of endometrial cancer from added progestogen was confirmed very early in our study as well as in others [12, 16, 22–25]. Progestogens induce the physical shedding of the endometrium each month, leaving behind fewer cells and glands to continue proliferation that may lead to cancer. In addition, otheractions of both natural progesterone and syntheticc progestogens are important. Progestogens decrease estrogen receptors in endometrial cells and induce estradiol dehydrogenase and isocitrate activity, which is the mechanism whereby these cells metabolize estrogens [25]. Because progesterone does not induce the cyclical shedding of breast cells, it is probable that the protective mechanism of progestogens operates at the intracellular level through changes in receptors and enzymatic activity. The presence of both estrogen and progesterone receptors in breast cancer tissue is related to a longer disease-free interval and decreased mortality. It is more predictive of a favorable response to endocrine manipulation with either ablative surgery or antiestrogen therapy [26].

If the increasing incidence of breast cancer by age is closely examined (Figure 1), the role of the female sex steroids can be somewhat clarified. The sharpest increase in breast cancer by age is between the late 30's and early 50's. At this time in a woman's life there is declining production of estrogens from ovaries as menopause is approached. Perhaps more important is the fact that many women become anovulatory in the late premenopausal years, resulting in an abrupt cessation of the cyclic progesterone levels that were present throughout most of the reproductive years. The incidence of breast cancer continues to increase throughout the postmenopausal years when estrogen is reduced but not absent. However, few postmenopausal women, if any, produce progesterone. If unopposed estrogens were the cause of breast cancer, then the incidence of this malignancy should peak in the 50's and 60's and decline thereafter, as does the incidence of endometrial cancer. Whatever the role of female sex steroids as cofactors or predisposing factors for carcinoma of the breast, progesterone deficiency seems to be one of the many factors in this multifactorial disorder. It may be that luteal dysfunction provides a state favorable to the induction of carcinoma in the susceptible mammary gland [27].

There is other evidence that progesterone deficiency may increase the risk for breast cancer. In a long-term follow-up of a group of infertility patients, those with progesterone deficiency had 5.4 times the risk of premenopausal carcinoma of the breast when compared with women in the nonhormone group whose infertility was caused by other factors [28]. The incidence of postmenopausal breast cancer did not differ significantly between the two groups; however, these patients were just reaching menopause. Another study of progesterone deficiency did observe an increased risk of postmenopausal breast cancer [29]. Chronic anovulation increased the risk of endometrial cancer 5-fold, and the risk of breast carcinoma after the age of 55 was increased 3.6-fold.

Numerous long-term studies of large numbers of postmenopausal women have failed to incriminate estrogen replacement therapy for any significantly increased risk of mammary malignancy [5, 6, 8, 9, 11–15]. There is increasing evidence that adding progestogen to the estrogen therapy significantly decreases the risk for breast cancer [7, 16, 19, 22]. In the 10-year double-blind study from New York, four carcinomas of the breast were diagnosed in the 84 placebo users while none were observed in the 84 estrogen-progestogen users, which was statistically significant with $P \leq 0.05$ [22]. The study from Germany observed a lower incidence of breast cancer in the estrogen (123:100,000) when compared to non-users (154:100,000) [16]. The incidence of mammary malignancy in the estrogen-progestogen users (109:100,000) was significantly lower ($P \leq 0.05$) when compared to either the estrogen users or the non-users. Long-term oral contraceptive use also decreases the risk for carcinoma of the breast, probably because of the combination of estrogen and progestogen in birth control pills [30]. Estrogen replacement therapy should not be withheld from postmenopausal women who are truly estrogen deficient since there is no evidence that estrogens increase the risk of breast cancer. Adding progestogen to estrogen replacement significantly reduces the risk for mammary malignancy, so combination estrogen-progestogen therapy should be given to women who have had hysterectomy if they are estrogen deficient.

References

[1] American Cancer Society: Cancer statistics, 1985. CA – A Cancer Journal for Clinicians 1985; 35:19.

[2] National Cancer Institute: Surveillance, Epidemiology, and End results (SEER). Bethesda, Biometry Branch of the National Cancer Institute, 1980, p 47.

[3] Vorherr, H., Messer, R. H.: Breast cancer: Potentially predisposing and protecting factors. Am J. Obstet. Gynecol. 1978; 130:335.

[4] Gutler, S. J., Young, J. L. Jr.: Third National Cancer Survey: Incidence Data. Natl. Cancer Inst. Monogr. 41, 1975, p 110.

[5] Kaufman, D. W., Miller, D. R., Rosen-

burg, L. et al.: Noncontraceptive estrogen use and the risk of breast cancer. JAMA 1984; 252:63.
[6] Ross, R.K., Paganni-Hill, A., Gerkins, V.R. et al.: A case-control study of menopausal estrogen therapy and breast cancer. JAMA 1980; 243:1635.
[7] Gambrell, R.D. Jr.: Breast Disease in the postmenopausal years. Sem Reprod Endocrinol 1983; 1:27.
[8] Bland, K.I., Buchanan, J.B., Weisberg, B.F. et al.: The effects of exogenous estrogen replacement therapy on the breast: Breast cancer risk and mammographic parenchymal patterns. Cancer 1980; 45:3027.
[9] Jick, H., Walker, A.M., Watkins, R.N. et al.: Replacement estrogens and breast cancer. Am. J. Epidemiol. 1980; 112:586.
[10] Jick, H., Watkins, R.N., Hunter, J.R. et al.: Replacement estrogens and endometrial cancer. N. Engl. J. Med. 1979; 300:218.
[11] Hoover, R., Gray, L.A. Sr., Cole, P. et al.: Menopausal estrogens and breast cancer. N. Engl. J. Med. 1976, 295:401.
[12] Hammond, C.B., Jelovsek, F.R., Lee, K.I. et al.: Effects of long term estrogen replacement therapy: II. Neoplasia. Am. J. Obstet. Gynecol. 1979; 133:537.
[13] Burch, J.C., Byrd, B.F., Vaughn, W.K.: Results of estrogen treatment in onc thousand hysterectomized women for 14,318 years. *In* van Keep, P.A., Greenblatt, R.B., Albeaux-Fernet, M. (eds.): Concensus on Menopause Research. Lancaster, England, MTP Press Ltd, 1976, p 164.
[14] Henderson, B.E., Powell, D., Rosario, I. et al.: An epidemiologic study of breast cancer. J. Natl. Cancer Inst. 1974; 53:609.
[15] Casagrande, J. Gerkins, V., Henderson, B.E. et al.: Exogenous estrogens and breast cancer in women with natural menopause. J. Natl. Cancer Inst. 1976; 56:839.
[16] Lauritzen, C., Meier, F.: Risks of endometrial and mammary cancer morbidity and mortality in long-term oestrogen treatment. *In* van Herendael, H. and B., Riphagen, F.E., Goessens, L., van der Pas, H. (eds.): The Climacteric. An Update. Lancaster, England, MTP Press Ltd, 1984, p 207.
[17] Volker, W.: Estrogen and estrogen-progestogen compounds: Is there a risk for the development of endometrial and breast cancer in the perimenopausal woman? *In* Pasetto, N., Paoletti, R., Ambrus, J.L. (eds.): The Menopause and Postmenopause. Lancaster, England, MTP Press Ltd, 1980, p 273.
[18] Vessey, M.P.: Exogenous hormones in the aetiology of cancer in women. J. Roy, Soc. Med. 1984; 77:542.
[19] Gambrell, R.D. Jr.: Studies of endometrial and breast cisease with hormone replacement therapy. In Studd, J.W.W., Whitehead, M. (eds.). Oxford, Blackwell Scientific Publications Ltd (in press).
[20] Mack, T.M., Pike, M.C., Henderson, B.E. et al.: Estrogens and endometrial cancer in a retirement community. N. Engl. J. Med. 1976; 294:1262.
[21] Gray, L.A. Sr., Christopherson, W.M., Hoover, R.N.: Estrogens and endometrial carcinoma. Obstet. Gynecol. 1977; 49:385.
[22] Nachtigall, L.E., Nachtigall, R.H., Nachtigall, R.B. et al.: Estrogen replacement: II. A prospective study in the relationship to carcinoma and cardiovascular and metabolic problems. Obstet. Gynecol. 1979; 54:74.
[23] Gambrell, R.D. Jr., Massey, F.M., Castaneda, T.A. et al.: Use of the progestogen challenge test to reduce the risk of endometrial cancer. Obstet. Gynecol. 1980; 55:732.
[24] Sturdee, D.W., Wade-Evans, T., Paterson, M.E.L. et al.: Relationships between bleeding pattern, endometrial histology and oestrogen treatment in menopausal women. Br. Med. J. 1978; 1:1575.
[25] Whitehead, M.L., Townsend, P.T., Pryse-Davies, J. et al.: Effects of estrogens and progestins on the biochemistry and morphology of the postmenopausal endometrium. N. Engl. J. Med. 1981; 305:1599.
[26] Clark, G.M., McGuire, W.L., Hubay, C.A. et al.: Progesterone receptors as prognostic factor in stage II breast cancer. N. Engl. J. Med. 1983; 309:1343.
[27] Korenman, S.G.: The endocrinology of breast cancer. Cancer 1980; 46:874.
[28] Cowan, L.D., Gordis, L., Tonascia, J.A. et al.: Breast cancer incidence in women with a history of progesterone deficiency. Am. J. Epidemiol. 1981; 114:209.

[29] Coulam, C. B., Annegers, J. F.: Chronic anovulation may increase postmenopausal breast cancer risk. JAMA 1983, 249:445.

[30] Gambrell, R. D. Jr.: Oral contraceptives, postmenopausal oestrogen-progestogen use and breast cancer. J. Obstet. Gynecol. 1984; 4:S121.

Prevention of endometrial abnormalities

M. I. Whitehead

Introduction

When subjected to prolonged stimulation by either endogenous or exogenous estrogens in the absence of progesterone or a progestogen, the endometrium of some pre – and postmenopausal women can become hyperplastic [1, 2]. It is not clear why some but not all women exhibit this abnormal response. Possible mechanisms include disordered estrogen metabolism; reduced plasma levels of sex hormone binding globulin (SHBG), whereby more of the circulating steroid becomes free to transfer into responsive cells [3]; and increased sensitivity of the endometrium to the estrogenic stimulation [4].

Hyperplasia can be considered as an abnormal increase in the amount of proliferative endometrium which exhibits varying degrees of architectural and cytological atypia. Two distinct forms are recognised: in cystic hyperplasia, the abnormalities are widespread although polypoid projections may form. The diameter of the epithelial glands varies widely and the lining epithelium, which is high cuboidal or columnar, may become multi-layered. The stroma appears hypercellular because the constituent cells are plump and closely packed.

Adenomatous hyperplasia is a term reserved for a spectrum of more marked changes that may be either focal or diffuse. In the affected areas, the glands are crowded together and may exhibit infolding and budding; the epithelium may show pseudostratification. These changes are exaggerated as the hyperplasia becomes more severe and, eventually, the epithelium may exhibit an eosinophilic pallor and form syncitium-like processes on the endometrial surface. Nuclear atypia is common and the stroma may be active or fibrotic. Sometimes, it is extremely difficult to differentiate between severe adenomatous hyperplasia and adenocarcinoma.

The histological distinction between cystic and adenomatous hyperplasia is of more than academic interest because of differences in the pre-malignant potential. With cystic hyperplasia, the subsequent conversion to adenocarcinoma is low, approximately 1% [5]: with adenomatous hyperplasia, the rate is higher and increases with time. Thus, 12% of adenomatous hyperplasias will have become carcinomas after 18 months and 30% will have undergone malignant change within 10 years [6]. Shanklin's data suggest that the development of adenomatous hyperplasia should be considered as "the point of no return" in the progression from normal, proliferative endometrium through hyperplasia to malignant endometrium [7]. In his series, every patient with adenomatous hyperplasia eventually developed endometrial carcinoma.

Endometrial response to postmenopausal estrogen therapy

American Experience: it is now almost 10 years since the first, retrospective, case-control studies published in America [8, 9, 10] linked unopposed, estrogen use with an increase in the incidence of endometrial cancer. Because of methodological flaws, these early studies were criticised and their conclusions were deemed unjustified by many other investigators. However, the subsequent publication of numerous, better controlled, epidemiological studies supporting the early reports [11, 12, 13] has, in the majority view, confirmed a causal relationship which appears to be both dose and duration dependent [14]. Certain aspects of this relationship still require elucidation. For example, it is still unclear if the duration-dependent increase in risk of endometrial cancer is linear or exponential [15]. Additionally, it is this author's opinion that other aspects of the relationship have been widely misinterpreted. Chu et al. [16] reported that women with endometrial cancer who had used unopposed estrogens had a significantly better survival that non-users and it is now often stated that estrogen-related cancers are associated with a low mortality. Robboy and Bradley have presented data [17] that although the 5 year and 10 year survival rates for estrogen users are higher than those for non-users, this difference disappears when the grade of the neoplasm is taken into account. Thus, the prognosis for estrogen-users with Grade 2, 3 or 4 neoplasms is NOT more favourable than for non-users.

To date, the long-term consequences of unopposed postmenopausal estrogen use have been investigated by only one group. Shapiro and his colleagues recently reported that women who had taken unopposed estrogens for at least 1 year remained at an increased risk for endometrial cancer for at least 10 years after discontinuing therapy. Long-term gynaecological surveillance was suggested [18].

Whilst the epidemiological data clearly state the risks for endometrial cancer, they do not provide information on the clinical consequences of unopposed, postmenopausal estrogen use in terms of gynaecological morbidity. Ettinger et al. [19] have recently reviewed their patients' records and have reported that the relative risk for abnormal vaginal bleeding and curettage were 7.8 and 4.9, respectively, in estrogen-users as compared to appropriately matched non-hormone exposed controls. During a 20 year period, the cumulative prevalence for hysterectomy was 5.3% in non-users but 28.2% in estrogen-users [19]. Thus, almost one woman in 3 receiving long-term, unopposed estrogens eventually required hysterectomy because of abnormal vaginal bleeding or the development of pre-malignant or malignant endometrial histology.

European Experience: the majority of the European data have been generated from prospective studies. Two London-based groups biopsied postmenopausal women at defined intervals during unopposed estrogen therapy and both reported that the development of hyperplasia was related to the estrogen dose [2, 20]. In our studies, the incidence of hyperplasia was 18% with conjugated equine estrogens (Premarin®/ Ayerst Laboratories) 0.625 mg daily or equivalent, and was 32% with conjugated estrogens 1.25 mg daily or equivalent, after a mean duration of therapy of approximately 16 months. Importantly, up to one third of the hyperplasias were of the more sinister adenomatous variety. Both groups also reported that the underlying endometrial status was not reflected by the pattern of bleeding per vaginam. Our bleeding data [21] are reproduced in Table 1. Regular withdrawal bleeding and no

Table 1 The patterns of vaginal bleeding with normal and hyperplastic endometrium during unopposed cyclical estrogen therapy. The data are presented as numbers of patients (percentages).

Type of therapy	Endometrial histology	Number of patients with withdrawal bleeding	Number of patients with breakthrough bleeding	Number of patients with no vaginal bleeding
Cyclical high-dose	Normal endometrium	14 (64%)	11 (69%)	22 (71%)
	Endometrial hyperplasia	8 (36%)	5 (31%)	9 (29%)
Cyclical low-dose	Normal endometrium	3	5 (31%)	23 (96%)
	Endometrial hyperplasia	1	4 (44%)	1 (4%)

Cyclical high dose = conjugated equine estrogens 1.25 mg, daily
piperazine oestrone sulphate 3.0 mg daily
estradiol valerate 2.0 mg daily
Cycical low dose = one half the high dose, daily.
Reproduced, with permission of the Editor from Whitehead M. I., Maturitas, 1:87, 1978 (ref 21).

bleeding per vaginam were both associated with endometrial hyperplasia and therefore these patterns of bleeding did not signify, as is often assumed, that endometrial pathology was not present. Abnormal vaginal bleeding was reported by 24% (25/106) of women during cyclical, unopposed, high or low-dose estrogen therapy. However, in only 9 of these women was endometrial hyperplasia diagnosed at biopsy. Confirmatory, American data on the unreliability of the bleeding pattern as an indicator of the underlying endometrial status are now available [22].

In summary, therefore, there is overwhelming evidence that unopposed, postmenopausal, estrogen use causes a high incidence of abnormal bleeding; an unacceptable incidence of endometrial hyperplasia, and increases the risk of endometrial cancer:

and there is one report that the risk of cancer may be increased for as long as 10 years after therapy has been discontinued. Although the increase in risk of adenocarcinoma is small it is not surprising that these data have resulted in a decline in estrogen use and have led to various suggestions regarding changes to the treatment schedule to minimise the risk of endometrial hyperstimulation.

Modifications to reduce endometrial hyperstimulation

Routine endometrial biopsy: we have reported that in postmenopausal women who have not received exogenous estrogens and who have not experienced abnormal vaginal bleeding, the incidence of cystic hyperplasia is 2–3%, and of atypical hyperplasia is 1% [23]. We have also reported that if women with pre-existing hyperplasia receive unopposed, cyclical estrogens, then the development of endometrial carcinoma can be rapid, within 12 months [23]. For these reasons, we believe that if cyclical estrogen therapy is to be prescribed then a pre-treatment biopsy should be seriously considered. Further biopsies should, most probably, be performed at approximately annual intervals during unopposed cyclical therapy irrespective of the bleeding pattern and for as long as therapy is prescribed. Hyperplasia may arise at least 2 years after the initiation of cyclical therapy with a previous biopsy, at the end of the first year of treatment, having been normal [24].

Whilst such an approach is likely to achieve the desired result of reducing the risk of endometrial cancer, it has two major disadvantages.

Firstly, it cannot be cost-effective because the detection rate for endometrial hyperplasia is low. Secondly, repeated endometrial biopsies, if performed as an in-patient procedure expose women to the risks of general anaesthesia. This can be overcome using an out-patient procedure but endometrial biopsy in conscious women can cause discomfort which some find unacceptable [25].

Reducing the estrogen dose: Logically, the most attractive modification would be to reduce the estrogen dose and thereby lower the risk of endometrial hyperstimulation. However, dosage reductions are now known to reduce the beneficial estrogen effects of relieving not only the physical and psychological symptoms due to ovarian failure, but also of conserving bone mass. The bone-conserving effects of estrogens are increasingly being recognised as the major indication for long-term use, not only because the consequences of postmenopausal osteoporosis in terms of morbidity, mortality and costs are so appalling [26], but also because adequate doses of estrogens are the most effective therapy for conserving bone mass [27, 28].

Both beneficial effects are now known to be dose-dependent. Reductions in the daily dose of estradiol from 4 mg to 2 mg to 1 mg daily are associated with a failure to relieve hot flushes completely, and the 1 mg dose exerts sub-optimal bone-sparing activity [29]. Almost identical data are available for conjugated estrogens. In our clinical experience, a lowering in dosage to 0.3 mg daily is associated with a loss of supression of vasomotor symptoms and does not appear to conserve bone mass as effectively as 0.625 mg daily [30]. Thus, the minimum effective bone-sparing dosages of estradiolvalerate and conjugated estrogens are 2 mg and 0.625 mg daily, respectively, and endometrial proliferation has been observed with these dosages [2, 21]. Smaller daily doses may control very mild climacteric symptoms effectively, but the physician and patient should be aware that conservation of bone mass is not likely to be achieved.

Avoiding estrone preparations: It has been suggested that because the retrospective, American, epidemiological studies associated mainly conjugated estrogens (65% of which is estrone sulphate) with an increase in risk of endometrial carcinoma, then this preparation must possess special carcinogenic properties [31] not present with other estrogen formulations containing estradiol or estriol. The assumption is that these latter preparations can be safely prescribed without a risk of endometrial hyperstimulation, but this assumption is incorrect. Conjugated estrogens were most closely linked with endometrial carcinoma because they are the most widely prescribed estrogen preparation in the United States. At equivalent doses, estradiolvalerate (Progynova®/Schering) causes the same degree of endometrial stimulation as conjugated estrogens with almost identical rates of hyperplasia [2].

Further evidence that estradiol-based preparations provoke endometrial stimulation similar to that of estrone-based formulations has come from biochemical investigations of endometrial tissue. Nuclear estradiol (REN) and cytoplasmic progesterone receptor (RPC) are induced by estrogen stimulation. Levels of these receptors have been measured in postmenopausal women receiving a variety of orally and parenterally administered estrogens [32]. Oral conjugated estrogens, 0.625 mg and 1.25 mg daily, oral estradiol valerate 2 mg daily, and oral piperazine estrone sulphate (Harmogen®/Abbott Laboratories) 1.5 mg daily, induced similar levels of REN and RPC: all receptor values were within the premenopausal, proliferative phase range implying that a potent stimulus was being applied to the postmenopausal endometrium [32]. It is stressed that even in postmenopausal women receiving estrone-based preparations, estradiol remains the predominant, intra-nuclear estrogen within the endometrium [33, 34]. Estradiol is a much more potent stimulator of cell biosynthesis than estrone [35] and therefore, estrogen formulations which selectively increase plasma estradiol values, such as estradiol implants, are likely to be associated with marked endometrial proliferation. Thus, the high incidence of hyperplasia, 56%, reported with estradiol implants [20] is not surprising.

Based upon the available epidemiological [8–13], histological [2, 20] and biochemical data [32–34], dosages of all estradiol and estrone-based formulations needed for the relief of climacteric symptoms and the conservation of bone mass are likely to provoke endometrial proliferation.

Prescribe estriol preparations: unlike the estrone and estradiol-based preparations, low doses of estriol, 2 mg daily, appear to have little proliferative effect upon the endometrium [36]. Estriol has, therefore been recommended as the ideal estrogen for postmenopausal use [37]. Whether such low doses of estriol actually impart an estrogenic stimulus is doubtful because, unlike all other estrogens studied to date, low-dose estriol does not appear to conserve bone mass and is not better than placebo in relieving acute vasomotor symptoms [38]. Estriol pharmacodynamics are different from those of estrone and estradiol: estriol is not strongly bound to plasma proteins and globulins but circulates largely as the glucuronide: rapid renal excretion is facilitated [39]. Thus, an oral dose of estriol is absorbed and largely excreted within 3 hours. When administered at 8-hourly intervals, estriol has been linked to the development of endometrial hyperplasia [39].

It has been suggested that the addition of estriol to another estrogen preparation may be beneficial in terms of reducing endometrial proliferation. Indeed, formulations in which a small dose of estriol (1 mg) is added to estradiol are widely used throughout Europe. The rationale for this addition is as follows. Certain experimental evidence suggested that estriol causes minimal endometrial proliferation because the intra-nuclear retention time is short [40, 41]. Therefore, estriol was classified as a short acting estrogen. Estriol possesses an affinity for the estrogen receptor, and it was argued that the addition of estriol might interfere with the binding of the receptor to the more potent estrogens, estradiol and estrone. In so doing, the overall estrogenic stimulus would be reduced [42], with estriol impeding receptor binding to estradiol.

Recently, we have tested this hypothesis. In a prospective, randomised, double-blind, cross-over study, postmenopausal women received either estradiol in combination with estriol and then estradiol alone, each for 3 months, or vice versa. Endometrial biopsies were performed after each course of treatment. The frequency of the various histological diagnoses was not significantly different between treatments (Table 2), and we were unable to demonstrate any protective effect for estriol [43]. Hence, we doubt the validity of the hypothesis and question the wisdom of estriol addition.

Progestogen addition: unlike the other strategies listed above, there is considerable evidence that the addition of a progestogen to the estrogen therapy is protective to the endometrium. Both London-based groups which have performed prospective, histological studies have reported a reduction in the incidence of hyperplasia with progestogen addition [2, 20]. In our studies, the incidence of hyperplasia was 18–32% with unopposed, cyclical estrogens and was significantly lowered to 3–4% when progestogens were added for 7 days each calendar month [2]. Extending the duration of progestogen administration to 10 days reduces the incidence of hyperplasia to 2% [20], and maximum protective effects are obtained with 12–13 days of progestogen exposure, the incidence of hyperplasia being zero [20, 44]. The

Table 2 Endometrial histology during estradiol or estradiol plus estriol therapy. Data are presented as numbers of samples (percentages).

Histological Diagnosis	Estradiol Therapy	Estradiol + Estriol Therapy
Proliferative	8 (57%)	7 (50%)
Non-secretory	2 (14%)	2 (14%)
Tissue insufficient for analysis	2 (14%)	3 (21%)
Hyperplasia	1 (7%)	2 (14%)
Secretory	1 (7%)	–

Reproduced, with permission of the Editor from Padwick M. L. et al., Brit. J. Obstet. Gynaecol. (In Press) (ref 43).

incidence of endometrial carcinoma with combined estrogen/progestogen regimens is also reduced, and not only to below that recorded with unopposed estrogens but also to below that observed in untreated women. The incidence rates for endometrial cancer in an untreated population between 1975 and 1979 in Texas was 242.2 per 100,000 women; in the estrogen users, the rate was 434.4 per 100,000 women, and with combined estrogen/progestogen therapies was 70.8 per 100,000 women [45]. The difference between the estrogen/progestogen-users and the estrogen-users was highly significant ($p<0.0001$).

Benefits and risks of progestogen addition

General considerations: with all forms of therapy, the benefits of treatment have to be weighed against the disadvantages. In addition to protecting the endometrium, there is increasing evidence that progestogen addition may enhance the bone-conserving effects of estrogens. It has been known for some years that unopposed estrogen therapy will conserve postmenopausal bone mass [46]. However, two prospective, placebo controlled studies have reported a small but significant increase in bone mass with combined estrogen/progestogen regimens started soon after menopause [27, 47, 48]. Most recently, Christiansen et al. [49] have reported that serum alkaline phosphatase and bone Gla protein increase during progestogen administration and have suggested that progestogens may enhance bone formation.

There can be no doubt that progestogens can also cause undesirable side-effects and, quite clearly, it is pointless adding a progestogen to prevent against endometrial hyperstimulation (and perhaps increase bone formation), if, by so doing, the physical and psychological well-being are adversely affected and/or the risk of other potentially fatal diseases is increased. It is important to emphasise that the frequency and severity of progestogenic side-effects will be modified by (i) the type of progestogen administered; (ii) the route of administration, and (iii) the daily/monthly dose.

Progestogens can be classified in a variety of ways. The classification based upon structure [50] seems most sensible because the chemical configuration appears to influence biological activity and thereby the type of side-effects. For example, the 19-nor-testosterone derivatives, norethisterone and dl-norgestrel adversely affect plasma lipid concentrations and lipoprotein metabolism [51, 52], but the halogenated progesterone derivatives, such as cyproterone acetate, do not. Although it was established many years ago that progesterone was well absorbed after rectal, vaginal and intra-muscular administration [53], few comparative, pharmacodynamic data are available. Ottosson et al. have reported serum levels of progesterone 2–3 times higher with the intramuscular route as compared to the oral route [54]. Routes of administration which permit good absorption so that the total administered progestogen dose is lowered without a loss of endometrial effect are likely to reduce the incidence of side-effects.

Because most progestogenic side-effects are dose-related, the minimum effective dose should be prescribed. Because progestogens are administered primarily to prevent against endometrial hyperstimulation, the minimum effective dose is the lowest which confers endometrial protection. This cannot be overstressed and before considering progestogenic side-effects further, the endometrial data will be reviewed.

Endometrial effects of progestogens

Progestogen effects on the estrogenised postmenopausal endometrium can be determined by histological and biochemical investigations.

Histological evaluation includes assessments with the conventional light microscope and also the transmission electron microscope. The latter is used to determine the presence or absence in postmenopausal endometrium of certain ultra-structural features which are known to be induced by endogenous progesterone between days 17–21 of the ovulatory cycle: these include sub-nuclear accumulations of glycogen, nucleolar channel systems and giant mitochondria. Biochemically, we have measured progestogen-induced suppression of DNA synthesis and nuclear estradiol receptor (REN); this suppression is evidence for the anti-mitotic or antiproliferative effect of progestogens. We have also determined progestogen induction of the enzymes estradiol-17-β-dehydrogenase and isocitrate dehydrogenase; this induction is evidence of the secretory effect of exogenous progestogens.

Our histological, ultrastructural and biochemical data for norethisterone and dl-norgestrel [32, 55]: oral progesterone (Utrogestan®/Laboratoires Besins Iscovesco)

[56]; dydrogesterone (Duphaston®/Duphar Laboratories) [57], and medroxyprogesterone acetate (Provera®/Upjohn) [58] have been published and have been reviewed [59]. In summary, good agreement was observed between the histological and biochemical assessments. Our interpretation of the data is that, when prescribed for 12 days each calendar month, the minimum effective daily dose of norethisterone (NET) is 0.7 mg; of oral progesterone is 300 mg; of dydrogesterone is 10–20 mg and of medroxyprogesterone acetate (MPA) is 10 mg. The dl-norgestrel data were more difficult to evalute: 75 mcg is clearly inadequate.

It is stressed that the above comments apply to estrogen/progestogen regimens in which the estrogen was administered continuously, for 365 days each year, and the progestogen was added for 12 days in each calendar month (sequential estrogen/progestogen therapy). With such treatment, vaginal bleeding is usually re-established. This appears to be well tolerated by women seeking treatment for relief of distressing symptoms. However, concern has been expressed that asymptomatic women, considering exogenous estrogens to prevent against postmenopausal bone loss, are much less likely to tolerate bleeding.

At adequate doses, progestogens suppress DNA synthesis and REN formation [32, 55–58], and thereby prevent endometrial proliferation. By administering the progestogen continuously, every day in combination with the estrogen (continuous estrogen/progestogen therapy), various workers have attempted to develop a therapy which induces amenorrhoea. The first report was by Staland [60] who administered tablets containing estradiol-17-β 2 mg, estriol 1 mg and norethisterone acetate (NETA) 1 mg, daily to 265 women for up to 52 months. Therapy was extremely effective in inducing an atrophic endometrium (> 96% of patients). However, Staland reported that approximately 40% of patients had irregular bleeding during the first treatment month and that approximately 10% were still bleeding irregularly during the fourth month of treatment. Thereafter, the incidence of abnormal bleeding fell with approximately 4% of patients bleeding between the fifth and twelfth month of therapy. Thirty per cent of patients had discontinued treatment by the end of one year [60].

An identical regimen was prescribed by Mattsson et al. [61] with very similar results. Light, breakthrough bleeding was not uncommon during the first 3 months of therapy: thereafter, however, bleeding was infrequent. Both Staland [60] and Mattsson et al. [61] reported less bleeding in post as compared to perimenopausal women.

The precise reasons for the frequent, but light, bleeding experienced during the first 3–4 months of therapy remain unclear. In 1983, Staland reported that plasma levels of NETA had returned to baseline 8 hours after administration of 1 mg NETA [62]. We wondered whether this rapid fall in plasma values might not be responsible for the breakthrough bleeding – the rapid decline in circulating progestogen levels inducing a "mini" progestogen withdrawal bleed. Therefore, we prescribed a

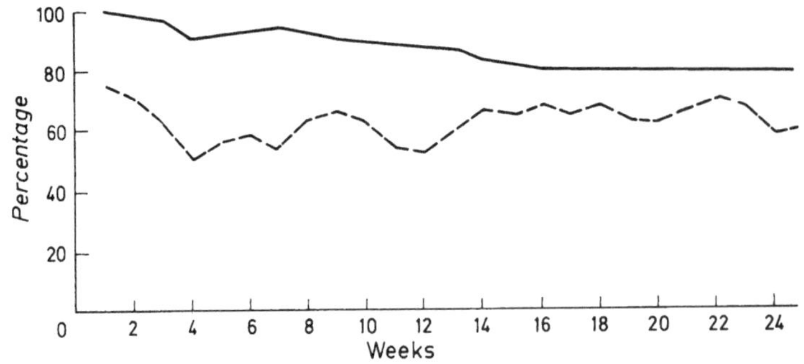

Fig. 1 – percentage of patients continuing on continuous estrogen/progestogen treatment (———): and percentage with amenorrhoea (------) expressed as a percentage of those initially recruited. See text for details of treatment regimen.

continuous regimen in which low doses of NET 0.35 mg or MPA 2.5 mg were administered twice daily in combination with conjugated estrogens 0.625 mg daily. Our data are presented in Figure 1: 73 patients were recruited and the figure illustrates the percentage continuing on treatment and the percent with amenorrhoea (expressed as a percentage of those recruited), week by week, for the first 6 months of therapy. Essentially, our results with twice daily progestogen administration are similar to those of Staland [60] and Mattsson et al. [61]. For example, at the end of 6 months, 18% of our patients had discontinued treatment because of irregular, but light, bleeding: 60% of those initially recruited had amenorrhoea.

A different approach was adopted by Magos et al. [63]. Two estrogen doses were prescribed – conjugated estrogens 0.625 mg or 1.25 mg daily. NET was commenced at doses of either 0.35 mg or 1.05 mg daily and the dose was increased at 3 monthly intervals if persisting breakthrough bleeding was reported. In general, fewer and lighter bleeding episodes were reported with the lower estrogen dose, and after 3 months of therapy significantly more women taking conjugated estrogens 0.625 mg daily had amenorrhoea (68%) than 1.25 mg daily (42%) ($p<0.05$). Amenorrhoea was eventually achieved in all women after 15 months of treatment: however, 35% of women had stopped therapy because of side-effects, mainly unacceptable vaginal bleeding. Using a similar protocol, the same group investigated continuous progestogen administration to patients receiving estradiol and testosterone implants (Organon): the results were much less encouraging with amenorrhoea being achieved in only 63% of women after 12 months [64].

Based on the data currently available for continuous estrogen/progestogen therapy, it is this author's opinion that the ideal regimen has not yet been developed: and that whilst such treatment can be prescribed in specialised menopause clinics which possess facilities for out-patient endometrial biopsy, it is extremely doubtful whether continuous estrogen/progestogen therapies can be widely prescribed by family physicians. Breakthrough bleeding, even if it is subsequently shown to arise from an atrophic endometrium, is a worrying sign for the patient and the family physician and demands appropriate investigation. The current continuous regimens cause too much breakthrough bleeding for widespread use.

Physical, psychological and metabolic effects of progestogens

The clinical implications of the endometrial data are that with sequential therapies, progestogens need to be prescribed for 12 days each calender month to afford optimal endometrial protection [20, 44]. It is clear that the doses of certain progestogens, such as NET and dl-norgestrel, can be reduced without a loss of protective effect [32, 55]. At present, we recommend the addition of NET 0.7 mg or dl-norgestrel 150 mcg [59]; or of oral progesterone 300 mg [56]; or of dydrogesterone 10–20 mg [57], or of MPA 10 mg [58] daily for 12 days each calender month. Are there differences between these doses of these progestogens in terms of adverse effects upon the physical, psychological and metabolic (including cardiovascular and bone) status of postmenopausal women? Additionally, what are the effects of NETA 1 mg when added to the estrogen therapy in a continuous fashion?

Regrettably, and somewhat surprisingly, there are few answers to these questions at present. Sequential estrogen/progestogen therapy incorporating 250 mcg levonorgestrel daily exerts a less beneficial effect on mood, mastalgia and breast size than estrogen alone [65, 66]. Our clinical experience would support these data because with dl-norgestrel 500 mcg daily, (equivalent to 250 mcg levonorgestrel), approximately 10% of our patients experience a pre-menstrual tension-like syndrome during the progestogen phase of treatment (unpublished observations). However, in our experience, reducing the dose to 150 mcg dl norgestrel daily results in a reduction in the frequency and intensity of these adverse changes. Sadly, there are no data from properly conducted, prospective studies on the physical and psychological changes caused by the doses of the progestogens that are currently recommended for addition to postmenopausal estrogen therapy.

More information is available on the effects of sequential and continuous estrogen/progestogen regimens on lipid and lipoprotein metabolism. The progestogen component of the oral contraceptive pill has been linked to an increase in incidence of arterial disease and hypertension [52, 67], an effect possibly mediated through suppression of high density lipoprotein (HDL)-cholesterol and elevation of low density lipoprotein (LDL)-cholesterol. Obviously, it is pointless adding a progestogen to protect against endometrial hyperstimulation if, by such an addition, the risk of death from arterial disease is increased and the beneficial effects of estrogens on the cardio-vascular system are negated [68].

The metabolic effects of progestogens are clearly dose-related [69, 70]. The early studies of sequential estrogen/progestogen regimens tended to use progestogen doses greatly in excess of those required for endometrial protection. For example, Hirvonen et al. [51] compared the effects of NET, 10 mg daily, with those of dl-norgestrel, 500 mcg daily and MPA, 10 mg daily. NET and dl-norgestrel caused significantly greater depression of HDL-cholesterol than MPA and therefore, it was argued that MPA was the progestogen of choice for addition to postmenopausal estrogens. We doubt the validity of this conclusion given that a lower dose of NET, 0.7 mg daily, appears to protect the endometrium: and NET, 1 mg daily, causes virtually no changes in HDL-cholesterol values [71]. Low doses of levo-norgestrel, 30 mcg daily, are similarly devoid of adverse effects on lipoprotein metabolism [72], but have not been shown to prevent against endometrial hyperstimulation. At higher doses, levo-norgestrel causes significant suppression of HDL-cholesterol, and in particular the HDL_2-cholesterol sub-fraction [73]. Unfortunately, no data are available as to whether 75 mcg of levonorgestrel, which appears to be the minimum effective dose for endometrial protection with sequential regimens, causes adverse lipid changes.

At present, controversy exists regarding the safety of MPA. Hirvonen et al. [51], Silferstolpe et al. [74], Mattsson et al. [75] and Notelovitz et al. [76] all reported that MPA did not interfere with lipoprotein metabolism. A more recent study by Ottosson et al. [77] reported significant suppression of HDL and HDL_2-cholesterol, the latter being depressed by 17% after 3 months of cyclical therapy with estradiol-valerate, 2 mg daily, and MPA, 10 mg daily, being added for 10 days each cycle. Ottosson et al. [77] suggested that the conclusions of certain of the previous studies [51, 74, 75] were based on comparatively few clinical observations. It is unlikely that this explanation can account for the differences reported by Ottosson et al. [77] as compared to Notelovitz et al. [76]. The latter study 20 postmenopausal women treated for 12 months with conjugated estrogens and MPA: a control group of 18 subjects was also included. Other explanations to account for these differences can be proposed: they include differences in laboratory methodology and dissimilarities in the type of estrogen prescribed. The latter will be considered further below.

There is general agreement that, at effective doses, oral progesterone causes few, if any, changes in lipid metabolism [73, 77]: no data are currently available for dydrogesterone.

Only one group has reported on lipid changes due to continuous estrogen/progestogen regimens. A combination of estradiol, 2 mg, estriol, 1 mg, and NETA, 1 mg, daily, reduces HDL-cholesterol but also lowers LDL-cholesterol [78]. Therefore, the HDL/LDL ratio is not altered by such therapy. The clinical implications of these data, in terms of altering the risk of arterial disease, are unclear.

It is now apparent that the estrogen component of sequential, and presumably continuous, estrogen/progestogen therapies influences the lipid status. Differences in lipid metabolism between dissimilar types of estrogens are well documented [79], and Jensen et al. have recently drawn attention to the influence that the estrogen dose may have upon overall changes in lipoprotein metabolism during sequential estrogen/progestogen therapy [80]. For example, the average increase in HDL-cholesterol was 13%, 9% and 2% with micronised estradiol 4 mg, 2 mg and 1 mg, daily, respectively: the corresponding mean decrease in LDL-cholesterol was 18%, 15% and 10%, respectively.

Summary

Exogenous estrogens are highly effective in relieving not only the acute symptoms of ovarian failure, such as vasomotor instability and vaginal dryness, but also in conserving postmenopausal bone mass. However, the estrogen doses needed to achieve these benefits also induce endometrial proliferation. The risk of endometrial hyperplasia and carcinoma are thereby increased and unopposed estrogen therapy is associated with a high incidence of abnormal vaginal bleeding requiring appropriate, invasive investigations. The cost-effectiveness of therapy and patient compliance are likely to be correspondingly reduced.

Various strategies have been proposed to try to overcome the risk of endometrial hyperstimulation and these strategies have been reviewed.

Based upon the available evidence, progestogen addition appears the most sensible and has been shown to be effective. It is now clear that progestogens should, in sequential therapies, be administered for 12 days each cycle for maximum protection. Concern has been expressed that the regular withdrawal bleed induced by sequential treatment will reduce patient compliance. Progestogens have, therefore, been added in a continuous fashion to try to prevent endometrial proliferation and thereby induce amenorrhoea. The ideal continuous, estrogen/progestogen regimen has not yet been developed: all those evaluated to date are associated with a high incidence of breakthrough bleeding which is likely to restrict their use.

Progestogens can cause undesirable physical, psychological and metabolic effects. The incidence and severity of side-effects will depend upon the type of progestogen prescribed, the route of administration, and the dose. Minimum effective daily doses of certain types of progestogens have now been established in terms of endometrial protection. Regrettably, few data are available on the physical and psychological effects of these progestogen doses: more information is available on lipid and lipoprotein effects but the data are confused and, at times, contradictory.

More research is urgently needed to determine which of these progestogens is most suitable for addition to postmenopausal estrogen therapy.

Acknowledgements

It is a pleasure to acknowledge the assistance of numerous colleagues in the Menopause Clinic, Academic Department of Obstetrics and Gynaecology, King's College School of Medicine and Dentistry; of Dr R. J. B. King, Hormone Biochemistry Department, Imperial Cancer Research Fund Laboratories, Lincoln's Inn Fields, London; and of Drs J. Pryse-Davies and T. Ryder at the Institute of Obstetrics and Gynaecology, Queen Charlottes Maternity Hospital. Hammersmith, London.

The financial assistance of the Imperial Cancer Research Fund Laboratories to the author is gratefully acknowledged.

The help of Miss J. Bennett and Mrs J. Horne in the preparation of this manuscript is much appreciated.

References

[1] Siiteri, P. K., Hemsell, D. R., Edwards, C. L., MacDonald, P. C.: Estrogens and endometrial cancer. In: Scow, R. O. (Ed) Proceedings of the Fourth International Congress on Endocrinology. Amsterdam, Excerpta Medica, pp 1237–1239, 1973.

[2] Whitehead, M. I., King, R. J. B., McQueen, J., Campbell, S.: Endometrial histology and biochemistry in climacteric women during oestrogen and oestrogen/progestin therapy. J. R. Soc. Med. 72:322, 1979.

[3] Davidson, B. J., Gambone, J. C., Lagasse, L. D. et al.: Free estradiol in postmenopausal women with and without endometrial cancer. Clin Endocrinol. Metab. 52:404, 1981.

[4] King, R. J. B., Whitehead, M. I., Campbell, S. Minardi, J.: Effect of estrogen and progestin treatments on endometria from postmenopausal women. Cancer Res. 39:1094, 1979.

[5] McBride, J. M.: Premenopausal cystic hyperplasia and endometrial carcinoma. J. Obstet. Gynaecol. Br. Commonwealth, 54:521, 1959.

[6] Gusberg, S.: The individual at high risk for endometrial carcinoma. Am J. Obstet. Gynecol. 126:535, 1976.

[7] Shanklin, D. R.: Endometrial carcinoma. Pathol. Annu. 2:233, 1978.

[8] Smith, D. C., Prentice, R., Thompson, D., Herrman, W.: Association of exogenous estrogens and endometrial cancer. N. Engl. J. Med. 293:1164, 1975.

[9] Ziel, H. Finkle, W.: Increased risk of endometrial carcinoma among users of conjugated estrogens. N. Engl. J. Med. 293:1167, 1975.

[10] Mack, T., Pike, M., Henderson, B. et al.: Estrogens and endometrial cancer in a retirement community. N. Engl. J. Med. 294:1262, 1976.

[11] Antunes, C. M. F., Stolley, P. D., Rosenheim, N. B. et al.: Endometrial cancer and estrogen use. Report of a large case-control study. N. Engl. J. Med. 300:9, 1979.

[12] Shapiro, S., Kaufmann, D. W., Slone, D. et al.: Recent and past use of conjugated oestrogens in relation to adencarcinoma of the endometrium. N. Engl. J. Med. 303:485, 1980.

[13] Jick, H., Watkins, R. N., Hunter, J. R. et al.: Replacement estrogens and endometrial cancer. N. Engl. J. Med. 300:218, 1979.

[14] Vessey, M. P., Bungay, G. T.: Benefits and risks of hormone therapy in the menopause. In Smith, A. (ed): Recent Advances in Community Medicine. Edinburgh: Churchill Livingstone, pp 77–94, 1982.

[15] Cramer, D. W., Knapp, R. C.: Review of

epidemiologic studies of endometrial cancer and exogenous estrogen. Obstet. Gynecol. 54:521, 1979.
[16] Chu, J., Schweid, A. I., Weiss, N. S.: Survival among women with endometrial cancer: A comparison of estrogen users and non-users. Am. J. Obstet. Gynecol. 143:569, 1982.
[17] Robboy, S. J., Bradley, R.: Changing trends and prognostic features in endometrial cancer associated with exogenous estrogen therapy. Obstet. Gnyecol. 54:269, 1979.
[18] Shapiro, S., Kelly, J. P., Rosenberg, L. et al.: Risk of localised and widespread endometrial cancer in relation to recent and discontinued use of conjugated estrogens. N. Engl. J. Med. 313:969, 1985.
[19] Ettinger, B., Golditch, I. M., Friedman, G.: Gynecologic consequences of long-term estrogen replacement therapy (In Press).
[20] Studd, J. W. W., Thom, MH., Paterson, M. E. L., Wade-Evans, T.: The prevention and treatment of endometrial pathology in postmenopausal women receiving exogenous estrogens. In Pasetto, N., Paoletti, R., Ambrus, J. L. (eds). The Menopause and Postmenopause. Lancaster, M. T. P. Press, pp 127–139, 1980.
[21] Whitehead, M. I.: The effects of oestrogens and progestogens on the postmenopausal endometrium. Maturitas, 1:87, 1978.
[22] Schiff, I., Sela, H. K., Cramer, D., Tulchinsky, D., Ryan, K. J.: Endometrial hyperplasia in women on cyclic or continuous estrogen regimens. Fertil. Steril. 37:79, 1982.
[23] Whitehead, M. I., Campbell, S.: Endometrial histology, uterine bleeding and oestrogen levels in menopausal women receiving oestrogen therapy and oestrogen/progestogen therapy. In: Brush, M., Taylor, R. W. T. and King, R. J. B. (eds) Endometrial Cancer. London, Balliere Tindall, pp 65–80, 1978.
[24] Campbell, S., McQueen, J., Minardi, J., Whitehead, M. I.: The modifying effect of progestogen on the response of the postmenopausal endometrium to exogenous oestrogens. Postgrad. Med. J. 54, (Suppl 2) 59, 1978.
[25] Siddle, N. C., Young, O., Sledmere, C. M., Reading, A. E., Whitehead, M. I.: A controlled trial of Naproxen Sodium for relief of pain associated with Vabra suction curettage. Brit. J. Obstet. Gynaecol. 90:864, 1983.
[26] Stevenson, J. C., Whitehead, M. I.: Postmenopausal osteoporosis. Br. Med. J. 285:585, 1982.
[27] Christiansen, C., Christensen, M. S., McNair, P., Hagen, C., Stocklund, E., Transbol, I.: Prevention of early postmenopausal bone loss. Controlled 2-year study in 315 normal females. Eur. J. Clin, Invest. 10:273, 1980.
[28] Lindsay, R., Hart, D. M., Maclean, A., Clarke, A. C., Kraszewski, A., Garwood, J.: Bone response to termination of oestrogen treatment. Lancet, i:1325, 1978.
[29] Christensen, M. S., Hagen, C., Christiansen, C., Transbol, I.: Dose-response evalution of cyclic oestrogen/progestogen in postmenopausal women. Placebo-controlled trial of its gynecologic and metabolic actions. Am. J. Obstet. Gynecol. 144:873, 1982.
[30] Genant, H. K., Cann, C. E., Ettinger, B., Gordan, G. S.: Quantitative computer tomograph of vertebral spongiosa: A sensitive method for detecting early bone loss after oophorectomy. Ann. Intern. Med. 97:699, 1982.
[31] Ziel, H. K., Finkle, W. D.: Association of estrone and the development of endometrial cancer. Am. J. Obstet. Gynecol. 124:735, 1976.
[32] Whitehead, M. I., Townsend, P. T., Pryse-Davies, J., Ryder, T. A., King, R. J. B.: Effects of estrogens and progestins on the biochemistry and morphology of the postmenopausal endometrium. N. Engl. J. Med. 305:1599, 1981.
[33] Whitehead, M. I., Lane, G., Dyer, G., Townsend, P. T., Collins, W. P., King, R. J. B.: Oestradiol: The predominant intranuclear oestrogen in the endometrium of oestrogen-treated postmenopausal women. Br. J. Obstet. Gynaecol. 88:914, 1981.
[34] King, R. J. B., Dyer, G., Collins, W. P., Whitehead, M. I.: Intracellular estradiol, estrone and estrogen receptor levels in endometria from postmenopausal women receiving estrogens and progestins. J. Steroid Biochem. 13:377, 1980.
[35] King, R. J. B., Mainwaring, W. I. P.: Steroid Cell Interactions. London. Butterworths. pp 288–378, 1974.

[36] Myrhe, E.: Endometrial response to different estrogens. In Lauritzen, C., van Keep, P. A. (eds) Frontiers of Hormone Research. Vol. 5, Estrogen Therapy, the Benefits and Risks. Basel, S. Karger, pp 126–143, 1978.
[37] Follingstad, A. J. Estriol: The forgotten oestrogen. JAMA 239:29, 1978.
[38] Lindsay, R., Hart, D. M., Maclean, A., Garwood, J., Clark, A. C., Kraszewski, A.: Bone loss during oestriol therapy in postmenopausal women. Maturitas, 1:279, 1979.
[39] Englund, D. E.: Oestrogen treatment and the menopause. Acta Univ. Upsaliensis. 335, 1979.
[40] Clark, J. H., Peck, E. J., Anderson, J. N.: Oestrogen receptor binding, relationship to oestrogen induced responses. J. Toxicol. Environ. Health, 1:561, 1976.
[41] Clark, J. H., Paszko, Z., Peck, E. J.: Nuclear binding and retention of the receptor oestrogen complex: Relation to the agonistic and antagonistic properties of oestriol. Endocrinology, 100:91, 1977.
[42] Lemon, M. H.: Clinical and experimental aspects of the anti-mammary carcinogenic activity of oestriol. In: Lauritzen, C., van Keep, P. A. (eds). Frontiers of Hormone Research, Vol. 5, Estrogen Therapy, the Benefits and Risks. Basel, S. Karger, pp 155–163, 1978.
[43] Padwick, M. L., Siddle, N. C., Lane, G., Endacott, J. A., Cooper, H., Pryse-Davies, J., Whitehead, M. I.: Oestriol with oestradiol versus oestradiol alone: A comparison of endometrial, symptomatic and psychological effects. Brit. J. Obstet. Gynaecol. (In press).
[44] Whitehead, M. I., Townsend, P. T., Pryse-Davies, J., Ryder, T., Lane, G., Siddle, N. C., King, R. J. B.: Effects of various types and dosages of progestogens on the postmenopausal endometrium. J. Reprod. Med. 27:8, 539, 1982.
[45] Gambrell, R. D.: Clinical use of progestins in the menopausal patient. J. Reprod. Med. 27:8, 531, 1982.
[46] Lindsay, R., Hart, D. M., Aitken, J. M., MacDonald, E. B., Anderson, J. B.: Long-term prevention of postmenopausal osteoporosis by oestrogen. Lancet, i:1038, 1976.
[47] Nachtigall, L. E., Nachtigall, R. H., Nachtigall, R. D., Beckman, E. M.: Estrogen replacement therapy. I. A 10-year prospective study in relationship to osteoporosis. Obstet. Gynecol. 53:277, 1979.
[48] Christiansen, C., Christensen, M. S., Transbol, I.: Bone mass in postmenopausal women after withdrawal of oestrogen/gestogen replacement therapy. Lancet, i:459, 1981.
[49] Christiansen, C., Riis, B. J., Nilas, L., Rodbro, P., Deftos, L.: Uncoupling of bone formation and resorption by combined oestrogen and progestogen therapy in postmenopausal osteoporosis. Lancet, ii:800, 1985.
[50] Brotherton, J.: Sex Hormone Pharmacology. London: Academic Press, pp 1–41, 1976.
[51] Hirvonen, E., Malkonen, M., Manninen, V.: Effects of different progestogens on lipoproteins during postmenopausal replacement therapy. N. Engl. J. Med. 304:560, 1981.
[52] Kay, C. R.: The happiness pill? J. R. Coll. Gen. Pract. 30:8, 1980.
[53] Nillius, S. J., Johansson, E. D. B.: Plasma levels of progesterone after vaginal, rectal or intramuscular administration of progesterone. Am. J. Obstet. Gynecol. 110:470, 1971.
[54] Ottosson, U. B., Carlstrom, K., Damber, J. E., von Schoultz, B.: Serum levels of progesterone and some of its metabolites including deoxycorticosterone after oral and parenteral administration. Br. J. Obstet. Gynaecol. 91: 1111, 1984.
[55] Whitehead, M. I., Townsend, P. T., Pryse-Davies, J., Ryder, T., Lane, G., Siddle, N., King, R. J. B.: Actions of progestins on the morphology and biochemistry of the endometrium of postmenopausal women receiving low-dose therapy. Am. J. Obstet. Gynecol. 142:791, 1982.
[56] Lane, G., Siddle, N. C., Ryder, T. A., Pryse-Davies, J., King, R. J. B., Whitehead, M. I.: Dose-dependent effects of oral progesterone on the oestrogenised postmenopausal endometrium Brit. Med. J. 287:1241, 1983.
[57] Lane, G., Siddle, N. C., Ryder, T. A., Pryse-Davies, J., King, R. J. B., Whitehead, M. I.: Effects of dydrogesterone on the oestrogenised postmenopausal endometrium. Brit. J. Obstet. Gynaecol. 93:55, 1986.
[58] Lane, G., Siddle, N. C., Ryder, T. A.,

Pryse-Davies, J., King, R. J. B., Whitehead, M. I.: Is Provera the ideal progestogen for addition to postmenopausal oestrogen therapy? Fertil. Steril. 45:345, 1986.
[59] Whitehead, M. I., Lane, G., Siddle, N. C., Townsend, P. T., King, R. J. B.: Avoidance of endometrial hyperstimulation in estrogen-treated menopausal women. Seminars in Reproductive Endocrinology 1:1, 41, 1983.
[60] Staland, B.: Continuous treatment with natural oestrogens and progestogens. A method to avoid endometrial stimulation. Maturitas, 3:145, 1981.
[61] Mattsson, L.-A., Cullberg, G., Samsioe, G.: Evalution of a continuous oestrogen-progestogen regimen for climacteric complaints. Maturitas, 4:95, 1982.
[62] Staland, B.: Absorption of an oestrogen/progestogen preparation. Maturitas, 5:85, 1983.
[63] Magos, A. L., Brincat, M., Studd, J. W. W., Wardle, P., Schlesinger, P., O'Dowd, T.: Amenorrhoea and endometrial atrophy with continuous oral oestrogen and progestogen therapy in postmenopausal women. Obstet. Gynecol. 65:496, 1985.
[64] Magos, A. L., Brincat, M., O'Dowd, T., Wardle, P., Schlesinger, P., Studd, J. W. W.: Endometrial and menstrual response to subcutanoeus oestradiol and testosterone implants and continuous oral progestogen therapy in postmenopausal women. Maturitas. 7:297, 1985.
[65] Dennerstein, L., Burrows, G. D., Hyman, G. J., Sharpe, K.: Some clinical effects of oestrogen/progestogen therapy in surgically castrated women. Maturitas, 2:19, 1979.
[66] Dennerstein, L., Burrow, G. D., Hyman, G. J., Sharpe, K.: Hormone therapy and affect. Maturitas, 2:247, 1979.
[67] Meade, T. W., Greenberg, G., Thompson, S. G.: Progestogens and cardiovascular reactions associated with oral contraceptives and a comparison of the safety of 50 and 30 μg oestrogen preparations. Br. Med. J. 280:1157, 1980.
[68] Ross, R. K., Paganini-Hill, A., Mack, T. M., Arthur, M., Henderson, B. E.: Menopausal oestrogen therapy and protection from ischaemic heart disease. Lancet, i:858, 1981.
[69] Larsson-Cohn, U., Wallentin, L., Zador, G.: Plasma lipids and high density lipoproteins during oral contraception with different combinations of ethinyl oestradiol and norgestrel. Horm. Metab. Res. 11:437, 1979.
[70] Notelowitz, M.: Carbohydrate metabolism in relation to hormonal replacement therapy. Acta. Obstet. Gynecol. Scand (Suppl) 106:51, 1982.
[71] Christiansen, C., Christensen, M. S., Grande, P., Transbol, I.: Low-risk lipoprotein pattern in post-menopausal women on sequential oestrogen/progestogen treatment. Maturitas, 5:193, 1984.
[72] Wren, B., Garrett, D.: The effect of low-dose piperazine oestrone sulphate and low-dose levo-norgestrel on blood lipid levels in postmenopausal women. Maturitas, 7:141, 1985.
[73] Fahraeus, L., Larsson-Cohn, U., Wallentin, L.: L-norgestrel and progesterone have different influence on plasma lipoproteins. Eur. J. Clin. Invest. 30: 447–453, 1983.
[74] Silferstolpe, G., Gustafsson, A., Samsioe, G., Svanborg, A.: Lipid metabolic studies in oophorectomised women: Effects on serum lipids and lipoproteins of three synthetic progestogens. Maturitas, 4:103, 1982.
[75] Mattsson, L., Cullberg, G., Samsioe, G.: Influence of esterified oestrogens and medroxyprogesterone on lipid metabolism and sex steroids. A study in oophorectomised women. Horm. Metab. Res. 14:602, 1982.
[76] Notelovitz, M., Gudat, J. C., Ware, M. D., Dougherty, M. C.: Oestrogen/progestin therapy and the lipid balance of postmenopausal women. Maturitas, 4:301, 1982.
[77] Ottosson, U.-B., Johansson, B. G., von Schoultz, B.: Subfractions of high-density lipoprotein cholesterol during oestrogen replacement therapy: A comparison between progestogens and natural progesterone. Am. J. Obstet. Gynecol. 151:746, 1985.
[78] Mattsson, L. A., Cullberg, G., Samsioe, G.: A continuous oestrogen/progestogen regimen for climacteric complaints: effects on lipid and lipoprotein metabolism. Acta. Obstet. Gynecol. Scand. 63:673, 1984.
[79] Ottosson, U.-B., Lagrelius, A., Rosing, U., von Schoultz, B.: Relative fatty acid

composition of lecithin during postmenopausal replacement therapy – a comparison between ethinyl oestradiol and oestradiol valerate. Gynecol. Obstet. Invest. 18:296, 1984.

[80] Jensen, J., Nilas, L., Christiansen, C.: Cyclic changes in serum cholesterol and lipoproteins following different doses of combined postmenopausal hormone therapy. Brit. J. Obstet. Gynaecol. (In press).

Estrogen/progestogen as a prophylactic treatment of postmenopausal osteoporosis

C. Christiansen

During the last few years, our Department of Clinical Chemistry has examined the pathophysiological mechanisms behind postmenopausal osteoporosis, in order to identify the optimal prophylactic treatment of this disease. To clarify the issue involved, we carried out two large-scale, controlled clinical investigations.

Study I comprised 315 women between 45 and 54 years old who had all just past the menopause. This study lasted 2 years: all women were examined at intervals of 3 months; that is, each woman was examined 9 times. Of the original group, 264 women, that is 85%, completed to the treatment program. The primary purpose of this study was to identify the optimal prophylactic treatment of osteoporosis.

Study II involved 213 normal women who were approximately 3 years postmenopausal, between 47 and 56 years old. The duration of this study was 1 year, and 94% of the participants completed the treatment. The main goal of Study II was to identify the optimal dose of the optimal prophylactic treatment.

The questions we wanted to answer with these two studies can be formulated as follows:

- Is there a prophylactic treatment for osteoporosis?
- Is it possible to identify the women who are predisposed for fractures immediately after the menopause?
- Does prophylactic treatment also work in the case of this high risk group of women?

Is there a prophylactic treatment of osteoporosis?

From our investigations, it can be concluded that estrogen/progestogen replacement therapy prevents the progression of bone mass reduction after the menopause [1–3]. After 3 years' estrogen treatment, the bone mineral content (BMC) increased by approximately 4%, while placebo treatment over the same period produced a loss in BMC of around 5.5 percent. Furthermore, the decline in BMC after estrogen treatment was withdrawn was completely parallel to that seen in the placebo group (Fig. 1).

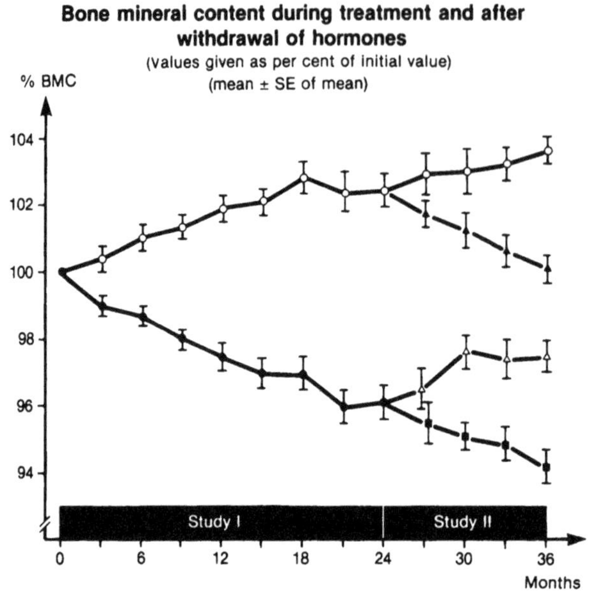

Fig. 1

We also investigated the effect of the following agents in addition to estrogens: thiazide diuretics, sodium fluoride, vitamin D_3 1α-hydroxy D_3, 1,25-dihydroxy D_3, and various combinations of these agents. Treatment with these agents in the doses given had no preventive effect on postmenopausal calcium loss [1, 4, 5] (Fig. 2). Similarly, there was no additive effect of thiazide diuretics or 1,25-dihydroxy D_3 in combination with estrogen (Fig. 3).

Is it possible to identify the women who are predisposed for fractures immediately after the menopause?

When a woman reaches the menopause, a number of factors in calcium metabolism are changed. Bone formation increases, but bone resorption is increased even more. This causes a negative calcium balance, which is reflected in increased calcium excretion in the urine. During estrogen replacement therapy, these metabolic processes are changed to levels similar to the premenopausal levels. It is possible to monitor postmenopausal women to measure loss of bone mass per unit of time. It appears that there are two characteristic groups:

1. Approximately 25% lose significant amounts of bone mineral, the so-called fast losers.
2. Approximately 75% lose only around 1% a year, the so-called normal losers.

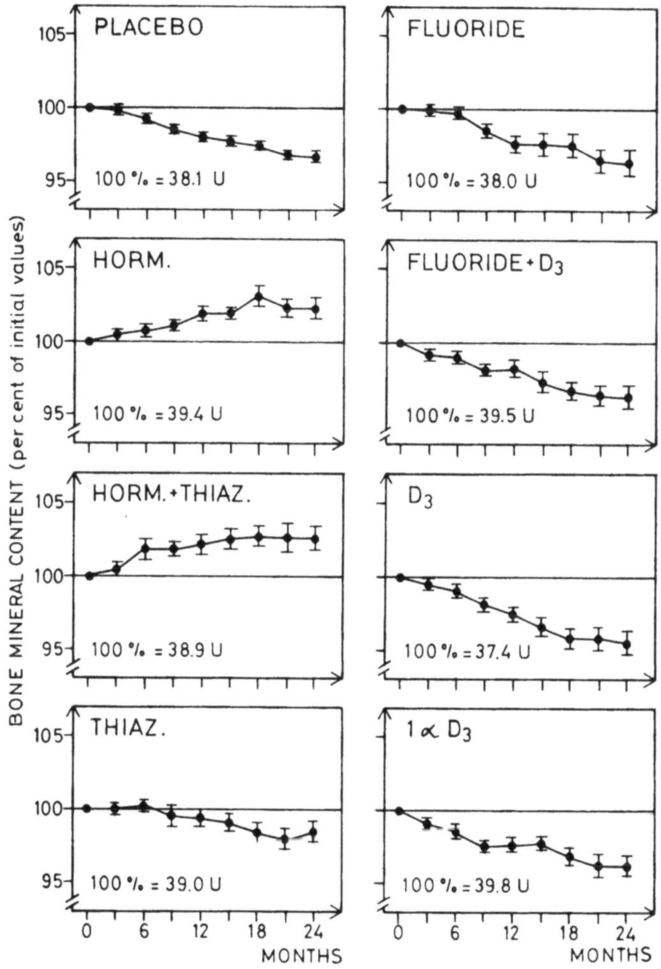

Fig. 2

Because it would be impossible to examine all postmenopausal women with costly techniques, we tried to find a method to predict which women will become fast losers by the use of simpler and less costly methods. We found that on the basis of a single blood sample, a specimen of urine, and the measurement of the woman's height and body weight, shortly after the start of her menopause it is possible to predict with some 80% certainty whether she will become a fast loser or a normal loser [6].

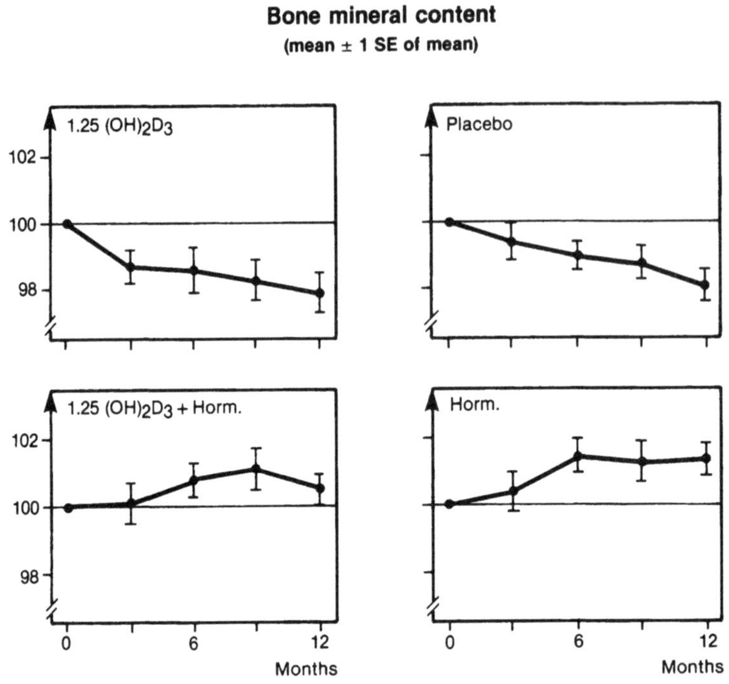

Fig. 3

Does prophylactic treatment also work in the case of this high-risk group of women?

Recent investigations by our department indicate that hormone treatment has the same effect on the high-risk group as on the low-risk group [7].

Conclusion

Osteoporosis is a considerable social problem, and the problem is aggravated partly because of the increased average duration of life in the world population and partly because of an inexplicable increase in the incidence of fractures that is not ascribably to increased average duration of life [8]. To the individual, it is a very debilitating condition. Today, we have no efficacious treatment of osteoporosis, once symptoms have appeared. Our investigations show, however, that we do have an efficacious prophylactic treatment, and that it is economically feasible to identify the high-risk group of women immediately after the menopause.

There is naturally a cost/benefit question to consider as to whether women after the menopause should be treated with hormones.

- It must now be considered as proven that estrogen replacement prevents osteoporosis and reduces the number of osteoporotic fractures.
- It similarly also appears to be proven – although the studies on which the conclusions are based are restrospective – that treatment with estrogen alone increases the woman's risk of developing cancer of the uterus. On the other hand, other investigations indicate that a combined estrogen/progestogen treatment does not increase this risk, and several investigations even indicate that the risk is smaller than in the case of untreated women [9].
- Sequential estrogen/progestogen treatment causes a regular withdrawal bleeding similar to menstruation.
- It is an established fact that estrogen treatment reduces subjective postmenopausal symptoms [10].
- Our studies indicate that natural estrogen reduces serum cholesterol and that this is caused by a reduction of the LDL cholesterol fraction [11]. Similarly, a significant reduction of blood pressure and body weight occurs during this treatment [12]. Other studies indicate a reduced rate of mortality from cardiovascular diseases in postmenopausal women receiving estrogen treatment [13].
- Prophylactic treatment of a large population over many years would naturally result in considerable economic cost. Furthermore, from a clinical-pharmacological point of view, all long-term prophylactic treatment of large populations should be monitored critically in order to identify possible undiscovered longterm side effects.

An overall assessment of benefits and risks may reasonably result in the conclusion that estrogen/progestogen prophylactic treatment can be recommended in the case of the high-risk group of women potentially liable to develop osteoporosis.

References

[1] Christiansen, C., Christensen, M. S., McNair, P., Hagen, C., Stocklund, K.-E., Transbøl, I.: Prevention of early postmenopausal bone loss: Controlled 2-year study in 315 normal females. Eur. J. Clin. Invest. 1980; 10:273–279.

[2] Christiansen, C., Christensen, M. S., Transbøl, I.: Bone mass in postmenopausal women after withdrawal of oestrogen/gestagen replacement therapy. Lancet 1981; i:459–461.

[3] Christiansen, C., Mazess, R.3B., Transbøl, I., Jensen, G. F.: Factors in response to treatment of early postmenopausal bone loss. Calcif. Tissue Int. 1981; 33:575–581.

[4] Transbøl, I., Christensen, M. S., Jensen, G. F., Christiansen, C., McNair, P.: Thiazide for the postponement of postmenopausal bone loss. Metabolism 1981; 31:383–386.

[5] Christiansen, C., Christensen, M. S., Rødbro, P., Hagen, C., Transbøl, I.: Effect of 1,25-dihydroxyvitamin D_3 in itself

or combined with hormone treatment in preventing postmenopausal osteoporosis. Eur. J. Clin. Invest. 1981; 11:305–309.
[6] Christiansen, C.: Prophylactic treatment for age-related bone loss in women. In "Osteoporosis", Copenhagen International Symposium on Osteoporosis June 3–8, 1984:587–593.
[7] Christiansen, C., Rødbro, P.: Does postmenopausal bone loss respond to estrogen replacement therapy independent of bone loss rate? Calcif. Tissue Int. 1983; 35:720–722.
[8] Wallace, W. A.: The increasing incidence of fractures of the proximal femur: an orthopaedic epidemic. Lancet 1983; i:1413–1414.
[9] Gambrell, R. D., Maier, R. C., Sander, B. E.: Decreased incidence of breast cancer in postmenopausal estrogen/progestogen users. Obstet. Gynecol. 1983; 62:435–443.
[10] Jensen, J., Christiansen, C.: Dose-response and withdrawal effects on climacteric symptoms after hormonal replacement therapy. A placebo-controlled therapeutic trial. Maturitas 1983; 5:125–133.
[11] Christiansen, C., Christensen, M. S., Grande, P., Transbøl, I.: Low-risk lipoprotein pattern in postmenopausal women on sequential oestrogen/progestogen treatment. Maturitas 1984; 5:193–199.
[12] Christiansen, C., Christensen, M. S., Hagen, C., Stocklund, K.-E., Transbøl, I.: Effects of natural oestrogen/gestagen and thiazide on coronary risk factors in normal postmenopausal women: A 2-year double-blind placebo study. Acta Obstet. Gynecol. Scand. 1981; 60:407–412.
[13] Ross, R. K., Paganini-Hill, A., Mack, T. M., Arthur, M., Henderson, B. E.: Menopausal oestrogen therapy and protection from death from ischaemic heart disease. Lancet 1981; i:858–860.

Discussion

Lachnit: I have one question: you mentioned that self-selection occurs in the group of hormone-treated women from higher socio-economic classes. As we know, class differences are even more pronounced in the UK than in other countries. In view of this, could the reason be a selection bias? For instance, other factors such as dietary factors – higher fat intake or something else – could be involved. Could that moderate increase in the relative risk possibly be explained by things like that?

Hunt: Yes, I am sure people are aware that there is a social class gradient in the incidence of breast cancer as there is for mortality. In fact, the gradient is slightly stronger for mortality than for incidence in the United Kingdom. It isn't possible to obtain good social class-specific/age-specific incidence rates for breast cancer in Britain, although we made an attempt to obtain them. We made a very crude adjustment for the social class distribution by taking proportional risk ratios, and this brought down the risk very slightly to about 1.55 as opposed to about 1.6. The reason I mentioned the points about our selected population is that it is sometimes so difficult in epidemiology to pin down the extent to which the population under study contributes to the results obtained. I think Dr. Gambrell was making some of the same points when he referred to the non-users in his own study. He pointed out that these women are probably quite different from the women who have taken opposed preparations and unopposed preparations. We have no information on dietary factors in our own study.

Greenblatt: You studied these patients for five and a half years. How many patients developed breast cancer in each individual year of the study?

Hunt: They had an average of five and a half years' therapy, and were follwed up for different periods. Offhand, I cannot tell you the numbers of cases which were diagnosed year by year. I should point out that our incidence data were analysed up to the end of 1982, since the method of notification of cancer incidence in Britain means that one has to leave a period of two or three years in order to the sure of complete ascertainment of cases. All I can say is that the vast majority of cases – in the order of 75% – were diagnosed between 1978 and 1982.

Greenblatt: The reason I asked is that it takes 7 to 8 years for a breast cancer to reach a palpable size of 1 cm. You studied these women for only five and a half years, so many of these cancers – the ones you diagnosed in the second or third years – had already developed before you started your hormone therapy.

Hunt: The five and a half years refers to the average duration of therapy for the whole five and a half thousand women. In fact, the women were observed for different periods – some of them for up to 20 years, since they entered the study retrospectively from some of the larger clinics such as Mr. Whitehead's. So we do have quite long periods of follow-up on some of the women, while others have been followed up for only about 3 years.

Gambrell: The special surveillance these days, and particularly the use of xero mammography, has changed the whole incidence of breast cancer. Hearing that yours are from 1982 removes a bit of that comment, because we are now finding so many early cancers – punctate calcification, as was stated in breast symposium the other day of the conference centre. If 50% are benign, then 50% are malignant. The American Cancer Society has recommended that every woman over the age of 50 should have a mammography every year. As Dr. Greenblatt has stated, it takes 7 or 8 years in Georgia and 2 years in California for a breast cancer, doubling every 60 to 70 days, to develop from one cell into a palpable lump. However, the diagnostic areas have changed tremendously as a result of xero mammography.

Ramcharan: In view of the fact that it is a highly selected group of women that you are following, I wonder at your assurance in using the national figures as your comparison group. I wonder how you come to terms with that.

Hunt: As I've explained before, the use of hormone replacement therapy is very low in Britain, and the availability of menopause clinics is quite restricted. Initially, we tried to have a control population of women who had been on hormone replacement therapy for a very short period of time – less than 6 months – and who had then discontinued. In fact, this proved to be an impossible control group to continue because so few women attending the clinics took therapy for such short periods. Furthermore, most of the menopause clinics are under considerable financial strain and therefore are able to see very few women who are not receiving long-term therapy. Because of this, we were unable to find an appropriate control group. As regards the mortality results, we adjusted for the social class distribution and found that it made very little difference to the overall mortality. We thought that the low overall mortality might be attributable to the high social class distribution, because women from social classes one and two experience a better mortality than women from lower social classes. With regard to the breast cancer and in answer to the first question, we made what crude adjustments could be made, but the data just aren't there to do any more. I accept that comparisons with national rates are not optimal, but we can only do research in the real world and those are the best statistics available to us. We've made all the adjustments we can.

Vessey: This question is for Dr. Gambrell. We found that people change their therapy. They start off by taking estrogens alone, but then they switch to estrogens and progestogens. The women who receive estrogens alone are those without uteri, and the women who receive estrogens and progestogens are those with uteri and ovaries. Whether or not you have ovaries is, of course, a powerful risk factor for breast cancer, and women whose ovaries are removed are at lower risk. It is very, very difficult to sort out all these different selective factors. As Dr. Hunt has stressed, we do not regard these results as in any way conclusive.

Ramcharan: Breast cancer is a multifactorial disease. The fact that you are using just a national figure for your comparison means that a whole lot of questions remain unaddressed. You may be controlling for social class, but there are all the other risk factors for breast cancer that you are not addressing at all. Because of this, I would think that the results must be extremely inconclusive.

Hunt: We don't have a control group. We abandoned the recruitment of a control group because it wasn't feasible in Britain. We operate in a very different situation from the one which you have in the United States, where you have so many more users of hormone replacement therapy that it is usually possible to conduct larger studies. However, it is important to note that most of Dr. Gambrell's significant results come, in fact, from comparisons with national rates similar to our own, and Dr. Gambrell himself pointed out that his own control group was probably an atypical group of women. Ours is the only long-term study being done in Britain. We wouldn't expect it to be a conclusive study because, as I interpret the literature, there is still some controversy about the effects of hormone replacement therapy on breast cancer.

Comment: I was surprised about your results regarding endometrial cancer in people on progestogens combined or on sequential therapy. I wonder whether this could be the result of masking the effect of a developing endometrial cancer, since you are expecting a bleeding. We know from the past that women on sequential treatments with oral contraceptives – for instance Serial, there are papers – developed endometrial cancer. Because of this, I think there is a real need to check these patients very carefully.

Lauritzen: Could you not have performed a separate evaluation of the percentage of patients who received estrogen/progestogen therapy, so that you could have risk values for this special group?

Hunt: You are asking about separating the opposed and unopposed users. We are, in fact, trying to do that at the moment. However, women tend to have changed from one type of therapy to another so many times that it is extremely difficult to look at the effect of treatment.

Lauritzen: This is not the case in our studies, where one doctor treated all the patiens. We used matched pairs, and I think this is the beste method for a successfull study.

Question: I would like to ask Dr. Gambrell how, in his analysis, he handled patients who started on estrogens alone and who later switched. Certainly in Britain, if you go back over a period of years you will be unable to find pure groups – unopposed estrogens and an opposed group. Once switching starts, it is very difficult to handle the statistics. I would like to know whether Dr. Gambrell had this problem and how he dealt with it statistically.

Gambrell: Yes, we certainly did have that problem. Unfortunately, the trend was in one direction – patients who had been on estrogens were adding progestogens to them. It was very rare for a patient to stop progestogen and go back to estrogen, although there were cross-overs from non-treatment to treatment and back to non-treatment again. That is why we used the patient years of observation method – which is, you will probably say, a poor method of analysing data. However, if the patient took an estrogen alone for 5 years, then that was 5 patient years of observation. If she then took progestogens for 2 years after that, then that was 2 years, and that is how we handled it. But, as you pointed out, there are so many different variables that it is very difficult to analyse these data.

Cohen, Amsterdam: I wonder why the incidence of breast cancer is so high in your control group – almost twice that given by the national cancer people.

Gambrell: We really do not know, because our study was set up to study endometrial carcinoma. We did not have the major risk factors for breast cancer on our data cards. I think a logical conclusion is that this group of women was a different group who were at higher risk for breast cancer to begin with. It may be that, because a mother or sister had breast cancer, they themselves chose not to use estrogen therapy, or that the physician evaluating a particular patient chose not to give estrogen therapy because of fibrosis disease or lumpy breasts. But it is certainly true that they were at higher risk – I cannot say exactly why, but I think that it was because they were a different group of patients.

Rauramo: I am very happy that we now quite agree with Dr. Gambrell, that estrogens are not dangerous and progestogens do not diminish the risk of cancer. I believe we are both thinking the same way now, although we have not always done that. My only question is: did I understand right, that the mortality for breast cancer is smaller in women using estrogens than in others?

Gambrell: Yes, the mortality is definitely decreased, primarily because of an early diagnosis but also, I think, because women on estrogen therapy have increased surveillance. Certainly improving diagnostic techniques detect the lesions earlier but, in addition to that, when we compare the same stage of disease with the non-users they still had a better prognosis. This has been found for estrogen therapy in nearly every study that has looked at it. When breast cancer does develop during estrogen therapy, there is certainly a better prognosis.

Lauritzen: In my experience, the patients who receive estrogen/progestogen and develop breast cancer are invariably receptor positive. This is an important point for the prognosis.

Gambrell: We are just putting this data together, but it does look like that – either estrogens alone unopposed or estrogen plus progestogen does increase not only oestrogen receptors, but progestogen receptors in the breast cancer terminus.

Christiansen: I wonder whether you have any information on the smoking habits of your patients. The reason I ask is that there have been publications showing that smokers have a lower risk of breast cancer. There is a paper in the last issue of the New England of Medicine which indicates that smokers have a lower risk of endometrial cancer. Furthermore, we have a paper coming out in the New England Journal of Medicine showing that smokers need twice the amount of estrogen to get the same serum concentration of the estrogens.

Gambrell: Unfortunately not, and I don't know whether any prospective studies have even started. There have always been factors that I wished I had started with, but we commenced this study in 1975 and that is one thing we did not think to look at, so we have no data whatsoever about this.

Lauritzen: Dr. Husmann, your theory is that cortisol concentrations are maintained while estrogens decline, which means that the ratio of catabolic to anabolic or to anticatabolic hormones changes. Now, I think it is important that adrenal dehydroepiandrosterone shows a decrease in the postmenopause. This is the hormone which, under normal conditions, counteracts the catabolic effect of cortisol to a great extent. Chris Nordin told me that he has studied this and was of the opinion that dehydroepiandrosterone also plays a role in the development of osteoporosis.

Husmann: The ratio of cortisol and estrogens is only one point. We are now investigating the role of dehydroepiandrosterone as well, but so far we have only examined the disturbed ratio between cortisol on the one hand and estrogens on the other.

Rauramo: Did I understand correctly, that the natural progesterone is the only progesterone that does not abolish the positive effect of estrogens on total mortality?

Husmann: Yes, progesterone and some of its derivatives – especially 17-hydroxy-progesterone – have no influence on lipid metabolism, at least in physiological concentrations.

Lauritzen: Dr. Husmann, you said that estrogens increase HDL. This is not, I think, the case with all estrogen medication since the effect on lipids is much less pronounced when estrogens are given parenterally, and completely absent on percutaneous transdermal administration.

Husmann: Quite right, it is a matter of the dosage and the route of administration.

Schwartz: I would like to add some pertinent observations from the literature regarding the combination of 17-hydroxy-progesterone dervivatives with estrogenes. Hammond* found no reduction of the positive estrogen effects on cardiovascular morbidity, while Nachtigall** reported a higher, although statistically insignificant overall survival rate than in controls.

Lachnit: As regards the lack of effect of estrogen on the HDL on transcutaneous administration, for example, it may be that the first liver passage – which we would

* Hammond, C. B., et al., Am. J. Obstet. Gynecol. 133:537, 1979.
** Nachtigall, L. E., et al., Obstet. Gynecol. 54:74, 1979.

like to avoid for other reasons – is necessary for the beneficial effect on lipid metabolism. Another point I would like to make is that we always refer to synthetic progestogens. There are, however, two types of synthetic progestogen. One line derives from 19-nortestosterone, and is clearly different from the hydroxyprogesterone derivatives. I think it will be shown in the next session that these derivatives, the C-21 steroids, actually have no untoward effect on lipid metabolism and do not interfere with the estrogen effect.

Lauritzen: What we need very urgently are studies into the effect of the combination of progestogen with estrogens in long-term treatment. We have such studies, but the numbers are very small and for a relatively short time. What about your numbers? You have a large number of patients with progesterone. Do you have any data on mortality, on vascular diseases or on heart disease?

Gambrell: We do not have any mortality data other than malignancy. We, too, have seen a decrease in ovarian malignancies, but the number is too small for any significance. In our studies we have not found any adverse effects even from the 19-norsteroids, although the C-12 compounds in combination with estrogen give the best induction of HDL cholesterol and the best reduction of VLDL and LDL.

Question: What do you think – from a theoretical point of view – of using CPA in combined therapy instead of a progestogen?

Whitehead: CPA is a very attractive substance because of its lack of androgenic effects, but I think some people have expressed anxiety about possible catabolic problems with it. We are currently studying a small group of patients on estrogen and continuous CPA. The initial results look encouraging. At present we are looking at the bleeding patterns. There is not much point in doing detailed, very expensive lipid studies until you have actually shown that the preparation is going to give you the desired effect on the endometrium.

Christiansen: Dr. Jensen in my department has looked at the lipids in our study with CPA. It is about ready for publication, and it shows that CPA added to estrogens does not change the beneficial effects of the estrogens.

Question: I missed a reference in Dr. Whitehead's lecture to cytological screening for endometrial cancer. Does he consider it too unreliable to be used in clinical practice?

Whitehead: I can only quote from the published data. I would say that cytological evaluation is most probably valuable – but only if you have a very good cytologist who is confident that what he is seeing in terms of cells is representative of histological change. If you do not have an experienced cytologist, then I think, it is a very dangerous procedure to introduce.

Tikkanen: I would like to go back to Mr. Whitehead's frightening vision of a lady falling like an ox because she had taken progestogens together with estrogens. You are, of course, right that progestogens have some adverse effects on lipids, such as lowering HDL cholesterol. This has been shown in many studies, and I have done a series myself. However, these studies were always designed to find a maximum effect of progestogen. They were short-term studies and were designed to ascertain the biochemical effects of progestogens. What we really need are studies that will answer the question of what the average effect on HDL is, during long-term combination therapy. Dr. Gambrell, for example, is carrying out such studies right now and I think we must wait until this kind of clinically relevant study becomes available before we start to get frightened.

Christiansen: The problem is that high doses of progestogen have this adverse effect, but that is not really the point. The question of clinical importance is what do small doses do on long-term ingestion. We shall be publishing this data in the near future, since we now have it all from a two-year period.

Lauritzen: The effect of progestogens on lipids is very clearly dependent on the compound, the dosage, the mode of administration and, perhaps, the diet. It is therefore very difficult to make a statement on this – you must specify what you are talking about.

Question: Returning to CPA, would you please specify the characteristics of this kind of treatment as far as the type of estrogen and the dosage and duration of treatment with estrogen and CPA is concerned. Have you any data on the endometrial response to such treatment?

Christiansen: The dose is 2 mg estradiol valerate given in combination with cyclical CPA, the dose of which is 1 mg daily for 10 or 11 days. There were about 30 women in each group, and all except one were bleeding regularly on that treatment. We have not done anything else in this field.

Brincat: I have always been a little worried about using hydroxyproline assessments – especially if you leave the skin collagen, which is 40% of the total body collagen, and the other 40% in the bone and assume that these are being lost at the same rate. This may be a wrong assumption. Urinary hydroxyproline represents only about 10% of the collagen break-down, and there is a big individual variation. It depends on tubular absorption and on how much of it is peptide-bound. So I worry because I think that urinary hydroxyproline represents only a small inaccurate fraction of the amount of collagen break-down that is actually occurring. The only use for this test is to assess the disease status and where you have a huge turnover. For subtle changes such as those occurring in postmenopausal osteoporosis, however, the test is just not good enough.

Christiansen: I would be delighted if you could give me a new test of bone resorption which is precise, accurate and easy to perform. The problem is that no such test exists. However, I am quite excited about what is going on in the United States at the moment, where they are trying to find new bone markers. We are testing some of these markers at the moment and I hope that some of them will come out – a specific marker for bone formation and another specific marker for bone resorption, possibly more specific than the markers which we have today. But I agree when you say that hydroxyproline is difficult to measure and not really precise.

Question to Mr. Whitehead: When you evaluated the various doses of progestogen, was this done in 6 months or a year? How much time did you allow to elapse before you evaluated the endometrium?

Whitehead: All our patients had been on therapy for a minimum of 6 months, and some had been on therapy for 3 or 4 years.

Question: Many women cannot accept the progestogen therapy and the bleeding every month, but might accept a withdrawal bleeding every second or third month. Would you recommend prolongation of the artificial cycle to 2 to 3 months or not?

Mr. Whitehead: People are always telling me that patients won't accept the withdrawal bleeding, but the compliance in our clinic is so high that I find this very difficult to believe. I accept totally that high doses of progestogens can produce undesirable psychological and physical effects. If you use low doses, however, patient compliance is increased. When we used a fairly high dose of estrogen, say 4 mg of estradiol valerate or 1.25 mg of conjugated estrogens, on a continuous basis, some patients were already experiencing some break-through bleeding by the second or third month and, what is more, when withdrawal bleeding occurred it was extremely heavy, which frightened them a great deal. I think you may get round this problem with a lower estrogen dose but, from Dr. Christiansen's data this morning, it seems that what is required for good bone conservation is 2 mg of estradiol per day or equivalent, and I would have thought that, with 2 mg continuously for 2 to 3 months, you would run into the same problems with break-through bleeding.

Lauritzen: I have a comment for Mr. Whitehead. You may have noticed that we maintain cyclical therapy, our hypothesis being that the treatment should be as close to the normal cycle as possible. You have shown in your slides that the incidence of hyperplasia is not affected by continuous cyclical therapy. We believe that a rest from proliferation of one week is essential and physiological. Complete shedding of the endometrium is only seen while estrogen levels are very low or decreasing. You have no complete shedding if you have permanently high estrogen levels, even if the progestogen is withdrawn. Treatment should therefore be cyclical and not continuous.

Whitehead: We took endometrial tissue from patients on the fifth or sixth day of their treatment-free week and looked at the receptor status. There is actually very little diminution in receptor levels during the week of treatment. You cannot make comparisons with the premenopausal woman because the postmenopausal woman who has been on oral estrogens has a vast pool of estrone sulphate which is quite unphysiological. The postmenopausal woman will almost certainly back-convert some of that estrone sulphate into estrone, then into estradiol, and you will maintain a sufficient stimulus for reasonable receptor levels even during the treatment-free week. If you did not have that continued stimulus, then I would agree that your arguments would be much more logical.

2.4 Special aspects in premenopausal women

Management of the premenstrual syndrome

A. L. Magos, J. W. W. Studd

Introduction

Menstruation and premenstrual malaise have been inexplicably linked since ancient times. Although the term 'premenstrual tension' was formally introduced as recently as 1931 (Frank, 1931), perhaps the most poignant description of the condition was made by Henry Maudsley over half a century before when he wrote '... The monthly activity of the ovaries which marks the advent of puberty in women has a notable effect upon the mind and body; wherefore it may become an important cause of mental and physical derangement ...' (1873). This statement is all the more important because Maudsley made the connection between cyclical premenstrual symptoms and cyclical ovarian activity.

Several years later, with a literature that is as controversial as it is extensive, much remains unknown concerning the aetiology, diagnosis and treatment of what has become known as the premenstrual syndrome (PMS). Nonetheless, there is now sufficient information to allow for a rational approach in the management of this distressing problem. Most attention will be focused on diagnosis and treatment, the two areas of most practical interest.

Definition

It typifies the PMS that not only is there no universally accepted definition of the condition but even the label 'PMS' is somewhat unsuitable. Confusion arises firstly because any definition has to be sufficiently broad to allow for great variability in symptomatology, severity and duration. Secondly, menstruation is not a prerequisite, as cyclical symptoms can continue following hysterectomy provided ovarian function is conserved (Backstrom et al., 1981). Thirdly, symptoms are not necessarily premenstrual, but can occur at other phases if the cycle (eg. around ovulation). Whithin these limitations, a working definition of the PMS is:

"Distressing physical, psychological and behavioural symptoms, not caused by organic disease, which regularly recur during the same phase of the menstrual (ovarian) cycle, and which significantly regress or disappear during the remainder of the cycle" (Magos and Studd, 1984a).

The essence of this definition is that the symptoms should be distressing and significantly cyclical in phase with the menstrual/ovarian cycle. While it is relatively obvious when symptoms wax and wane regularly with menstruation, it is more difficult to be determine whether the changes seen are non-random and not merely reflecting chance day-to-day variation. This is an important limitation on any definition that does not include an objective measure of the degree of change in symptoms, a problem that can only be addressed by statistical analysis.

Symptoms

The manifestations of the PMS are so protean that it is a hopeless task to attempt to list all the possible symptoms. Indeed, a list can be counter-productive as it has the effect of setting unneccessary diagnostic limits on symptomatology. Thus, the 160 or so symptoms listed by Moos represent the tip of an infinite iceberg and should be considered as such (Moos, 1969). It is more realistic to consider that any symptom involving any body system can fluctuate with the ovarian cycle and thus be responsible for cyclical morbidity.

Looking at the prevalence of symptoms is a more informative exercise. Although in no way an indication of pathogenesis, symptoms can be classified as physical, psychological and behavioural. Physical symptoms such as breast tenderness and swelling, abdominal bloating, oedema, weight gain and headache appear to be the most common (Morton, 1950), while psychological symptoms including depression, anxiety tension and tiredness account for the most distress (Rees, 1953). Behavioural changes such as suicide attempts, criminal behaviour, lowered cognitive performance and proneness to accidents are more controversial as they are often isolated events. As noted by Parlee, stress itself has important effects on the menstrual cycle, and in particular it can precipitate menstruation; such an effect may falsely perpetuate a direct relationship between these behavioural phenomena and the premenstrual phase of the cycle (1982).

Attempts have been made to divide PMS into several sub-syndromes according to particular symptom combinations (eg. Abraham, 1980). However attractive such an approach seems both from a pathophysiological and therapeutic aspect, in reality most women are affected by their own unique and seemingly unrealted mix of complaints. For instance, in our prospective study of 145 women with PMS, 86.2% were found to have characteristic premenstrual exacerbations of physical, psychological and behavioural symptoms, while 32% showed these changes for all symptom clusters studied (Magos et al., 1986a). It may prove more useful to 'grade' complainers according baseline post-menstrual symptomatology, and thus into those who are symptomatic essentially only premenstrually as opposed to those with chronic symptoms that are exaggerated prior to menstruation.

Diagnosis

Correct diagnosis is a prerequisite for successful therapy. Unfortunately, the fundamental diagnostic dilemma with the PMS is the absence of a biological marker, and this is arguably the major confounding factor limiting our understanding. In this it resembles psychiatric conditions and is unlike endocrine disorders. As with most psychiatric pathologies, diagnosis is therefore based out of necessity on the assessment of symptoms, symptoms that are not only subjective but for which there are generally no satisfactory objective measures.

Symptoms are assessed by a variety of means that can be:

Retrospective or Prospective
Unstructured or Structured
Not evaluated or Evaluated

The simplest, and at the same time essential initial approach, is to consider the history (retrospective/unstructured/not evaluated) and see if it is consistent with the definition of PMS, such as the one given above. The history may immediately exclude the diagnosis in favour of other conditions such as dysmenorrhoea, anxiety state, depression, and cyclical oedema, which may be the result in a large proportion of women (eg. Wood & Jakubowicz, 1980). If the history is suggestive of the PMS, it has generally been recommended that further confirmatory evidence should be sought. Techniques proposed vary from the relatively straight forward to the extremely complex, but mostly involve structured questionnaires which are applied either retrospectively

eg. Menstrual Distress Questionnaire (Moos, 1968)
Research Diagnostic Criteria (Steiner et al., 1980)
Premenstrual Assessment Form (Halbreich et al., 1982)

or prospectively

eg. Profile of Mood States and Social-Sexual Activities Log (Ablanalp et al., 1979)
Visual Analogue Scales (Rubinow et al., 1984)
Menstrual Symptom Questionnaire (Freeman et al., 1985)
PMT-Cator (Magos & Studd, 1986b)

The traditional teaching has been that prospective daily assessment using a symptom check list, preferably over more than one menstrual cycle, is the optimum method of diagnosis of the PMS. This view developed from the results of several studies showing a poor correlation between the recall of menstrually related phenomena and prospective recordings (eg. McCance et al., 1933; Ablanalp et al., 1979). Further evidence against retrospective symptom reporting came from the neat experiment of Ruble (1977), and the studies looking at the role of 'social expectancy' and 'experimental demands' (Ruble & Brooks-Gunn, 1979; AuBuchon & Calhoun, 1985). However, all these reports suffer from one major drawback which puts in question the validity of their conclusions with respect to the PMS – normal, relatively asymptomatic women invariably formed the study group. Symptomatic women, specifically complaining of premenstrual distress, may have behave totally differently. The results of our study would support the latter.

We studied 150 women referred to our PMS Clinic who gave a convincing history of the PMS and monitored their symptoms daily by means of a modified Moos Menstrual Distress Questionnaire; analysis of the data by trend analysis showed that 145 (96.3%) had symptom trends consistent with the syndrome for at least one of the six adverse symptom clusters studied, with over half (52.7%) having this pattern for at least five of the clusters and almost one third (32%) for all six (Magos et al., 1986a). It seems that in this group of selected clinic attenders, a complaint of

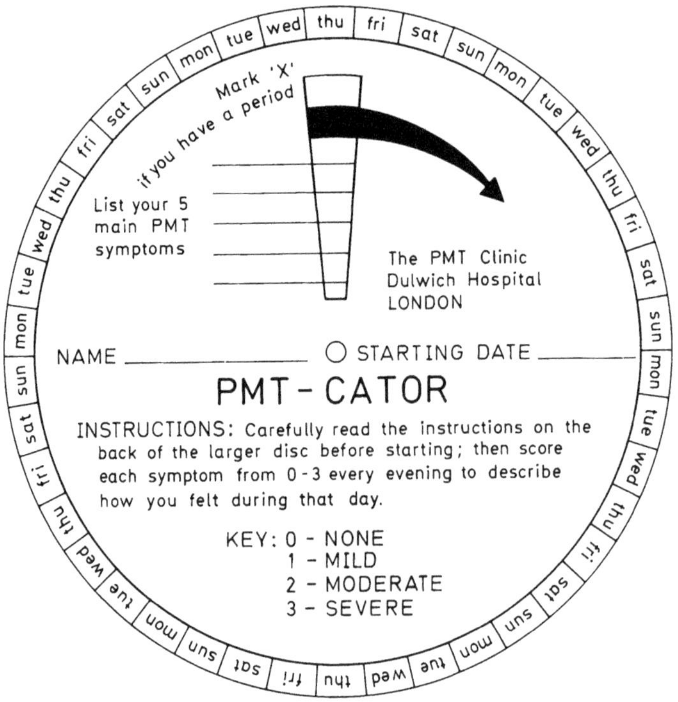

Fig. 1 The Dulwich PMS Clinic 'PMT-Cator'.

the PMS that satisfies the definition given above is usually sufficient proof of significant exacerbation of at least some symptoms prior to menstruation. In this population of women, made aware of the menstrual cycle by adverse complaints, retrospective reporting is a more accurate index of cyclical symptoms than in the case of healthy subjects who are perhaps less motivated.

The above result, if confirmed in a non-clinic population, has practical implications for the treating physician for it means that a careful history is sufficient to make a diagnosis of the PMS. However, in cases where there is some doubt, prospective proof is essential. While the more complex questionnaires clearly provide detailed information, they are time consuming and probably unsuited outside the specialist clinic. Alternatively, a simple diagnostic disc ("PMT-Cator", marketed by Rocket of London, Figure 1) has proved both easy to use and sufficiently sensitive for this purpose (Magos & Studd, 1986b).

Trend analysis

Detailed prospective symptom assessment is also integral to research into the PMS, whether relating to pathophysiology or therapy. However, the evaluation of these subjective physical, psychological and behavioural data is difficult and represents yet another area of confusion. Numerous methods have been suggested in the literature, ranging from simply the presence or absence of certain common complaints (Robinson et al., 1977) to the grading of the severity of symptoms using scores or linear analogue scales (Rubinow et al., 1984). Numerical methods allow for statistical analysis of the measurements, and simple but arbitrary formulae have been proposed (Muse et al., 1984), as well more complex mathematical models adapted (Sampson & Jenner, 1977). The validity of all these techniques for the assessment of menstrual cycle data and for the detection of non-random events is questionable.

The specific statistical approach to chronological data, that is observations made sequentially in time, is time series analysis. Daily symptom ratings are ideally suited to this approach, and we have adapted one such technique, namely Trigg's trend analysis, for the study of the prospective symptom ratings used in the evaluation of the PMS (Magos & Studd, 1986a). The method can be used to (1) identify and classify symptom patterns, (2) provide a mathematical definition of the PMS in terms of statistically significant symptoms trends at definable times in the cycle, (3) quantify symptoms, and (4) give a global index of menstrual cycle morbidity which we have defined as the menstrual cycle ratio. The analysis can be applied to any psychometric tool which quantifies symptoms (eg. Moos' Menstrual Distress Questionnaire applied daily), and is easily standardised to allow for comparison of research reports. Inconsistancies of patient populations are central to the mass of contradictory data concerning the PMS, and it is only by the use of reproducible and statistically valid methods of symptom assessment that we can hope to untangle the web that we have created.

Aetiology

The precise cause of the PMS remains unknown. In the absence of universally agreed diagnostic criteria for the PMS, such ignorance is not unexpected. Biological, psychological, social and genetic theories abound, often contradictory in nature, but none has been proven to be solely relevant to the genesis of symptoms (Table I). Indeed, the multisymptom nature of the condition makes it unlikely that a single pathophysiological mechanism is responsible.

Five observations, however, appear to be salient to our understanding (Magos and Studd, 1984b):

1. The PMS is associated with cyclical ovarian activity and does not occur before puberty, during pregnancy and after the menopause;

Table I Pathophysiological mechanisms implicated in the PMS

Biological	
Female sex hormones	Estrogen excess
	Progesterone deficiency
	Estrogen/progesterone ratio
	Falling estrogen/progesterone
Glucocorticoids	
Androgens	
Prolactin	
Fluid retention	Sex hormones
	Renin-angiotensin-aldosterone axis
	Prolactin
	Vasopressin
	Dietary factors
Vitamin deficiency	B6
	A
Hypoglycaemia	
Endogenous hormone allergy	
Magnesium deficiency	
Prostaglandins	
Melatonin	
Neurotransmitters	Cholinergic
	Catecholamines
	Serotonin
Neurointermediate lobe peptides	
Psychological	
Social and evolutionary	
Genetic	

2. As already noted, menstruation itself is incidental as cyclical symptoms continue following hysterectomy provided ovarian function is conserved (Backstrom et al., 1981);
3. Most healthy women report adverse symptoms prior to menstruation (Taylor, 1979);
4. Extensive metabolic and psychological studies have failed to find a specific abnormality in the PMS; and
5. The condition exhibits a considerable placebo response (Mattson & von Schoultz, 1974).

While factors involved in placebo responsiveness are extremely complex and clearly involved, the other overwhelming conclusion from the above observations is that cyclical ovarian activity plays a primary role in pathogenesis of the PMS. That ovarian activity can be associated with such profound effects should not be surprising. Numerous (>200) physical, psychological and behavioural variables normally fluctuate during the ovarian cycle (Magos & Studd, 1985). Furthermore, the PMS is only one of many (>70) disorders that regularly fluctuate with ovarian activity; other examples include migraine, rheumatoid arthritis, asthma, epilepsy, and diabetes (Magos & Studd, 1985).

With such widespread associations, it would be surprising if women did not normally experience regular symptom changes during the ovarian cycle. The logical extension of this rationale is that women complaining of the PMS are unusually sensitive to these changes, perhaps secondary to psycho-social factors or as yet undetermined central mechanisms, and experience exaggerated symptoms (Figure 2). Such a model is consistent with our present knowledge, and in particular explains the non-specific nature of premenstrual symptomatology.

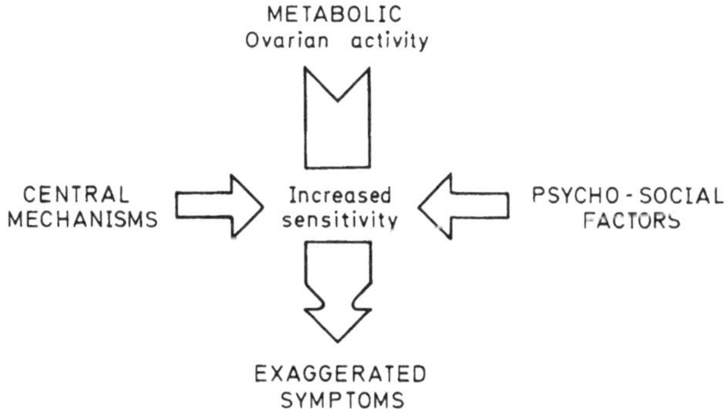

Fig. 2 Model for the premenstrual syndrome

Treatment

The management of the PMS is as variable as the symptomatology. Therapies are based on theoretical considerations, symptoms, personal dogma or desperation (Table II)! When assessing any treatment, it is essential to appreciate the massive placebo responsiveness reported by controlled studies, such that uncontrolled reports are impossible to interpret. For instance, Mattson and von Schoultz found a placebo response rate of 89%, while in our recently completed study of estradiol implants combined with cyclical norethisterone, the initial response to placebo was 94% (Magos et al., 1986 b). Surprisingly, there is virutally no information concerning the duration of this response, and yet this should be an important consideration when assessing active therapy. Thus, most therapeutic trials suffer from being too short as well as including too few cases, both these factors encouraging negative findings with respect to efficacy (Type II statistical error). As an indication of the duration of the placebo response, we found in our 10 months controlled study of estradiol implants that the placebo effect had generally worn off by the end of the study as judged by prospective daily symptom scores, but not when assessed by retrospective visual analogue scales (Magos et al., 1986 b).

Table II Treatments for the PMS

Pharmacological	
Sex hormones	Progesterone/Progestogens
	Androgens
	Combined oral contraceptive pill
	Danazol
	Gonadotropin-releasing hormone
	Estradiol implants
Diuretics	
Bromocriptine	
Psychoactive drugs	Tranquillisers
	Anti-depressants
	Lithium
	'Bellergal'
Vitamins	B6
	A
Prostaglandin mediators	Prostaglandin synthetase inhibitors
	Gamma-linolenic acid
Magnesium	
Diet	
Desensitisation	
Psychological and social support	
Physical activity	
Hypnosis	
Meditation	
Yoga	

Table III Plan of management of the premenstrual syndrome

Mild
Explanation and reassurance
Psychological and social support
'Placebo'
Severe
Manipulation of the ovarin cycle

Realising the self-imposed limitations of most controlled studies into the PMS, it is perhaps not unexpected that no single therapy has been shown to be convincingly superior to placebo, at least in terms of reproducibility (Magos & Studd, 1984 a). Many of the 'traditional' and still widely used therapies belong in this category, including progesterone, progestogens, diuretics, vitamins and psychotropics. Although some of the apparent treatment failures may be the victims of study design, it would seem unlikely on theoretical grounds that therapies aimed at specific (and hypothetical) abnormalities, which constitute the majority of therapeutic approaches, would be effective in a condition characterised by non-specific complaints. Thus, while explanation and reassurance, psychosocial support or even the many therapies which are probably little more than harmless placebos, may be sufficient in mild cases, a more direct approach is required when symptoms are severe and disruptive (Table III).

If one accepts the model of the PMS summarized in Figure 2, logical therapy should be aimed at suppressing cyclical ovarian activity, thereby abolishing cyclical symptoms. This can be achieved by several manoeuvres:

(1) The combined contraceptive pill may not only be contra-indicated in this age group but, although the definitive study has still to be carried out, is probably only effective in half the cases (Goldzieher et al., 1971). This may be because the benefits of anovulation secondary to the estrogen component are negated by progestogenic side-effects which are similar to the typical complaints of the PMS (Hammarback et al., 1985; Magos et al., 1986 c). Furthermore, the cyclical nature of the Pill regimen is itself associated with hormone swings.

(2) Ovarian function can also be inhibited by danazol. Recent trials have reported favourably on certain symptoms (Gilmore et al., 1985). However, danazol appears to be poorly tolerated because of androgenic and other side effects and may be unsuitable for the majority of patients.

(3) Gonadotropin-releasing hormone agonist has been used to produce "medical ovariectomy" and relief of premenstrual distress (Muse et al., 1984). As pointed out by the authors, the suppression of ovarian estrogen production precludes its long-term use.

(4) Anovulation can be achieved by six-monthly subcutaneous implants of estradiol (Greenblatt et al., 1977), treatment being combined with cyclical oral progestogen to ensure regular withdrawal periods and prevent the development of endometrial hyperplasia (Studd & Thom, 1981). Theoretical advantages of this approach over the ones discussed above include that (a) the treatment is safe in an older age group; (b) progestogen is not administered continuously; (c) plasma estrogen concentrations are maintained in the normal follicular range (Magos et al., 1984).

A pilot retrospective study demonstrated that this combination of estradiol implants and cyclical progestogen appeared to be both effective and well-tolerated (Magos et al., 1984). The results of our recently completed prospective double-blind, placebo controlled study, involving 68 women with severe PMS, have confirmed the efficacy of this mode of treatment (Magos et al., 1986b). Analysis of the prospective symptom ratings showed a significant superiority of the active treatment for all six adverse symptom clusters of Moos' Menstrual Distress Questionnaire after the first two months of therapy, despite the considerable benefits of placebo already mentioned. This is the first treatment subjected to a large-scale, controlled investigation that has been found to benefit all the typical symptoms of the PMS.

Conclusions

Although the light at the end of the aetiological and therapeutic tunnel seems to be in sight, much work remains. Unfounded dogma must be abandoned in favour of science. Useful progress will only be made by means of an objective and standardised approach to definition, diagnostic criteria, symptom assessment and therapy. Only then will we truly understand the aetiological complexities of this most complex of conditions.

References

Ablanalp, J. M., Donnelly, A. F., Rose, R. M.: Psychoendocrinology of the menstrual cycle: I. Enjoyment of daily activities and mood. Psychosom. Med. 1979; **41**:587–604.

Abrahams, G. E.: The premenstrual tension syndrome. Contemp Ob/Gyn Nursing 1980; **3**:170–184.

AuBuchon, P. G., Calhoun, K. S.: Menstrual cycle symptomatology: the role of social expectancy and experimental demand characteristics. Psychosom. Med. 1985; **47**:35–45.

Backstrom, T., Boyle, H., Baird, D. T.: Persistence of symptoms of premenstrual tension in hysterectomized women. Br. J. Obstet. Gynaecol. 1981; **88**:530–536.

Frank, R. T.: The hormonal basis of premenstrual tension. Arch. Neurol. Psychiatry 1931; **26**:1053–1057.

Freeman, E. W., Sondheimer, S., Weinbaum, P. J., Rickels, K.: Evaluating premenstrual symptoms in medical practice. Obstet. Gynecol. 1985; **65**:500–505.

Gilmore, D. H., Hawthorn, R., McKay, Hart, D.: A placebo-controlled double-blind cross-over study of danazol 400 mg per day for the premenstrual syndrome. XIth World

Congress of Gynaecology and Obstetrics, West Berlin, 1985.

Goldzieher, J. W., Moses, L. E., Averkin, E., Scheel, C., Taber, B. Z.: Nervousness and depression attributed to oral contraceptives: a double-blind, placebo-controlled study. Am. J. Obstet. Gynecol. 1971; **111**:1013–1020.

Greenblatt, R. B., Asch, R. H., Mahesh, V. B., Bryner, J. R.: Implantation of pure crystalline pellets of estradiol for conception control. Am. J. Obstet. Gynecol. 1977; **127**:520–527.

Halbreich, U., Endicott, J., Schacht, S., Nee, J.: The diversity of premenstrual changes as reflected in the Premenstrual Assessment Form. Acta Psychiat. Scand. 1982; **62**:46–65.

Hammarback, S., Backstrom, T., Hoslt, J., von Schoultz, B., Lyrenas, S.: Cyclical mood changes as in the premenstrual tension syndrome during sequential estrogen-progestagen postmenopausal replacement therapy. Acta Obstet. Gynecol. Scand. 1985; **64**:393–397.

Magos, A. L., Studd, J. W. W.: The premenstrual syndrome. In: 'Progress in Obstetrics and Gynaecology, Volume 4' (Ed: Studd, J. W. W.). Edinburgh, Churchill Livingstone 1984a: 334–350.

Magos, A. L., Studd, J. W. W.: PMS – A new approach to cause and cure. Contemp Ob/Gyn 1984b; **24**:85–91.

Magos, A. L., Studd, J. W. W.: Effects of the menstrual cycle on medical disorders. Br. J. Hosp. Med. 1985; **33**:68–77.

Magos, A. L., Studd, J. W. W.: Assessment of menstrual cycle symptoms by trend analysis. Am. J. Obstet. Gynecol. 1986a (in press).

Magos, A. L., Studd, J. W. W.: A simple method for the diagnosis, of the premenstrual syndrome using a self-assessment disc. Br. Med. J. 1986b (submitted).

Magos, A. L., Brincat, M., Studd, J. W. W.: Trend analysis of the symptoms of 150 women complaining of the premenstrual syndrome. Am. J. Obstet. Gynecol. 1986a (in press).

Magos, A. L., Brincat, M., Studd, J. W. W.: Treatment of the premenstrual syndrome by subcutaneous oestradiol implants and cyclical oral norethisterone: a placebo controlled study. Br. Med. J. 1986b (in press).

Magos, A. L., Brewster, E., Singh, R., O'Dowd, T., Brincat, M., Studd, J. W. W.: The effects of norethisterone in postmenopausal women on oestrogen replacement therapy: a model for the premenstrual syndrome. Br. J. Obstet. Gynaecol. 1986c (submitted).

Magos, A. L., Collins, W. P., Studd, J. W. W.: Management of the premenstrual syndrome by subcutaneous implants of oestradiol. J. Psychosom. Obstet. Gynecol. 1984; **3**:93–99.

Mattson, B., von Schoultz, B.: A comparison between lithium, placebo and a diuretic in premenstrual tension. Acta Psychiat. Scand. 1974; **Suppl. 255**:75–84.

Moos, R. H.: Typology of menstrual cycle symptoms. Am. J. Obstet. Gynecol. 1969; **103**:390–402.

Morton, J. H.: Premenstrual tension. Am. J. Obstet. Gynecol. 1950; **60**:343–352.

Muse, K. N., Cetel, N. S., Futterman, L. A., Yen, S. S. C.: The premenstrual syndrome. Effects of "medical ovariectomy". N. End. J. Med. 1984; **311**:1345–1349.

Parlee, M. B.: The psychology of the menstrual cycle: biological and physiological perspectives. In: "Behavior and the menstrual cycle", (Ed: Friedman, R. C.), New York: Marcel Dekker; 77–99.

Rees, L.: The premenstrual tension syndrome and its treatment. Br. Med. J. 1953: **i**:1014–1016.

Robinson, K., Huntington, K. M., Wallace, M. G.: Treatment of the premenstrual syndrome. Br. J. Obstet. Gynaecol. 1977; **84**:784–788.

Rubinow, D. R., Roy-Byrne, P., Hoban, C., Gold, P. W., Post, R. M.: Prospective assessment of menstrually related mood disorders. Am. J. Psychiatry 1984; **141**:684–686.

Ruble, D. N.: Premenstrual symptoms: a reinterpretation. Science 1977; **197**:291–292.

Ruble, D. N., Brooks-Gunn, J.: Menstrual symptoms: a social cognition analysis. J. Behav. Med. 1979; **2**:171–194.

Sampson, G. A., Jenner, F. A.: Studies of daily recordings from the Moos menstrual distress questionnaire. Br. J. Psychiatr. 1977, **130**:265–271.

Steiner, M., Haskett, R. F., Carroll, B. J.: Premenstrual tension syndrome: the development of research diagnostic criteria and new rating scales. Acta Psychiat. Scand. 1980; **62**:177–190.

Studd, J. W. W., Thom, M. H.: Oestrogens and endometrial cancer. In: 'Progress in Obstetrics and Gynaecology, Volume 1' (Ed.

Studd, J. W. W.). Edinburgh, Churchill Livingstone 1981:182–198.
Taylor, J. W.: The timing of menstruation-related symptoms assessed by a daily symptom rating scale. Acta Psychiat. Scand. 1979; 60:87–105.
Wood, C., Jakubowicz, D.: The treatment of premenstrual symptoms with mefenamic acid. Br. J. Obstet. Gynaecol. 1980; 87:627–630.

Contraception in premenopausal age

U. Schwartz

Introduction

Despite an ever increasing amount of information on the different modalities of contraception in general, the current state-of-knowledge concerning their use of contraceptives in premenopausal women must frankly be characterized as a state of relative ignorance. Data regarding the risks and benefits of the various methods in this age group is not only limited and incomplete, but often ambiguous and contradictory. This applies in particular to the real and imagined hazards of oral contraceptives (OC). Unfortunately, imprudent overinterpretation of still inconclusive results has been sensationalized by the mass media and, thus, has bred irrational fears in the public and exerted undue pressure on governmental health agencies. This brief review cannot provide clear-cut guidelines on premenopausal contraception, but will address some of the major areas of concern with special emphasis on the "pill controversy".

Contraceptive needs

Undoubtedly, there is a necessity for birth control in the more mature woman who has completed her family. The majority of premenopausal women between 40 and 50 years of age lead an active and satisfying sex life with unreduced libido (55%), an average coital frequency of more than twice per week (64%) and orgasmic responses (94%; [1]). The individual decline in fertility varies considerably, and permanent natural sterility is difficult to predict [2]: 95% of women with regular menses ovulate consistently and even 34% of women with oligomenorrhea ovulate in every cycle. Also, ovulation may occur regardless of previous documentation of elevated FSH. Statistically, the rising incidence of luteal deficiency is connected with a diminished overall chance of pregnancy, yet the individual risk remains quite real. Table 1 shows the relatively high number of pregnancies in English women over 40; this survey does not include spontaneous abortions, which follow premenopausal conception in about 26% of the cases [3]. Almost half of all pregnancies were terminated; the resultant moral, emotional and social problems are obvious. In this context, it should be pointed out that legal abortions in English women above 35

Table 1 Births and legal abortions above age 40 in Great Britain, 1981 [3].

Age	Live births	Stillbirths (% of total births)	Legal abortions (% of conceptions*)
40–44	6170	89 (1·4%)	4835 (43·6%)
45–49	640	10 (1·5%)	549 (45·8%)
50+	50	1 (2·0%)	15 (22·7%)
All ages	634 492	4207 (0·7%)	128 581 (16·8%)

*Excluding spontaneous abortions

increased by 17% within less than a year after the 1977 report by the Royal College of General Practitioners (RCGP) on cardiovascular mortality among OC users [4]. Such observations illustrate the striking and immediate impact of epidemiologic studies which are expounded by the lay press. The need for contraception in this age group is underscored by the steep elevation of perinatal mortality and congenital anomalies as well as the alarming six fold rise in maternal mortality (Figure 1; [3]). It has, therefore, been recommended that some form of birth control be practiced for one year after the last menstrual period [5].

Criteria of method comparison

While many different methods are available, none can be regarded as the single best for the premenopause. Every modality must be evaluated in terms of contraceptive efficacy, risks and benefits as well as acceptability for the individual couple. It has been suggested that the failure rates of all techniques approach zero in women above 40 due to declining fertility; however, this appears to be rather speculative. Safety assessment is quite often reduced to the comparison of method-related mortality rates in healthy users, even though death associated with birth control is fortunately an extremely rare occurrence. The quantitatively more important influence on morbidity is seldom assessed; the health status and life style of the users are frequently neglected; and noncontraceptive benefits are widely ignored, especially by the lay media.

A relatively refined, yet controversial estimate of the overall risks associated with reversible fertility regulation was presented by Tietze and Lewit [6]. Table 2 indicates that after age 40 the mortality of pill-takers who smoke is three times higher than the mortality related to pregnancy and delivery, which, in turn, is almost equal to the mortality of non-smokers on high-dose preparations, while IUD-associated deaths are observed at a very low level. This data suggests that the use of

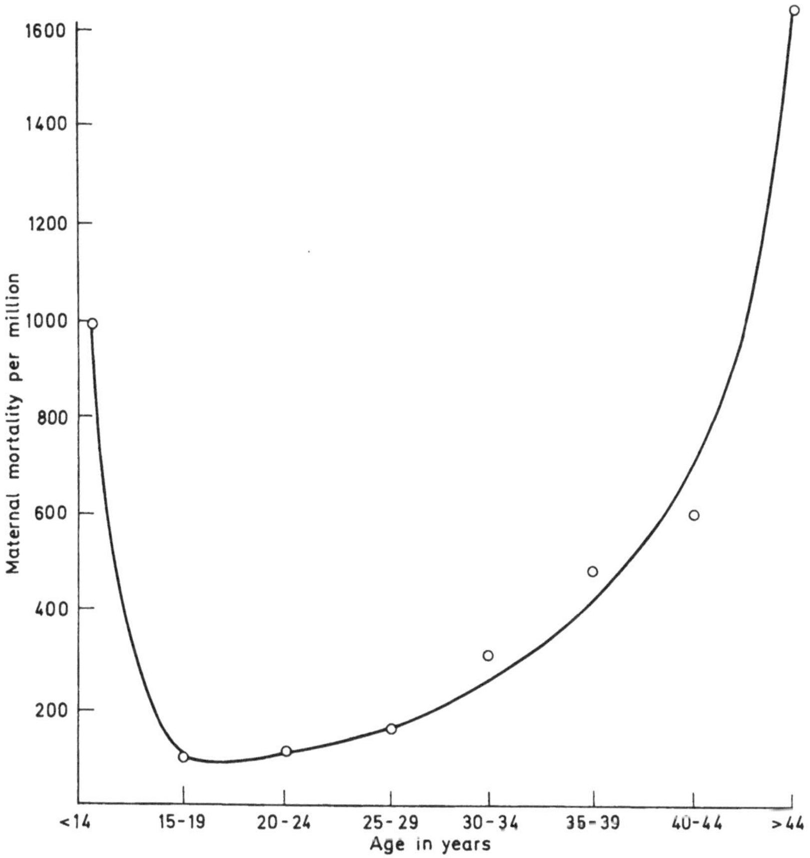

Fig. 1 Maternal mortality per million births plotted against maternal age in years ([3], adapted from Beard 1981).

barrier techniques backed up by early termination in case of failure should be far the best approach – that is, if the ethical and psychological problems of abortion could simply be discounted.

Combined oral contraceptives

Until the late 1970's the use of combined oral contraceptive was widely accepted by premenopausal patients and their doctors because it both controlled climacteric symptoms and prevented pregnancy most reliably. However, a dramatic change in attitude took place after several large epidemiologic investigations indicated a positive association between pill administration and circulatory fatalities. Yet, the results have always been inconsistent. For instance, in the three major prospective studies, the English RCGP and Oxford/Family Planning Studies found a relationship

Table 2 Annual mortality rates per 100,000 women associated with reversible fertility regulation [6].

Deaths, by Regimen	Age (years)
	40–44
No	
Birth-related	21.6
Abortion only	
Method-related	1.7
OCs only/nonsmokers	
Birth-related	0.4
Method-related	17.7
Total	18.1
OCs only/smokers	
Birth-related	0.4
Method-related	60.9
Total	61.3
IUDs only	
Birth-related	0.4
Method-related	1.4
Total	1.8
Barrier methods only	
Birth-related	4.0
Barrier methods plus abortion	
Method-related	0.2

with myocardial infarction and thrombotic stroke which was not evident in the American Walnut Creek Study, although the Walnut Creek Study demonstrated an association with subarachnoid hemorrhage. It is beyond the scope of this presentation to review all investigations either supporting or rejecting the claim that combined preparations predispose to cardiovascular death. Two contradictory examples will have to suffice. In 1981 the RCGP reported a four-fold rise of fatal circulatory disease in users of high-dose OCs [7]. The annual excess mortality for non-smoking women between 35 and 44 was estimated at 1 per 6,700 with a further increase after age 45 (Tabel 3). This figure roughly corresponds to the life risk of an English car driver [4]. The RCGP study further emphasized that the major hazard

Table 3 Annual excess cardiovascular mortality in users of oral contraceptives [7].

age of OC users (years)	nonsmokers	smokers
–34	1:77,000	1:10,000
35–44	1: 6,700	1: 2,000
45–	1: 2,500	1: 500

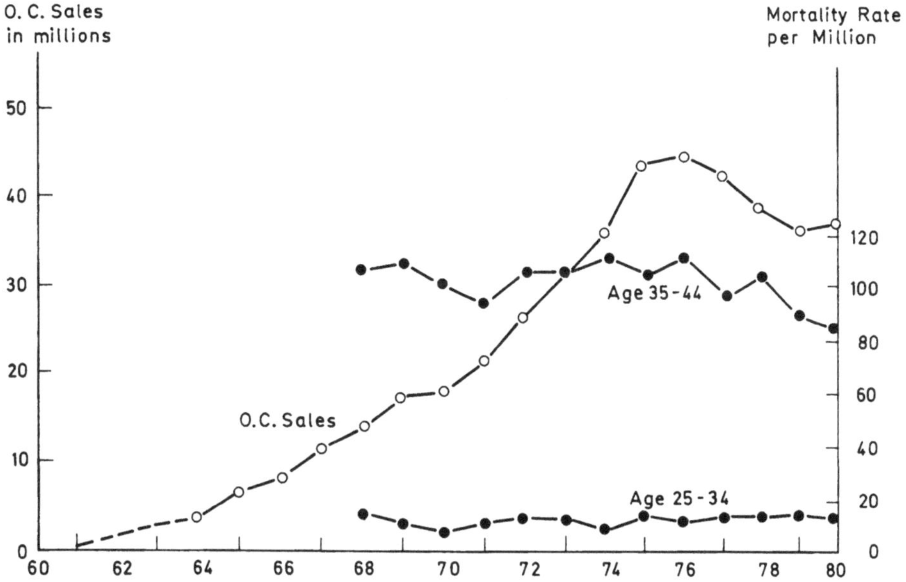

Fig. 2 Oral contraceptive sales in the UK and ischemic heart disease mortality rates in women per 1,000,000 population [8].

occurred in smokers. On the other hand, a recent analysis of vital statistics by Wisemann [8] showed that the mortality rates for ischemic heart disease in women between 35 and 44 actually decreased from 1960 to 1980 – a trend that was not correlated to the sales of oral contraceptives in Britain (Figure 2); similar observations applied to subarachnoid and cerebral hemorrhage rates.

The early epidemiologic data linked the circulatory risks primarily to the estrogen component of combined preparations. This assumption was based on the 1970 finding by Inman et al. that the incidence of thromboembolic disease rose with increasing doses of ethinylestradiol and mestranol (Figure 3; [9]). The notion of a causal relationship was later questioned when the application of modern technology revealed that the clinical diagnosis of venous thrombosis was incorrect in almost 80% of pill users [10]. In view of the assumed risk, drugs containing more than 50 µg of synthetic estrogen were withdrawn from the market in most countries. Despite the lower estrogen content of current products, however, some of the adverse vascular effects seemed to persist.

In the late 1970s attention was focussed on the potential hazards of the progestin component when another RCGP analysis revealed that the occurrence of hypertension, although minor and reversible, was related to the dose of norethisterone acetate (Figure 4; [11]). However, reports to the British Committee on Safety on Medicine in 1980 failed to confirm this finding [12]. Further epidemiologic research

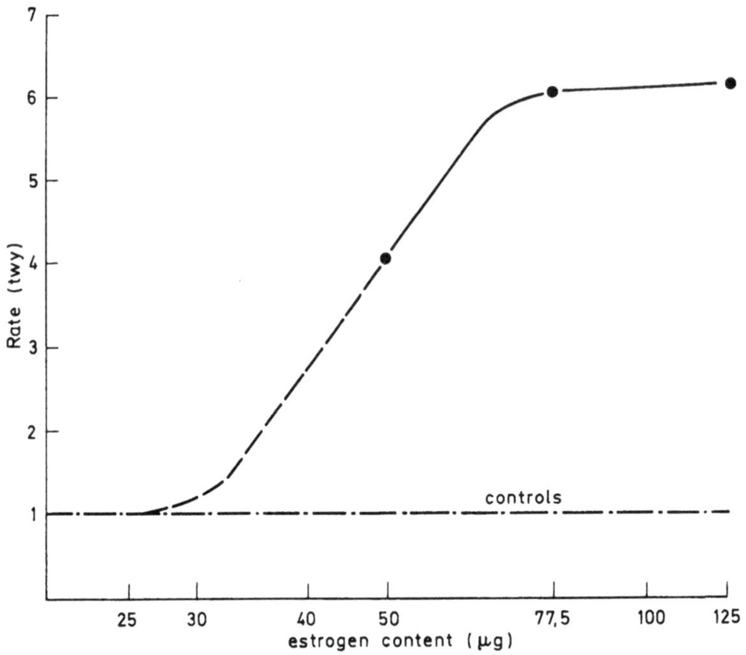

Fig. 3 Thromboembolic disease rates per 1,000 women years (twy) associated with estrogen content of oral contraceptives ([33], adapted from RCGP 1974 and Andrews 1979).

on progestin influence was, and is, confounded by the fact that combination drugs contain varying amounts of various progestins, each with its own spectrum of biological effects, and varying amounts of estrogen.

The association between total arterial disease and progestins, independent of estrogen activity, was supported by a subsequent RCGP study [13]. The results indicated higher rates of ischemic heart disease, cerebrovascular disease and peripheral vascular disease with larger amounts of norethisterone acetate and levonorgestrel (Figure 5). Attention was also drawn to the observation that both 19-nortestosterone derivatives caused a dose-related reduction of the "atheroprotective" high-density lipoprotein (HDL) cholesterol fraction [14]. At present it is believed that the development of circulatory disease may be accelerated by an accumulation of progestin effects such as alterations of lipid metabolism, elevation of blood pressure and modifications of carbohydrate metabolism, e.g. glucose intolerance, insulin resistance and hyperinsulinemia. However, this subject is by no means settled. Thus, a 1985 study of German oral contraceptive users with myocardial infarction was unable to demonstrate the presence of any of these atherogenic risk factors or actual coronary sclerosis [15]. Biochemical investigations have shown that the undesirable lipoprotein changes may be minimized or even averted by reducing progestin content and using step-up regimens. In a very recent

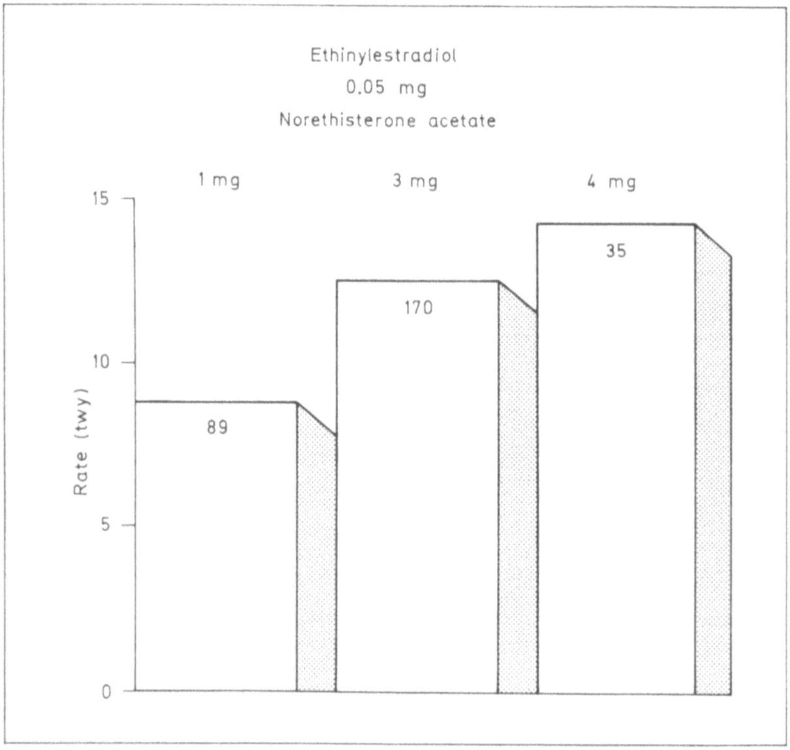

Fig. 4 Hypertension rates per 1,000 women years (twy) associated with progestin content of oral contraceptives [11].

prospective study from Israel, 100 women between age 41 and 49 were treated with a low-dose triphasic drug combining ethinylestradiol and levonorgestrel; after three years a significant decrease of atherogenic low-density lipoprotein cholesterol was evident, while the protective HDL fraction had increased (Figure 6; [16]). Finally, it has been suggested that the adverse impact on lipid metabolism may be further diminished by administration of 17-hydroxyprogesterone rather than 19-nortestosterone derivatives [17]. It remains to be seen whether such findings are of clinical significance.

Most epidemiologic data stems from analyses of high-dose oral contraceptives. It has always been speculated that the apparent risks would decrease with the introduction of low-estrogen drugs. So far, no clear picture has emerged. A Swedish investigation documented the decline in sales of high-dose brands after 1968 and the rising market share of preparations containing 50 and 30 μg (Figure 7; [18]). The morbidity from venous thromboembolic episodes fell drastically during that period (Figure 8); however, the frequency of coronary and cerebral arterial complications remained constant. In contrast, an American study reported a continuing positive

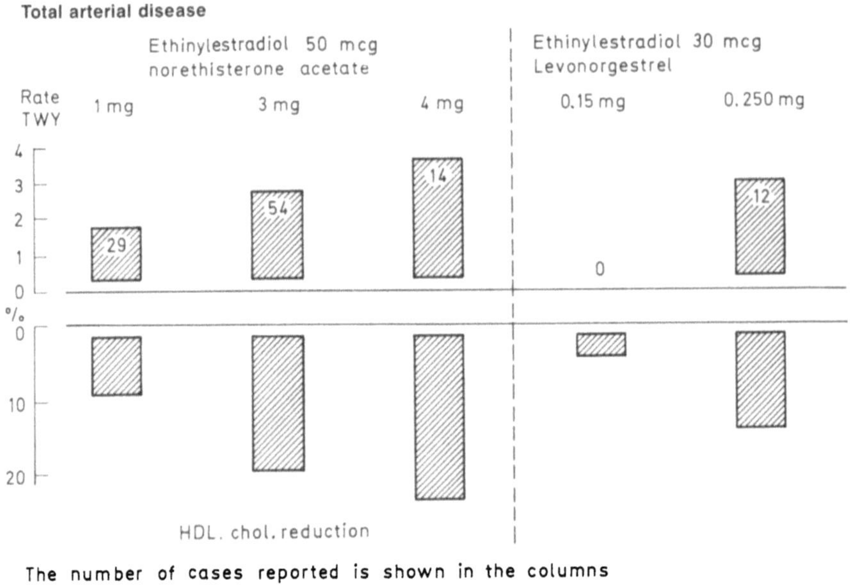

Fig. 5 Total arterial disease rates per 1,000 women years (TWY) and HDL cholesterol reduction associated with progestin content of oral contraceptives [13, 14].

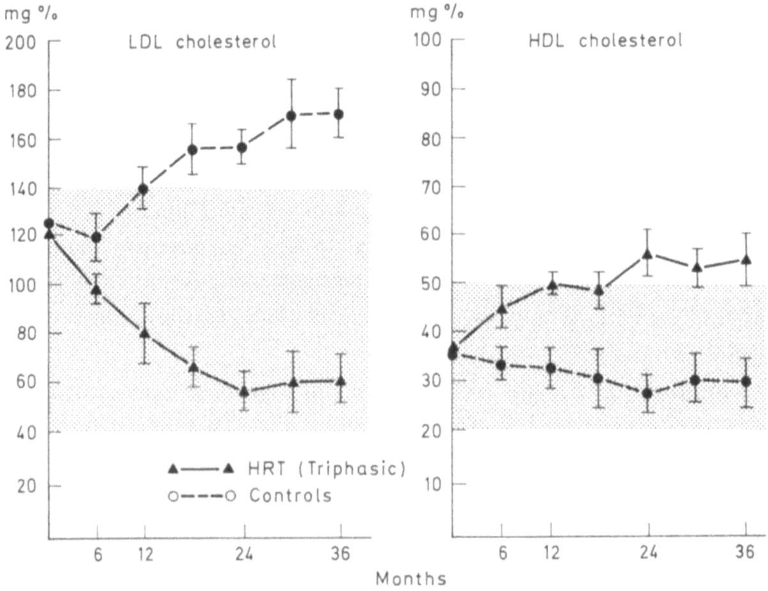

Fig. 6 Lipoprotein changes induced by a low-dose triphasic oral contraceptive in women between age 41 and 49 ([16]; HRT = hormone replacement therapy, shaded area = normal range).

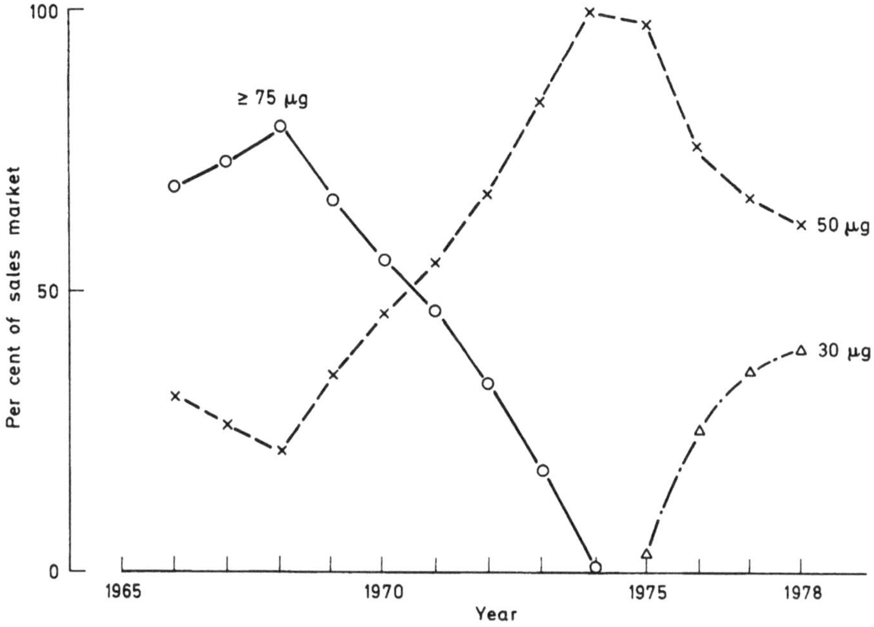

Fig. 7 Market share of high-estrogen and low-estrogen oral contraceptives in Sweden [18].

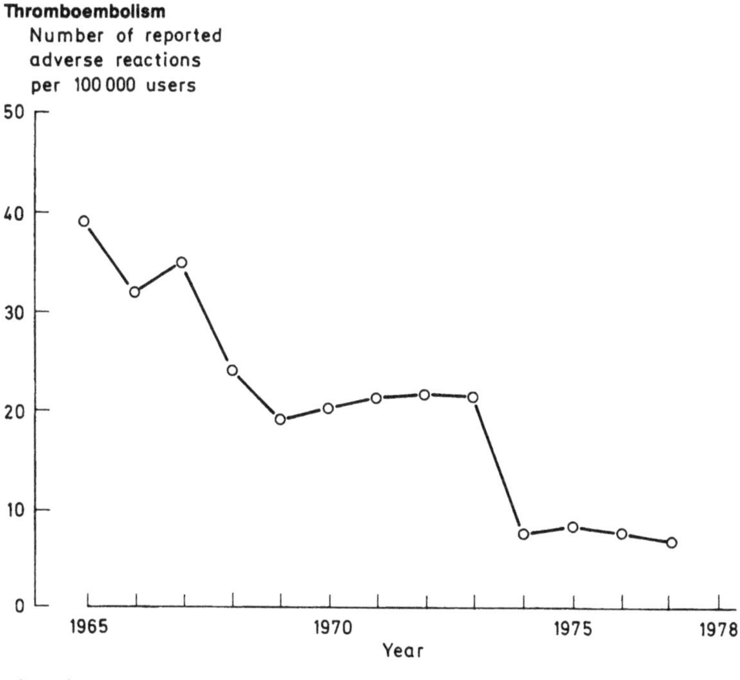

Fig. 8 Thromboembolic episodes reported to the Swedish Adverse Drug Reaction Committee [18].

association with venous thromboembolism, but not with myocardial infarction and stroke [19]. Perhaps this reflects the impact of unaltered progestin doses which masked the advantages of estrogen reduction. Another yet unresolved point of controversy involves the increased and longlasting residual risk of ischemic heart disease related to the duration of OC use which was suggested by Slone et al. [20], but not confirmed by the 1981 RCGP report [7]. Similarily, a linkage to the development of hepatomas remains to be conclusively proven.

While epidemiologic data on excess mortality associated with oral contraceptives is voluminous, data concerning morbidity is rather limited and does not differentiate between the various age groups. Vessey made a crude comparison of reversible birth control methods with regard to morbidity patterns (Table 4; [21]). He calculated an annual excess of 458 hospital admissions per 100,000 OC users due to nonobstetric and obstetric morbidity resulting from contraceptive failures; the estimates for users of IUDs and the diaphragm were considerably higher, i.e. 2,245 and 5,000, respectively. Theoretically, however, hospitalization for pregnancy-related reasons should markedly decrease in premenopausal women and, thus, reduce the relative advantage of OC's.

Patient counselling must not only include a prudent appraisal of the infrequent hazards, but also provide adequate information about the more common health benefits of oral contraceptives. These benefits include a lower incidence of iron deficiency anemia, benign breast disease, functional ovarian cysts, pelvic inflamma-

Table 4 Estimation of annual excess hospital admissions in users of oral contraceptives (OC), intrauterine devices (IUD) and diaphragms [21].

reason for admission	method-related hospital admissions per 100,000 users per year		
	OC	IUD	diaphragm
nonobstetric (total):	118	250	0
stroke	35		
venous thromboembolism	70		
myocardial infarction	10		
hepatoma	3		
uterine perforation		50	
pelvic inflammatory disease		200	
obstetric (total):	340	1,995	5,000
spontaneous abortion	45	775	640
termination	94	605	1,295
ectopic gestation	1	120	20
term birth	200	495	3,045
Total Morbidity	458	2,245	5,000

Table 5 Estimation of annual prevention of hospital admission in users of oral contraceptives ([24]; rate = per 100,000 pill users).

Disease	Rate	No.
Benign breast disease	235	20,000
Ovarian retention cysts	35	3,000
Iron-deficiency anemia[1]	320	27,200
Pelvic inflammatory disease (first episodes)		
Total episodes[1]	600	51,000
Hospitalizations	156	13,300
Ectopic pregnancy	117	9,900
Rheumatoid arthritis[1]	32	2,700
Endometrial cancer[2]	5	2,000
Ovarian cancer[2]	4	1,700

Except where noted, figures refer to hospitalizations prevented among the estimated 8.5 million current users of oral contraceptives in the United States.
1 Episodes prevented regardless of whether hospitalizations occurred.
2 Based on an estimated 39 million U.S. women who have ever used oral contraceptives.

tory disease and ectopic pregnancy. OC usage may also protect against rheumatoid arthritis, endometrial cancer and ovarian cancer, although these findings are still suggestive rather than absolute. It should be added that a study from the American Centers for Disease control [22] provided no support for the highly publicized allegation by Pike et al. [23] that OC's increase the risk of breast cancer. Ory has estimated that 50,000 hospital admissions are averted each year among current and past OC-takers in the United States alone (Table 5; [24]). The prospective study from Israel documented additional advantages for premenopausal women who received hormone replacement with a low-dose triphasic contraceptive: prevention of bone loss, elimination of hot flashes, improvement of psychofunctional disturbances and sex life [16]. During the three-year period, no adverse changes occurred in lipid and carbohydrate metabolism, coagulation factors or blood pressure.

So where do we stand in 1985 when assessing the risk-benefit ratio of oral contraceptive use in premenopausal women? In view of the conflicting data, a causal relationship between cardiovascular disease and OC cannot be drawn at present. Epidemiologic studies can never, by themselves, provide the ultimate truth due to their well-known inherent inadequacies. Although inconclusive, many results are disturbing and must be taken seriously, even when the number of patients actually affected by fatal and nonfatal disease is extremely small. Current confusion is reflected by the divergent recommendations concerning the maximum age for OC usage: they range from 35 [25] to 45 [7] and even 52 years [26]. It is our personal opinion that low-dose preparations, preferably triphasic, may be prescribed up to age 45 provided that risk factors such as smoking, hypertension, obesity, hyperlipidemia and diabetes are absent, that informed consent has been obtained and that continuous monitoring, especially of blood pressure and weight, is guaranteed. Since currently available laboratory tests fail to reliably predict which patient will suffer a cardiovascular incident [27], the costly routine screening of coagulation factors, lipid and carbohydrate metabolism is not recommended.

Other methods of contraception

No large-scale studies on age-related effects of the other hormonal birth control methods have been published. The experience is scanty, uncontrolled and mostly anecdotal. Progestin-only pills and injectable depot progestins provide nearly 100% security in this age group. Although they supposedly elicit only minor metabolic changes, a significant suppression of HDL cholesterol has recently been demonstrated for both methods [28, 29]. The estrogen-free approach has severe practical disadvantages: it may result in either amenorrhea, which can induce fear of pregnancy, or erratic bleeding patterns necessitating curettage. Postcoital interception should be regarded as an emergency measure and only be used in women with still regular menses following unprotected midcycle exposure [30]. It remains to be confirmed that the innovative replacement regimens combining oral or parenteral administration of natural estrogens with continuous or sequential low-dose progestin in addition are able to reliably prevent pregnancy in premenopausal women [31, 32].

Non-hormonal alternatives for fertility regulation must always be considered. In this age group, all rhythm methods are insecure due to the unpredictability of ovulation when menstruation becomes irregular. Barrier techniques with concomitant application of spermicides are quite appropriate in view of their increasing effectiveness with age, the absence of systemic risks and the protection against veneral disease. The intra-uterine device is especially suited for the more mature woman who has completed her family, for whom steroid contraceptives are contraindicated or who opposes sterilization. Figure 9 illustrates that the incidence of adverse effects such as pregnancy, expulsion and removal for bleeding or pain steadily falls with advancing age [33]. The risk of pelvic inflammatory disease is also diminished in older multiparous patients. Preliminary results suggest that the insertion of progestin-releasing devices may reverse endometrial hyperplasia, reduce menstrual blood loss and decrease the hazard of salpingitis [3, 34].

For couples desiring permanent contraception, vasectomy is the safest technique;

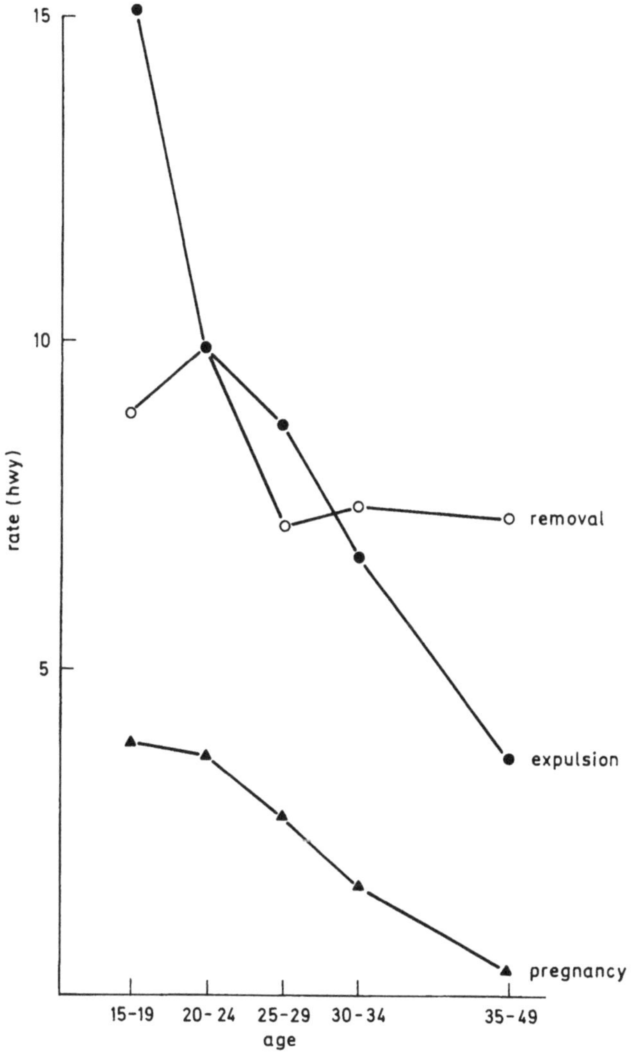

Fig. 9 Adverse effects per 100 women years (hwy) of intrauterine device in different age groups ([33], adapted from Population Reports 1979).

however, for sociocultural reasons, it is still not accepted in many countries. Female sterilization by laparoscopic tubal occlusion constitutes an effective procedure with low, non-recurrent morbidity that is justified once a stable motivation has been established [35]. Hysterectomy should not be performed for the sole purpose of sterilization since it is associated with a distinctly higher rate of complications such as febrile morbidity, hemorrhage requiring transfusion, unintended major surgery, rehospitalization and even death (Table 6; [36]).

Table 6 Complications associated with laparoscopic tubal occlusion and vaginal hysterectomy among women of reproductive age [35,36].

complication	complication rate: per 100 procedures: laparoscopic sterilization (n = 3,500)	vaginal hysterectomy (n = 568)
febrile morbidity	0.2	15.3
transfusion	0	8.3
unintended major surgery	1.1	5.1
rehospitalization	0.5	1.8
death	0	0.2
one or more complications	1.7	24.5

Conclusion

The need for reliable, safe and acceptable contraception during the premenopause is undisputed, while the selection of an appropriate method remains highly controversial. At present we are all caught in a dilemma that has been quite adequately described by Goldzieher [10]: "The benefit/risk ratio is not something that can be calculated in a vacuum. It is the moment of truth when the physician must take off his critical scientist's hat and put on his doctor's hat: the point at which all of the scientific doubts and questions must be resolved face-to-face with one particular human being whose unique problem must be dealt with right then and there. The multiplicity of factors which influence the final judgement in that particular instance represent a situation which the practicing physician deals with every day, but it is beyond the ability of computers and probably outside the ken of epidemiologists. Therein lies much of the difficulty and much of the confusion." None of us can evade the personal responsibility of converting the current ambiguities into operational decisions for our premenopausal patients.

References

[1] Bottiglioni, F., De Aloysio, D.: Female sexual activity as a function of climacteric conditions and age. Maturitas 4:27, 1982.

[2] Editorial: Have I stopped ovulating yet? Lancet 1:477, 1979.

[3] Guillebaud, J.: Contraception for the older woman. J. Obstet. Gynaecol. 5 (Suppl. 2):S 70, 1985.

[4] Law, B.: Kontrazeption bei der Frau über 35 Jahre. In: Hammerstein, J. (ed.): Aktuelle Aspekte der hormonellen Kontrazeption, p 155. Excerpta Medica, Amsterdam 1982.

[5] Bowen-Simpkins, P.: Contraception for the older woman. Br. J. Obstet. Gynaecol. 91:513, 1984.

[6] Tietze, C., Lewit, S.: Life risks associated

with reversible methods of fertility regulation. Int. J. Gynaecol. Obstet., 16:456, 1979.

[7] Royal College of General Practitioner's Oral Contraception Study: Further analyses of mortality in oral contraceptive users. Lancet 1:541, 1981.

[8] Wiseman, R. A.: Absence of correlation between oral contraceptive usage and cardiovascular mortality. Int. J. Fertil. 29:198, 1984.

[9] Inman, W. H. W., Vessey, M. P., Westerholm, B., Engelund, A.: Thromboembolic disease and the steroidal content of oral contraceptives. Br. Med. J. 2:203, 1970.

[10] Goldzieher, J. W.: Interpretation of data by the clinician. Int. J. Gynaecol. Obstet. 16:535, 1979.

[11] Royal College of General Practitioners' Oral Contraception Study: Effect on hypertension and benign breast disease of progestogen component in combined oral contraceptives. Lancet 1:624, 1977.

[12] Meade, T. W., Greenberg, G., Thompson, S. G.: Progestogens and cardiovascular reactions associated with oral contraceptives and a comparison of the safety of 50- and 30-µg oestrogen preparations. Br. Med. J. 280:1157, 1980.

[13] Kay, C. R.: Progestogens and arterial disease-Evidence from the Royal College of General Practitioners' study. Am. J. Obstet. Gynecol. 142:762, 1982.

[14] Briggs, M. H.: Recent biological studies in relation to low dose hormonal contraceptives. Br. J. Fam. Plann. 5:25, 1979.

[15] Engel, H. J., Engel, E., Lichtlen, P.: Koronarsklerose und Herzinfarkt bei jungen Frauen. Münch. med. Wschr. 127:415, 1985.

[16] Shargil, A. A.: Hormone replacement therapy in perimenopausal women with a triphasic contraceptive compound: A three-year prospective study. Int. J. Fertil. 30:15, 1985.

[17] Hirvonen, E., Mälkönen, M., Manninen, V.: Effects of different progestogens on lipoproteins during postmenopausal replacement therapy. N. Engl. J. Med. 304:560, 1981.

[18] Böttiger, L. E., Boman, G., Eklund, G., Westerholm, B.: Oral contraceptives and lowering of oestrogen content. Lancet 1:1097, 1980.

[19] Porter, J. B., Hunter, J. R., Jick, H., Stergachis, A.: Oral contraceptives and nonfatal vascular disease. Obstet. Gynecol. 66:1, 1985.

[20] Slone, D., Shapiro, S. Kaufman, D. W., Rosenberg, L., Miettinen, O. S., Stolley, P. D.: Risk of myocardial infarction in relation to current and discontinued use of oral contraceptives. N. Engl. J. Med. 305:420, 1981.

[21] Vessey, M. P.: Contraceptive methods: risks and benefits. Br. Med. J. 3:721, 1978.

[22] The Centers for Disease Control Cancer and Steroid Hormone Study: Long-term oral contraceptive use and the risk of breast cancer. JAMA 249:1591, 1983.

[23] Pike, M. C., Henderson, B. E., Krailo, M. D., Duke, A., Roy, S.: Breast cancer in young women and use of oral contraceptives: possible modifying effect of formulation and age at use. Lancet 2:926, 1983.

[24] Ory, H. W.: The noncontraceptive health benefits from oral contraceptive use. Fam. Plann. Perspect. 14:182, 1982.

[25] Wissenschaftlicher Beirat der Bundesärztekammer: Hinweise zur Verordnung oraler Kontrazeptiva. Dtsch. Äbl. 81:3170, 1984.

[26] Haspels, A. A.: Round table. In: Haspels, A. A., Rolland, R. (eds.): Benefits and risks of hormonal contraception, p. 184. MTP Press, Lancaster 1982.

[27] Mammen, E. F.: Oral contraceptives and blood coagulation: a critical review. Am. J. Obstet. Gynecol. 142:781, 1982.

[28] Wynn, V., Niththyananthan, R.: The effects of progestins in combined oral contraceptives on serum lipids with special reference to high-density lipoproteins. Am. J. Obstet. Gynecol. 142:766, 1982.

[29] Howard, G., Blair, M., Fotherby, K., Trayner, I., Hamawi, A., Elder, M. G.: Some metabolic effects of long-term use of the injectable contraceptive norethisterone oenanthate. Lancet 1:423, 1982.

[30] Yuzpe, A.: Postcoital contraception. Int. J. Gynaecol. Obstet. 16:497, 1979.

[31] Magos, A. L., Brincat, M., Studd, J. W. W., Wardle, P., Schlesinger, P., O'Dowd, T.: Amenorrhea and endometrial atrophy with continuous oral estrogen and progestogen therapy in postmenopausal women. Obstet. Gynecol. 65:496, 1985.

[32] Greenblatt, R. B.: Contraception for middle-aged women. In: Muldoon, T. G.,

Mahesh, V. B., Perez-Ballester, B. (eds.): Recent advances in fertility research. Part A, p. 287. Alan Liss, New York 1982.

[33] Rabe, R., Runnebaum, B.: Kontrazeption, p. 249. Springer, Berlin 1982.

[34] Volpe, A., Botticelli, A., Abrate, M., Dalla Vecchia, E., Mantovani, M., Carani, C., Grasso, A., Mazza, V., DiRenzo, G. C.: An intrauterine progesterone contraceptive system (52 mg) used in pre- and perimenopausal patients with endometrial hyperplasia. Maturitas 4:73, 1982.

[35] Destefano, F., Greenspan, J. B., Dicker, R. C., Peterson, H. B., Strauss, L. T., Rubin, G. L.: Complications of interval laparoscopic tubal sterilization. Obstet. Gynecol. 61:153, 1983.

[36] Dicker, R. C., Greenspan, J. R., Strauss, L. T., Cowart, M. R., Scally, M. J., Peterson, H. B., Destefano, F., Rubin, G. L., Ory, H. W.: Complications of abdominal and vaginal hysterectomy among women of reproductive age in the United States. Am. J. Obstet. Gynecol. 144:841, 1982.

Discussion

Question: What was the age of your series?

Magos: It was about 37 for both groups. The range was about 28 to 47.

Question: I was wondering if you are not treating climacteric complaints?

Magos: No, although the symptoms in one of the clusters included hot flushes. There were not really the problem to them. It was water retention, irritability and depression which were the big problems. And anyway, they were the wrong age group for climacteric problems.

Question: How did the patients accept the implants?

Magos: Very well, but it is obviously a short study. We have, in fact, got a much bigger group which has been treated for several years – up to 10 years – with implants, and they are very acceptable.

Question: I have a comment and a question for Dr. Magos. I think it would be inaccurate to state that there are no criteria for the premenstrual syndrome. Certain women with premenstrual tension or premenstrual syndrome have a definite and significant hyperprolactinaemia, and these women responded very well to bromocriptine. The fact that they did not respond to anything else prompted me to mention this here. How do you see LH-RH working in these women?

Magos: There is no universal definition of the PMS. I am sure that there are very small subgroups of patients who have raised prolactin levels and who would therefore probably benefit from bromocriptine. But I do not think that the majority has raised prolactin levels, and I do not think that they would benefit from bromocriptine. We are trying to achieve the same effect as with LH-RH. The big difference is that we are maintaining estrogen levels in the physiological range and there is therefore no reason why our treatment should not be long-term measure. With LH-RH, on the other hand, you have potential menopausal problems because of the low estrogen levels, which means it may not be suitable for long-term therapy. However, most of these patients require long-term therapy.

Lauritzen: I believe that the premenstrual syndrome is not an etiological or pathogenetic unity. No one therapy will help all patients, so we must try to find a suitable therapy for the individual patient, and there will not be a helpful therapy in all cases. Apart from this, I believe that a great percentage of these patients is neurotic.

Magos: People have looked at the psychological profile of women with the premenstrual syndrome, or with what they define as the premenstrual syndrome, which may not be the same as our definition. There doesn't seem to be a universal correlation between complaining of the PMS and being neurotic, so I disagree with you there. As far as response is concerned, all our patients with the implant responded. It was a genuine 100% response to the implant; the response to the placebo was almost 100%, but only initially for the first 2 to 4 months depending on the symptoms we were looking at. I would therefore suggest that a treatment does exist that is as universally successful as was LH-RH.

Question: Dr. Magos, what mean serum levels of estradiol or estrone do you find with estradiol implants?

Magos: We haven't actually measured levels in this particular study, but in our long-term retrospective look at this treatment over about 10 years the levels remained almost invariably within a physiological range.

Question: This is for Dr. Schwartz. Do you regard a previous history of smoking as a risk factor – for example, a patient aged 42 years who doesn't smoke at the present time but who was a heavy smoker until a few years ago? Do you consider this a contraindication to oral contraception or not?

Schwartz: I do not think I would consider it a contraindication. I would agree with Dr. Vessey, who said that, if you are over 35 and are a smoker, you either give up smoking and you may then use a low-dosed pill, or you continue smoking and then you had better discontinue the pill.

Vessey: I would like to comment briefly on Dr. Schwartz's paper becaue I have a lot of sympathy with what he said. However, I think he perhaps highlighted the controversy about some of the cardiovascular disease data by picking the most extreme discrepancies that there are. I believe that, if you sit down and review the total literature, bearing in mind the amount of data, sampling variation and factors such as duration of use and type of preparation, you can produce a rather more uniform answer. However, I think one of the most important things is that, almost without exception, the very large number of epidemiological studies dealing with cardiovascular disease relate to pills that we are no longer using. I feel that we need data relating to pills that we are using at the present time. Certainly, one of the things I am hoping to do in the U.K. – if I can get funding – is to undertake a new three-year case-control study of deaths amongst British women from cardiovascular disease, where we would, of course, be looking at modern pills. This is because I suspect that, whatever the variations you may see from study to study, the risks with modern pills used in a modern way are very, very tiny.

Schwartz: May I add that I totally agree with you, Professor Vessey. I chose these extremes purely for didactic purposes. I would also support your contention that what we need are prospective studies using the low-dosed preparations – and not only in one country, but in many different countries. As you all know, the incidence of cardiovascular disease varies from continent to continent, and I think we also know that the metabolism of synthetic steroids varies from country to country – to mention just two factors. I therefore believe that prospective epidemiological studies are needed for the countries involved.

Closing remarks

P. G. Crosignani

In Queen Victoria's time, menopause was not a problem for Europe and similarly in 1956 life expectancy for a chinese woman was 42 years, so there was no problem of menopause. But within a few years, as we heard during the Congress, there will be 700 million women over 45. This indicates the size of the problem. There are other important facts worth noting: 40% of women have osteoporosis-related fractures before the age of 70, while for women 45 years-old, more myocardial infarctions are reported in menopausal than in premenopausal subjects. It is thus reasonable to assume that in the near future menopause will be an important primary care problem and even today an increasing number of women ask to be protected against osteoporosis, urinary complaints and cardiovascular disease. Attempts at replacement therapy started 40 years ago, 20 years after the first replacement therapy for diabetes, as observed by Dr. Greenblatt. Today a series of questions are still not fully answered: how to select the patients to be treated? How to treat them? When to start the treatment? How long to continue the treatment?

At this meeting, yesterday and today, we have heard and discussed a lot of interesting physiological, clinical and epidemiological data on this subject. I personally enjoyed this quite useful review of the current knowledge. A comprehensive overview is always required as a basis for future advancement. At this point, Dr. Lachnit joins me in thanking all the many people involved in organizing the Congress, and particularly Mrs. Heithecker.

Last but not least, I wish to express warm thanks to Schering for their generous hospitality. I am sure that all of you join me in these thanks.

Epilogue

Before bringing this symposium to a close let me again express the indebtedness of the speakers and chairpersons to Schering-Berlin for making this event possible. The opportunity of sharing our experiences and discussing with you – the audience – the problems that confront us, helps all of us to understand what is, and what is not, the menopause and who should be treated – why, when, and with what.

It is hoped that the collected wisdom of experts gathered from eight different countries for this event will help defuse the indifference, the skepticism, and fears regarding hormones still extant in many parts of the world. I recall my attendance at a meeting in early 1946 where an elderly professor of Obstetrics and Gynecology spoke on the worthlessness of hormones in the treatment of the menopause. He declared that he had not used estrogens for 20 years because he found that bromides and phenobarbital yielded just as good results. I ebulliently rose to discuss his paper and reminded the good professor that 20 years before 1946 the only preparations available were ovarian residue. These preparations had no estrogenic activity. They were merely placebos and it is little wonder that he found bromides and phenobarbital just as useful. I reminded him "Old age hath yet his honor and his toil and ere t'is too late some work of noble note may yet be done" (Tennyson). I urged him to try the potent estrogens available to him and not to close the book on HRT.

The decade of the 1930's saw the dawn of a new era for womankind and I might add that the scientists at Schering made monumental contributions to the development and availability of potent estrogenic agents. Although the medical profession now has had more than a half century of experience with the use of estrogens, many physicians still do not accept their use; they still cling to the concept that the menopause is a natural physiologic process representing merely an adjustment to what Robert Browning depicted as "the last of life for which the first was made". They regard any attempt to correct the estrogen deficiency as a meddlesome intrusion into a normal aging process. Their attitude, not necessarily one of benign neglect, is that much may be accomplished by homespun psychology, encouragement, and simple sedatives. Then again, a good proportion of physicians, intimidated by alarming reports dealing with the hazards of estrogen therapy, are reluctant to offer hormone replacement therapy. In avoiding such therapeutic measures, they are relieved of responsibility if a gynecic cancer (breast or uterus) should develop. Brave new world – to do no harm should not be a mandate not to try to do good.

The difficulties of the postmenopausal period – the imbalance of the autonomic nervous system, the psychogenic disorders, the metabolic disturbances – continue in mild to severe degree to the end of life. Many women cannot adjust to them. Although their hormonal environment can be improved, they envision goals that must remain inaccessible. Simone de Beauvoir, in *"Le Deuxième Sexe"*, justly points to the menopausal woman's states of depression when she writes: "Inner illuminations fade and moments of exalation give way to hours of melancholic gloom." In those who have staked everything on femininity, the pathetic urge to turn back the clock contributes to the crisis. Hormones will not stay the aging process, efface the wrinkled brow or lift the sagging breast. It is, however, unrealistic to withhold measures that may prevent disabling pathologic processes or help a woman make the transition smoother during the difficult years. The proper use of gonadal steroids (estrogens, androgens, progestogens) may enable her to obtain fulfillment without interrupting her quest for a continuum of physical and mental health. She can grow old with grace and dignity, glowing with the radiance of the turning leaves of fall. Such was the vision of John Dunne, 16th C. poet and Dean of St. Paul's Cathedral of London, when he penned these lines:

No spring nor summer hath such grace
As I have seen in one autumnal face.

Robert B. Greenblatt
Honorary President
International Menopausal Society

List of contributors

Brincat, Dr. M. MRCS, LRCP, Honorary Registrar, King's College Hospital Medical School, Denmark Hill, London SE5 9RS, Great Britain

Cardozo, Dr. L. D., MB, ChB, MRCOG, Senior Registrar, Obstetrics and Gynaecology, Menopause Clinic, Dulwich Hospital, East Dulwich Grove, London SE22 8PT, Great Britain

Christiansen, Prof. C., MD, Glostrup Hospital, Dept. of Clinical Chemistry, University of Copenhagen, Nordre Ringvej, DK-2600 Glostrup

Crosignani, Prof. P. G., MD, Clinica Ostetrica e Ginecologica III, Facolta di Medicina, Via M. Melloni, I-20129 Milano

Don Gambrell Jr., Prof. R., MD, Clinical Professor, Medical College of Georgia, School of Medicine, Dept. of Endocrinology, Augusta, GA 30912, USA

Hannse, Dr. rer. nat. H., Mitglied des Vorstandes der Schering AG, Müllerstr. 170–178, D-1000 Berlin 65

Hunt, Dr. K., MD, Gibson Laboratories Building, Radcliffe Infirmary, Oxford ox 2 6 HE, Great Britain

Husmann, Prof. Dr. med. F., Chefarzt, Klinik am Malerwinkel, Wasserstr. 3, D-4772 Bad Sassendorf

Larsson-Cohn, Prof. U., MD, Dept. of Obstetrics and Gynaecology, University Hospital, S-581 85 Linköping

Lindsay, Prof. R., MB, ChB, PhD, FRCP, Director of Research, Helen Hayes Hospital, Route 9W, West Haverstraw, New York, NY 10993, USA

Magos, Dr. A. L., BSC, MB, BS, Registrar, Dept. of Obstetrics and Gynaecology, Dulwich Hospital, East Dulwich Grove, London SE22 8PT, Great Britain

Nocke, Prof. Dr. med. W., Leiter der Abt. Endokrinologie, Universitäts-Frauenklinik, D-5300 Bonn

Notelovitz, Prof. M., MD, PhD, The Center for Climacteric Studies, University of Florida, The Professional Center, 901 NW 8th Avenue, Suite B-1, Gainesville, FL 32601, USA

Schneider, Prof. Dr. med. H. P. G., Direktor der Universitäts-Frauenklinik, Albert-Schweitzer-Str. 23, D-4400 Münster

Schwartz, Prof. Dr. med. U., Irschenhauser Str. 11, D-8000 München 70

Studd, J. W. W., MD, MB, ChB, MRCOG, Consultant Obstetrician and Gynaecologist, Dulwich Hospital, East Dulwich Grove, London SE22 8PT, Great Britain

Tikkanen, Prof. M. J., MD, Third Department of Medicine, University of Helsinki, SF-00290 Helsinki

Utian, Prof. W. H., MD, PhD, Associate Professor of Reproductive Biology,The Mt. Sinai Hospital of Cleveland, Dept. of Obstetrics and Gynaecology, One Mt. Sinai Drive, University Circle, Cleveland, OH 44106, USA

Versi, Dr. E., MA, MB, Bch, Registrar, Menopause Clinic, Dulwich Hospital, East Dulwich Grove, London SE22 8PT, Great Britain

Vessey, Prof. M. P., MA, MD, MB, BS, FRCGP, FMCM, Lecturer, Gibson Laboratories Building, Radcliffe Infirmary, Oxford OX2 6HE, Great Britain

Wenderlein, Prof. Dr. med. J. M., Universitäts-Frauenklinik, Prittwitzstr. 43, D-7900 Ulm

Whitehead, M. I., MB, BS, MRCG, LRCP, MRCOG Senior Lecturer/Honorary Consultant Gynaecologist, Dept. of Obstetrics and Gynaecology, King's College School, Hospital Medical School, Denmark Hill, London SE5 8RX, Great Britain

Bei Fragen zur Produktsicherheit wenden Sie sich bitte an:
If you have any questions regarding product safety,
please contact:

Walter de Gruyter GmbH
Genthiner Straße 13
10785 Berlin
productsafety@degruyterbrill.com